AF767655

WRITTEN BY:
Stacey Lane

ILLUSTRATED BY:
Stacey Lane
Dan Lang
Christopher Ulrich
Dan Hennenberger

The illustrators of this book were carefully chosen by its author. Finding a team of artists who understood the walk of Skinny Miss S. was critical. For every voice in Skinny's head, there is an illustrator who contributed to these pages. Each having their own style and working in their own mediums, yet still coming together to coordinate and give flow to *Skinny Miss S. Was Very Depressed.* Some of the paintings are on canvas and others are uniquely done in a way which Christopher Ulrich brought to the collaborative table in its early stages. These paintings were done backwards on glass. The technique mirrored the mind's ability to reverse reality into what could result in a mental twist or simply the journey that was made to achieve purposeful results... only in a *different* way.

Skinny Miss S. Was Very Depressed
www.SkinnyMissS.com

Copyright © 2008 by Stacey Lane

All rights reserved. No part of this book may be reproduced by or transmitted in any form or by any means, electronic or mechanical, including photocopying, recording or by any information storage and retrieval system without written permission from the publisher, except for the inclusion of quotations in a review.

Published in 2009 by:
Aviva Publishing
2301 Saranac Avenue, Ste. 100
Lake Placid, NY 12946
518-523-1320

Library of Congress Control Number: 2009905461

ISBN: 978-1-890427-11-5

For the many who take their daily pills,
But also for those who find the humanity in the mentally ill.
We apologize, for we not always know what we do.
This book is dedicated to all of you.

Author

In my practice as a clinical psychologist, it is not unusual to work with patients for brief periods of time, nor is it unusual for treatment to span years. My work with Stacey Lane began in the spring of 1993. She had just turned twenty one years of age. When she presented in my office she seemed to have no body. She seemed to float into the room. She was nothing but eyes. Had I not known better I would have guessed she was maybe twelve years old. She was five foot three and weighed eighty five pounds. It became quickly obvious that she was in the midst of a severe episode of major depression with secondary anorexia nervosa.

I began a standard treatment approach: medication (prescribed by her psychiatrist), cognitive/behavioral and psychodynamic "talk" therapy. Cognitive behavioral techniques can quickly help patients feel in control. These techniques stop negative thinking and generalizations. I taught her relaxation exercises. She was compliant with treatment. She attended regularly. She did her homework. As treatment progressed, some of her symptoms reduced. She reported less depression. She revealed a history of chaos and maltreatment that had been a part of her developmental years. We had mutual trust, the so called "therapeutic alliance", BUT SHE DID NOT EAT. WORSE, SHE LOST MORE WEIGHT.

When she defiantly refused hospitalization, I in turn defiantly threw out all the techniques and in exasperation asked, "What will you eat?" In a small quiet voice she responded, "I like French fries, but my mom doesn't think they are good for me." I instantly sent her out for french fries and hoped her mother wouldn't hate me too much. Thereafter, she rapidly improved on all parameters. We discussed termination, and she then began a classic textbook episode of mania. This was not a surprise, as when therapy is about to end, a patient with abandonment issues will worsen. Without hesitation she agreed to in-patient treatment. She was diagnosed with bipolar disorder I. She was soon stabilized with medication and released. For a time, she continued treatment with me on an as needed out-patient basis. Whatever had triggered the mania seemed resolved. It was now the fall of 1996 and she relocated out of the area.

In the summer of 2008 we met again. Stacey reported to have had good therapy and much healing during her absence. She was emotionally stable and appropriately medicated. She was experiencing difficulty in her close relationships, had family of origin issues, and was appropriately grieving the sudden death of her father; all she wished to explore more fully. I saw her weekly, but then because she improved, I saw her less often. As part of her treatment and in pursuit of her own healing, she had begun writing an illustrated book. She soon reported the book was almost finished. She asked me to write the foreword. Without much thought, I agreed. Later that evening I began to have second thoughts. What was a "foreword"? I had never written one. I quickly began a search of my library for examples. I found a few and read them. The message was simple, "First, read the book!" I did so. *Skinny Miss S. Was Very Depressed* is a page turner, and as I read I knew exactly what it was I wanted to say.

There is no adequate adjective to describe this book. It is simply…awesome! Strictly adhering to child-like language and poetic phrasing, Lane has captured the world of the traumatized child. She has created life-like characters from her "voices" within. She allows their dialogue tell her story. In so doing escapes from utter madness and heals. As the next step in the construction of the book, Lane ties the subjective felt experience to the cold clinical language of the Diagnostic Studies Manual. This is a crucial move as it demonstrates for the uninformed, afraid, and untreated patient how to access support. It demonstrates for the reader that symptoms can occur in the absence of maltreatment as children. Major life stressors can trigger symptoms. We are all vulnerable.

Foreword

Finally, and perhaps most gratifying of all, Lane and her collaborators have brought to life her "voices" in breath-taking vivid art. In crisp dynamic color and exquisite detail, the art stands as a perfect example of the phrase, "A picture is worth a thousand words." In Otto Rank's masterpiece, "Art and Artist" (first published by Knopf, 1932) he asserts, "When you can no longer accept the collective solution to the problem of existence, you find your own. The artist's work is his own projection." The art is Lane's projection. It is her solution and gift. The art elicits our projection as well, and does so similarly as a Rorschach Test. It allows for our projected unknown selves to be exquisitely revealed. All who read this book may find parts of themselves or even new parts to explore. The book is "up close and personal". Art is exactly that, and in this up close and personal book, it is the "glue" that holds the disparate portions of the book together. Lane has crafted a masterly synthesis of three essential elements: subjective felt experience, clinical information, and visual expression. These three elements when taken together define the world of the mentally challenged. In addition, the elements of this book create a metaphor about the courage it takes to find a healing path. Lane shows us we cannot fix the world, but we can find a way to live in it.

Memory

I would like to comment a brief word about memory. When the patient comes into the therapist's office, so does "memory". They bring their remembered and unremembered history. In the telling and retelling of their history, new memory can surface. This can occur without any particular effort on the part of the therapist. Memory is what we "work" with, but patient and therapist take caution as memory is fallible. A memory may be accurate or inaccurate. It may be traces of dreams, television programs, fairy tales, and more all jumbled together. A constructed memory can result from a fragment of memory, but of all memory, trauma memory must be taken with a proverbially grain of salt. These memories are often misleading. Dr. Louise Gaston Ph.D. asserts, "It is too simple and outright misleading to assess memory accurately…from the information reported of complex events such as abuse or when memory is retrieved by interrogation."

In addition, the fact that a person reports a memory in great detail and vivid clarity does not mean the memory is accurate. Emotionally revealed memory, whether negative or positive is not guarantee of accuracy of the information, nor should it be assumed that confidence in a memory reflects accuracy. Most importantly hypnotically "recovered" memories are the most questionable of all memory. When clients are hypnotized they are highly suggestible, and in unskilled hands can be led to create notoriously "false memories". Memories can be lost. Memories can be created and memories can be spontaneously recovered. Psychotherapists must exercise caution even when memories are spontaneously recovered. Still the question remains: if we are not our remembered selves, then who are we?

Reader

Who should read this book? This exceptional and courageous book deserves to be read by psychiatrists, psychologists, LCSWs, NFTs, RNs, MDs, the general public, and above all else the mentally challenged. Additionally this book serves as a textbook and belongs in the classroom for the student of psychology, the psychology professor, and also for the artist and art instructor. This indeed is a heroic work and will stand the test of time.

Charlene Trueman-Crothers, Ph.D.
Thousand Oaks, California

May I Introduce Ourselves...

This is a story of one girl finding what works for her in a world she struggles to exist in and another girl telling her story in order to give both a path to follow. I use definitions defined by boxes, questions encapsulated in bubbles, medical book references to inform, a book in a book to metaphor inner transformation, story randomly placed on the page, and inconsistent visual art to vibrate the unspoken color that may. May what? Whoever knows what the mind unfolds. Images in different styles portrayed, colors vibrating on each page…it's up to you what you receive from this version of us. This book is an *experience* and answers may come as mysteriously as the questions of your life go. If you care for everything to make sense, you may miss the breath that carries the messages sent. Just mine, Miss Stacey Lane…and hers, my Skinny Miss S.

Many people do not believe in taking medication for conditions they cannot see. I am not one of those people. I do believe there are times when those suffering from mild depression may correct their moods with mind over matter and a healthy lifestyle, although I am not addressing mild depression, and who is to say where mild depression ends? Not even I can tell objectively after living with bipolar all of my years.

Depression comes like a demon in the night and it is prepared to fight. As any inner conflict which presents itself this strongly to change our personality, moods, mental clarity, and most importantly our bio-chemical mental health, we must gain control of it, simultaneously being gentle on ourselves. We are at war within ourselves, but it only needs to be for a time. In order to correct its affects we must use every tool which is available for this intense challenge. This includes medical care. Clinical depression and all mental illnesses for that matter are imbalances in brain chemistry and deserve medical attention in order to soften the fight. Unless your goal is to suffer as much as possible as you wrestle with the voices in your head, you will not get out of crisis without the supervision of a psychiatrist and the benefits of medication, returning you to mental balance.

Many people believe seeing a therapist, counselor, or life coach to be an excuse to wallow in our tears. These unawares do not know the benefit of honoring our past, listening to our pain, or developing skills to rise above in the arena of being heard. I am beyond a firm believer in therapy of any form. It creates awareness, compassion for oneself, and long term healing for the fight against any mental challenge.

Many people judge support groups as a collection of disturbed individuals who concentrate on their past or pain. These people may say we don't do anything to change our condition. They say we merely talk about it too much and being around such energy only drags one down. I disagree. Expressing our grief and difficulties with loving supporters gives us freedom to clear our minds and hope to move out of our expressions. Supporting others as we watch each other suffer the same war helps us to band together, lifting each other out of the pit of darkness. We are nothing without the touch of others.

I feel that some belief systems are limiting and can be damaging to the healing process if out of balance. I reference my own struggles to free myself from the doctrine of Catholicism. For my own reasons I found the Catholic Church to be a dysfunctional family in which it was necessary to lovingly close the door to. In no way am I telling others not to rely on their higher power; I rely on my version. I am saying the rules and boundaries of what is morally good and bad should not be defined by anyone other than ourselves in our personal missions of finding inner healing and health. If our belief systems are not working for us then I propose they should change, and with all truth in higher powers considered, we must thank ourselves for the work we do to find peace in our lives. There are those who rely solely on their higher power or there are those who acknowledge they are a part of the higher power they create. I challenge you to honor and create your highest power as being a part of your life's work.

We, survivors of our over-brilliant minds, are feeling, thought-filled, imaginative, creative, and incredibly strong people who create our own mythology as opposed to believing in what an outside source insists. We are willing to stand as warriors and witnesses to our inner conflicts. We are living saints, for anyone who has unwillingly or willingly gone to the dark ends of their minds and lived to fight their way home to balance is a saint and deserves to be honored. Let us honor our process of healing and use all of the tools we can to survive.

There is a formula to a deserving light at the end of a black tunnel. Skinny Miss S. adventures to find a way to recreate what subconsciously stirs in her in order to consciously live the way she desires…I hope you will too. Survivor? Saint? Yes, *YOU.*

Cautionary Notice

Do not attempt what Skinny attempts in her home, in your home.
Skinny Miss S. Was Very Depressed is a fictional book written and illustrated with a twist in hopes to trigger mentally ill persons to seek help from the appropriate mental health professionals, not from dolls.

If you exhibit symptoms of any number of the illnesses chosen to be included in this book, be advised to seek a psychiatric professional as soon as humanly possible. DSM-IV diagnostic criteria definitions are not complete and could be taken out of context without the proper professional guidance.

Do not take on mental illness alone. Do not attempt to diagnose yourself. Do not attempt to medicate yourself without a doctor's order.

If you are in an emergency emotional crisis call The National Suicide Prevention Lifeline which is a 24-hour, toll-free suicide prevention service which is available to anyone in suicidal crisis. This is a nationwide hotline for IMMEDIATE care.

If you need help, please dial 1-800-273-TALK (8255). You will be routed to the closest possible crisis center in your area. With more than 130 crisis centers across the country, their mission is to provide immediate assistance to anyone seeking mental health services. Call for yourself, or someone you care about. Your call is free and confidential.

You are not alone. There are real people who understand you.
Reach out now. Seek your right to live happily ever after.

You are welcome to email the creator of Skinny Miss S. any and all of your expressions at: SomethingToSay@SkinnyMissS.com where your comments will be heard and incorporated into the future writings of Stacey Lane on the topic of living with mental challenges with total confidentiality.

This book in not intended for anyone under 18 years of age.

Mental Illness

noun
Any of various conditions characterized by impairment of an individual's normal cognitive, emotional, or behavioral functioning, and caused by social, psychological, biochemical, genetic, or other factors, such as infection or head trauma. Also called emotional illness, mental illness, mental disease, mental disorder.
Any disease of the mind; the psychological state of someone who has emotional or behavioral problems serious enough to require psychiatric intervention.

DSM-IV Medical Reference Book for Mental Disorders

The Diagnostic and Statistical Manual of Mental Disorders (DSM) is an American handbook for mental health professionals that lists different categories of mental disorders and the criteria for diagnosing them, according to the publishing organization the American Psychiatric Association. It is used worldwide by clinicians and researchers as well as insurance companies, pharmaceutical companies and policy makers. It has attracted controversy and criticism as well as praise.[2]

Major Depressive Episode

[according to DSM-IV Reference Book for Mental Disorders]

A. Five (or more) of the following symptoms have been present during the same 2-week period and represent a change from previous functioning; at least one of the symptoms is either (1) depressed mood or (2) loss of interest or pleasure.

Note: Do not include symptoms that are clearly due to a general medical condition, or mood-incongruent delusions or hallucinations.

(1) depressed mood most of the day, nearly every day, as indicated by either subjective report (e.g., feels sad or empty) or observation made by others (e.g., appears tearful). Note: In children and adolescents, can be irritable mood.

(2) markedly diminished interest or pleasure in all, or almost all, activities most of the day, nearly every day (as indicated by either subjective account or observation made by others).

(3) significant weight loss when not dieting or weight gain or decrease or increase in appetite nearly every day. Note: In children, consider failure to make expected weight gains.

(4) insomnia or hypersomnia nearly every day.

(5) psychomotor agitation or retardation nearly every day (observable by others, not merely subjective feelings of restlessness or being slowed down).

(6) fatigue or loss of energy nearly every day.

(7) feelings of worthlessness or excessive or inappropriate guilt (which may be delusional) nearly every day (not merely self-reproach or guilt about being sick).

(8) diminished ability to think or concentrate, or indecisiveness, nearly every day (either by subjective account or as observed by others).

(9) recurrent thoughts of death (not just fear of dying), recurrent suicidal ideation without a specific plan, or a suicide attempt or a specific plan for committing suicide.

B. The symptoms do not meet criteria for a Mixed Episode.

C. The symptoms cause clinically significant distress or impairment in social, occupational, or other important areas of functioning.

D. The symptoms are not due to the direct physiological effects of a substance (e.g., a drug of abuse, a medication) or a general medical condition (e.g., hypothyroidism).

E. The symptoms are not better accounted for by Bereavement, i.e., after the loss of a loved one, the symptoms persist for longer than 2 months or are characterized by marked functional impairment, morbid preoccupation with worthlessness, suicidal ideation, psychotic symptoms, or psychomotor retardation.[3]

Skinny Miss S. Was Very Depressed

voices

noun

1. the sound or sounds uttered through the mouth of living creatures speaking, shouting, singing, etc; *to loose one's voice.*

2. the condition or effectiveness of the voice for speaking or singing: *to be in poor voice.*

3. something likened to speech as conveying impressions to the MIND; *the voice of nature, the voice of the wind.*

4. an expressed opinion or choice; *a voice for compromise.* [which insinuates sacrifice of choice]

5. an expressed will or desire; *the voice of the* [inner] *'people'.*

-Idiom the still, small voice, the conscience: *She was only occasionally troubled by the still, small voices in her head.*

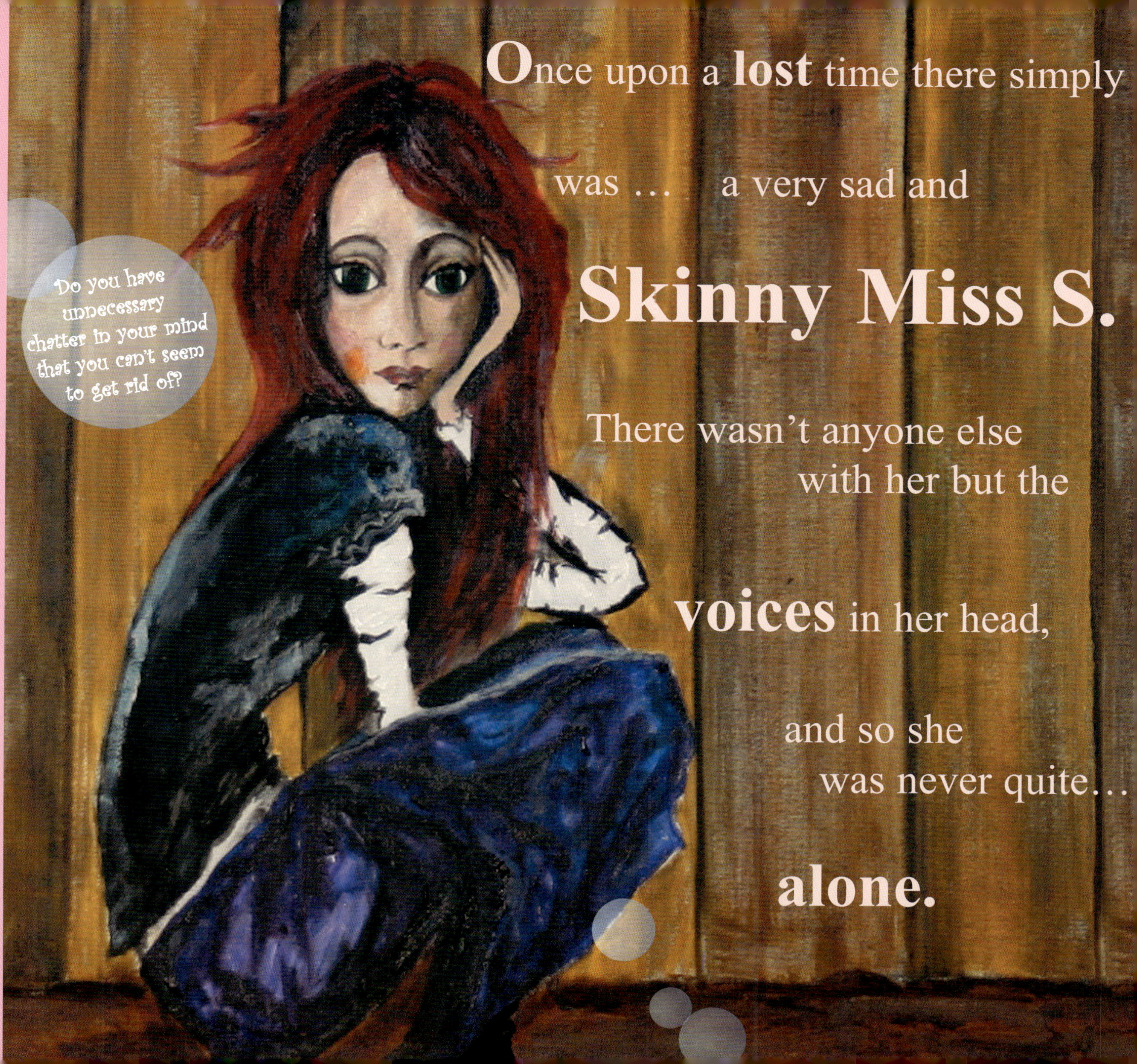
Do you have unnecessary chatter in your mind that you can't seem to get rid of?

Once upon a **lost** time there simply was … a very sad and

Skinny Miss S.

There wasn't anyone else with her but the **voices** in her head, and so she was never quite…

alone.

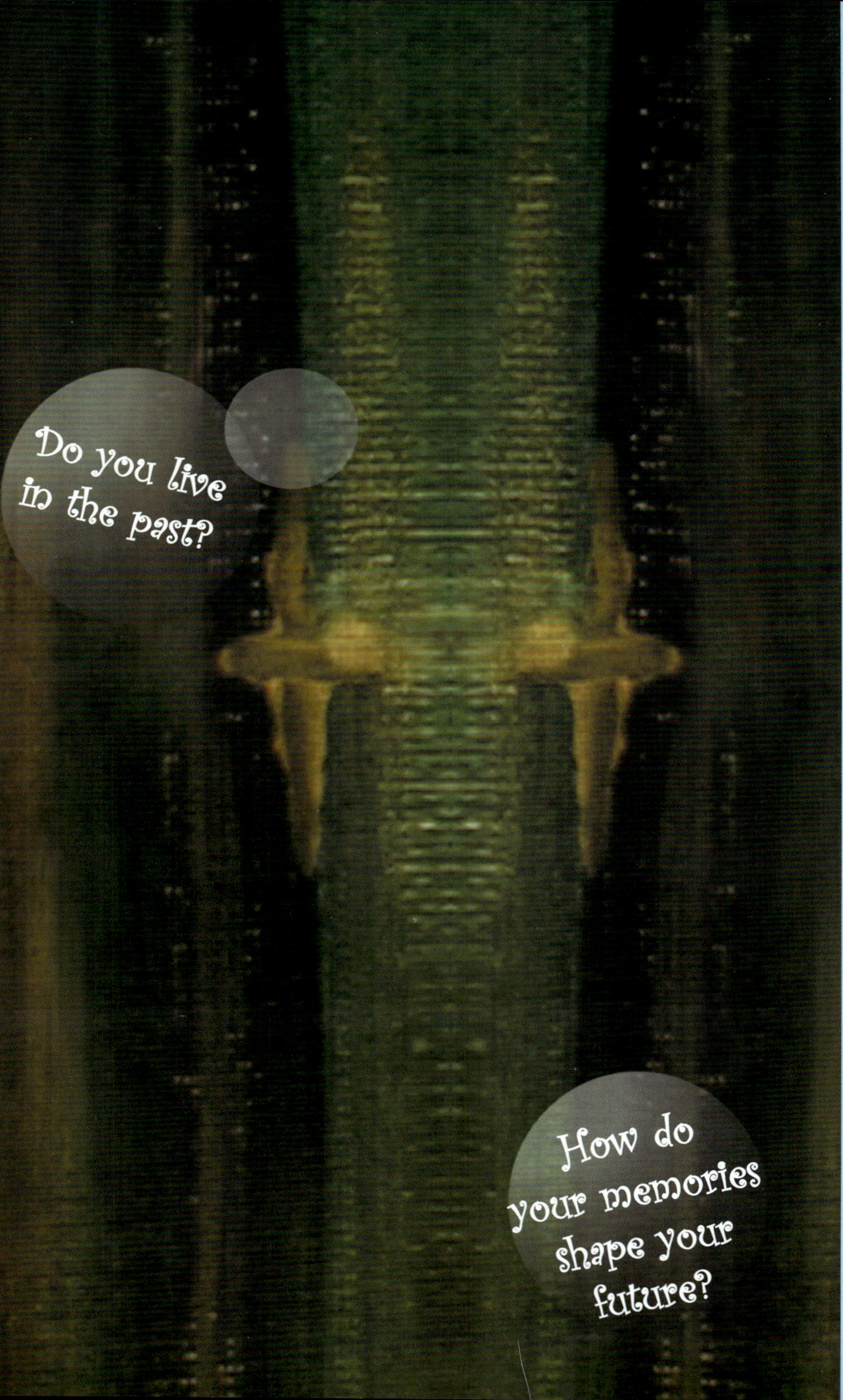
Do you live in the past?
How do your memories shape your future?

memory

noun

1. the mental capacity or faculty of retaining and reviving facts, events, impressions, etc., or of recalling or recognizing previous experiences.

2. this faculty as possessed by a particular individual [Lonely Miss C.]; *to have a good memory.*

3. the act or fact of retaining and recalling impressions, facts, etc.; *remembrance; recollection; to draw from memory;*

4. a mental impression retained; a recollection: one's earliest memories; *spent the afternoon lost in memory.*

5. the ability of certain materials to return to an original shape after deformation.
It hasn't happened in my memory.

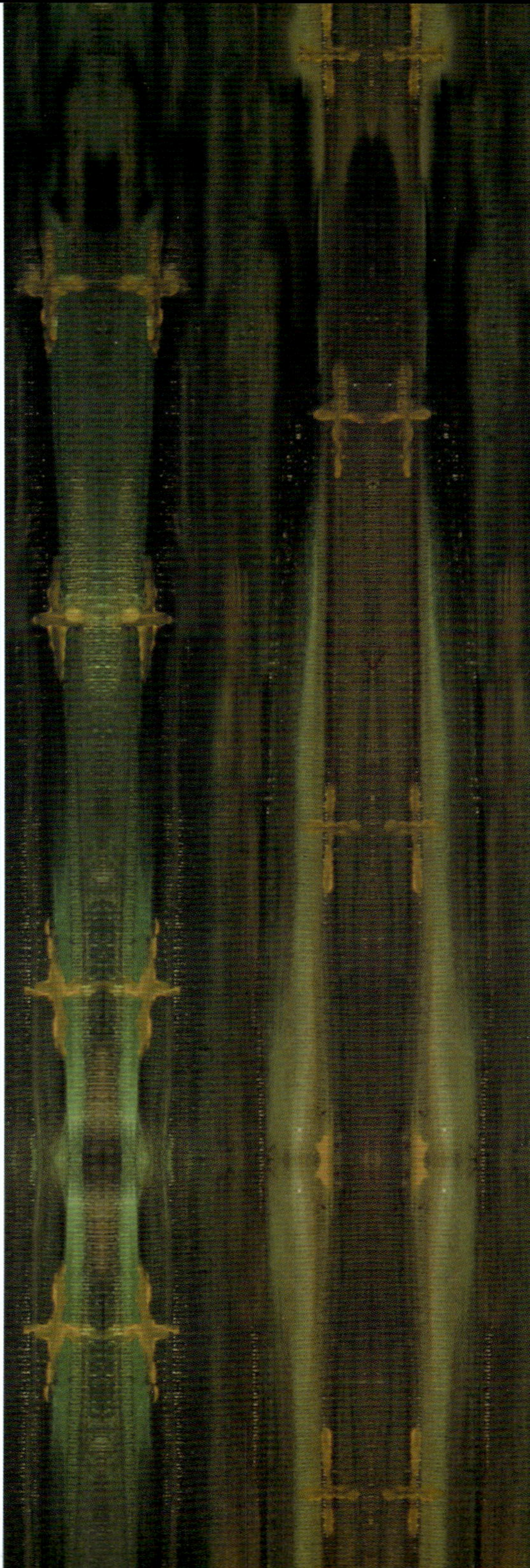

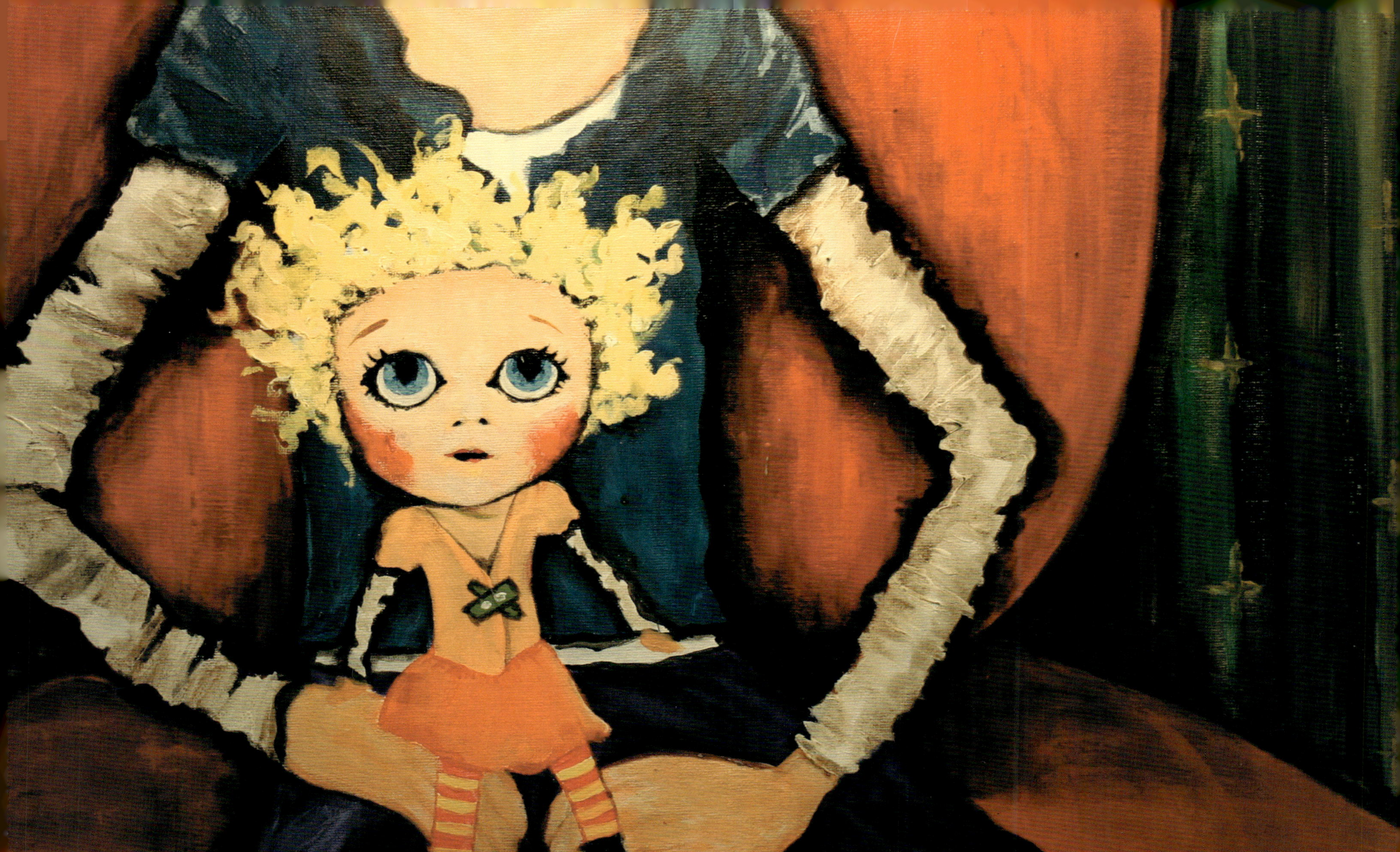

Lonely Miss C. was her favorite doll. She had been with her from the beginning of time and remembered things that Skinny's old memory had forgotten, but Skinny Miss S. was very depressed and Lonely Miss C. could never seem to help, try as she may.

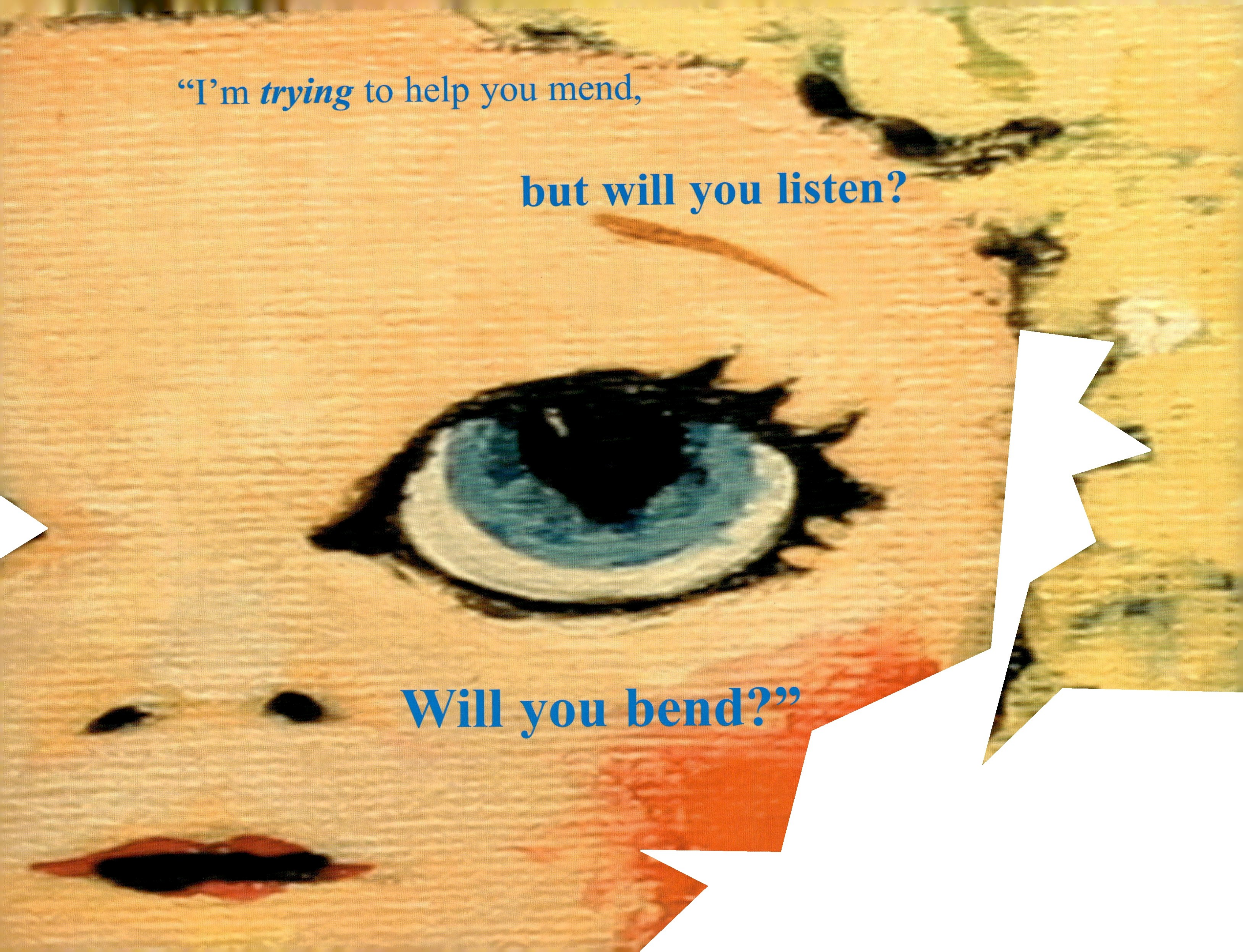

"I'm ***trying*** to help you mend,

but will you listen?

Will you bend?"

trying
adjective

1. severely straining the powers of endurance; *a trying experience.*
2. requiring great or extreme bodily, mental, or spiritual strength.

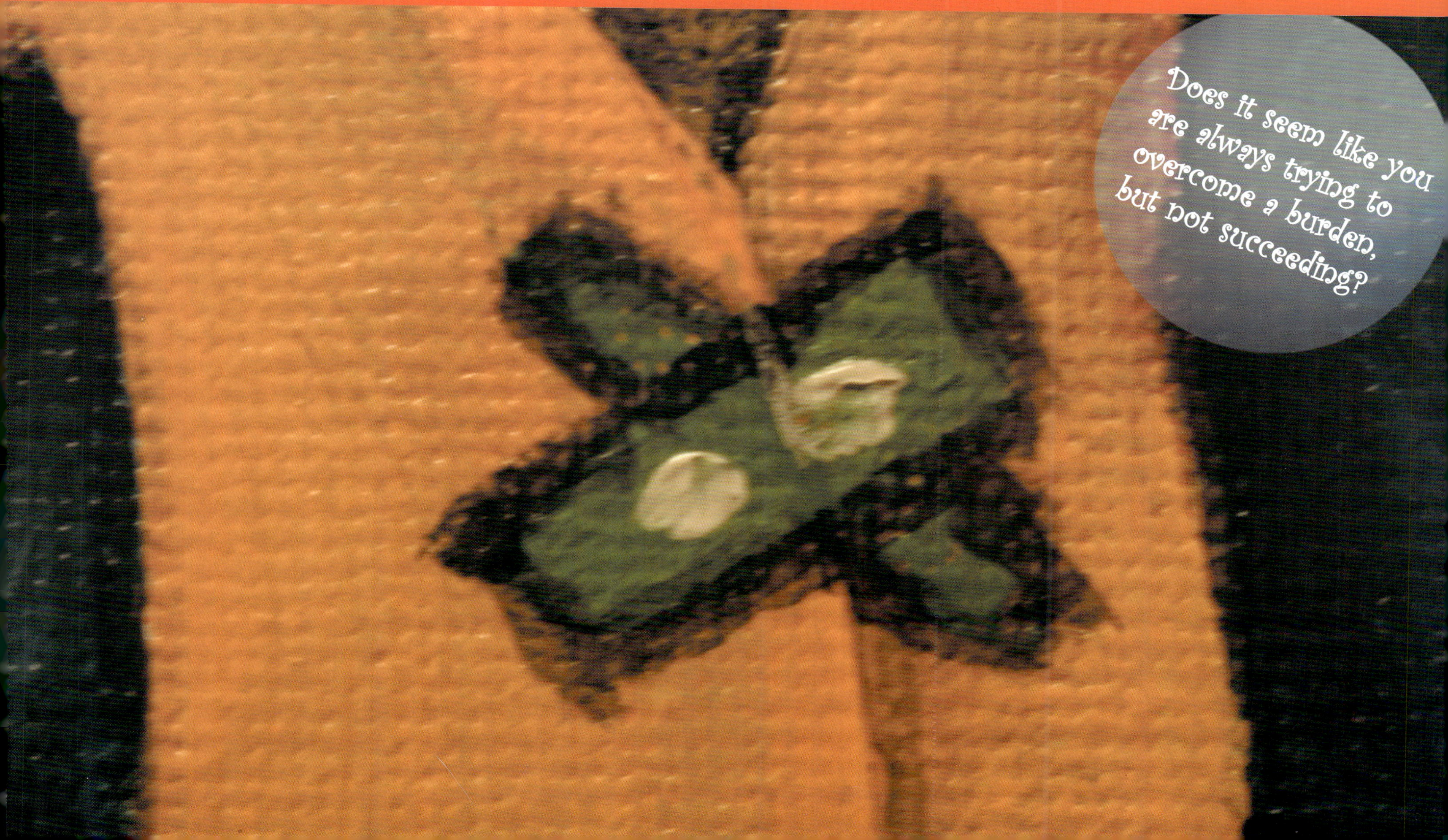
Does it seem like you are always trying to overcome a burden, but not succeeding?

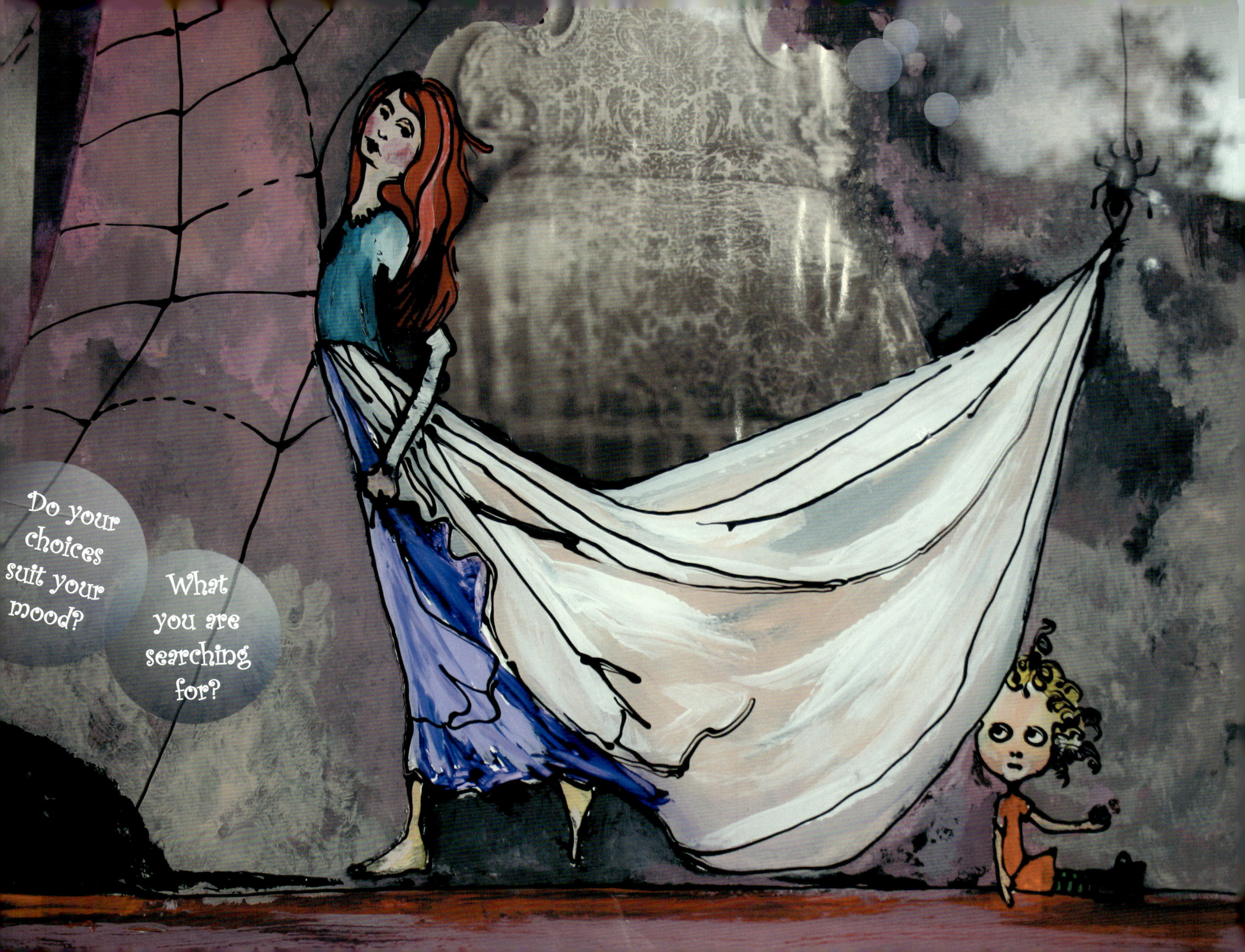
Do your choices suit your mood?
What you are searching for?

"Lonely C, don't bother me!
I need to get dressed for our daily cup of tea!" said Skinny Miss S.

"That's all you can expect of me."

Skinny always wore the same shabby clothes. If it wasn't her long heavy purple skirt, it was her striped jammie pants. She searched for something more, but Skinny Miss S. was locked in her comfort zone and old and comfortable clothes were all she chose.

Skinny Miss S. had clutter all around her. She was such a mess and didn't know where to begin to get undressed! An uninvited visitor, Sir Grouchy Spider, thought he knew the **way**, although doing it his way meant there would be hell to **pay**. "I made a list of what's wrong with you. These flaws you must fix and here is what you should do. If you put those things there… and these things here…you'd be able to see.
You should always make it a point to
listen to me!"

Sir Grouchy Spider thought he knew.

Are you hard on yourself?

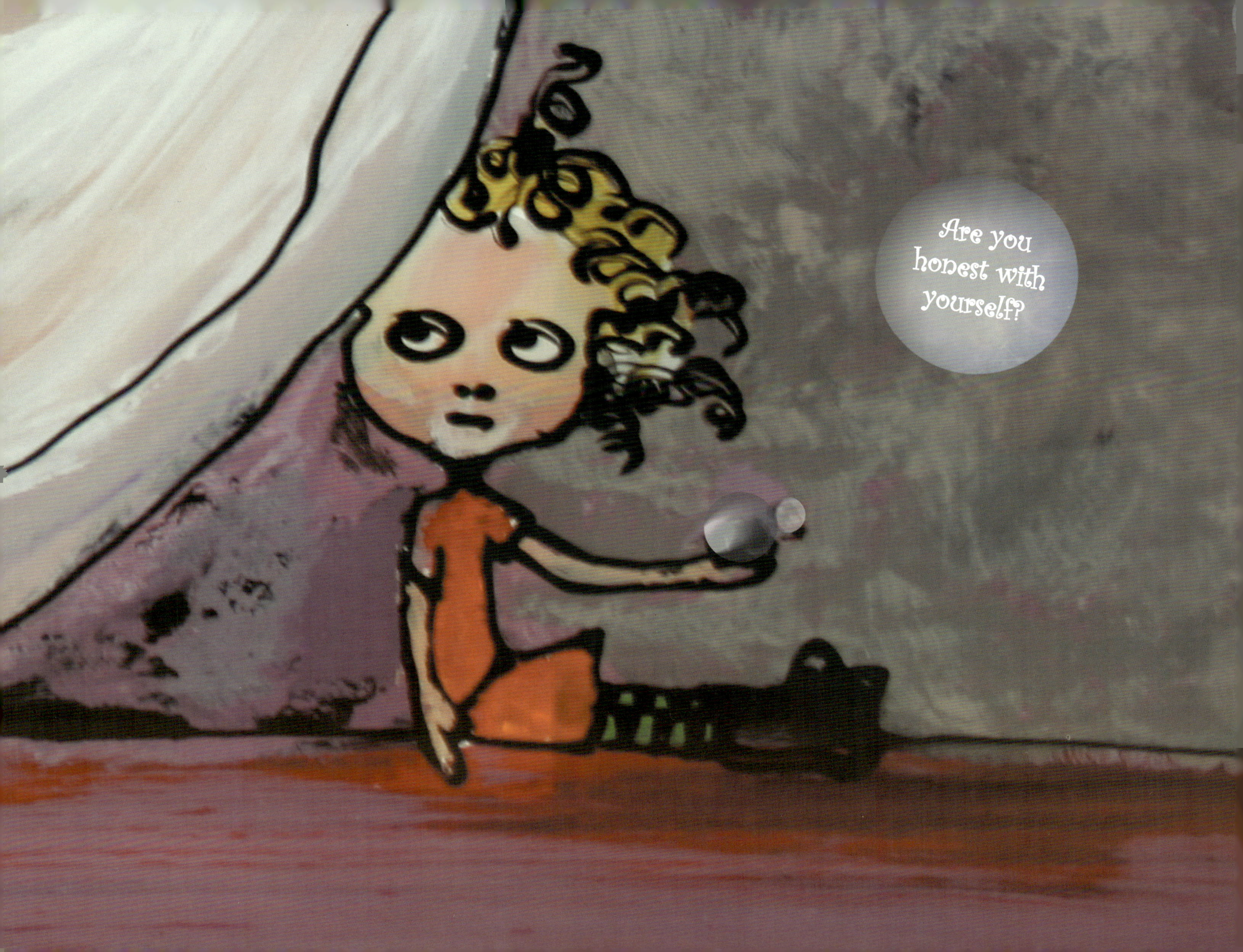
Are you honest with yourself?

"Skinny, don't listen to him!

He'll spin you into denial.

He is not a *real* doll,

but *really* a spider.

Just stomp him out.

He's merely a **liar!**" said Lonely Miss C.

denial
noun

1. refusal to satisfy a request or desire.

2. refusal to admit the truth or reality.

3. refusal to acknowledge a person or a thing.

4. self-denial.

5. negation in logic.

6. a psychological defense mechanism in which confrontation with a personal problem or with reality is avoided by denying the existence of the problem or reality —in denial: refusing to admit the truth or reality of something unpleasant; *a patient in denial about her mental health problems.*

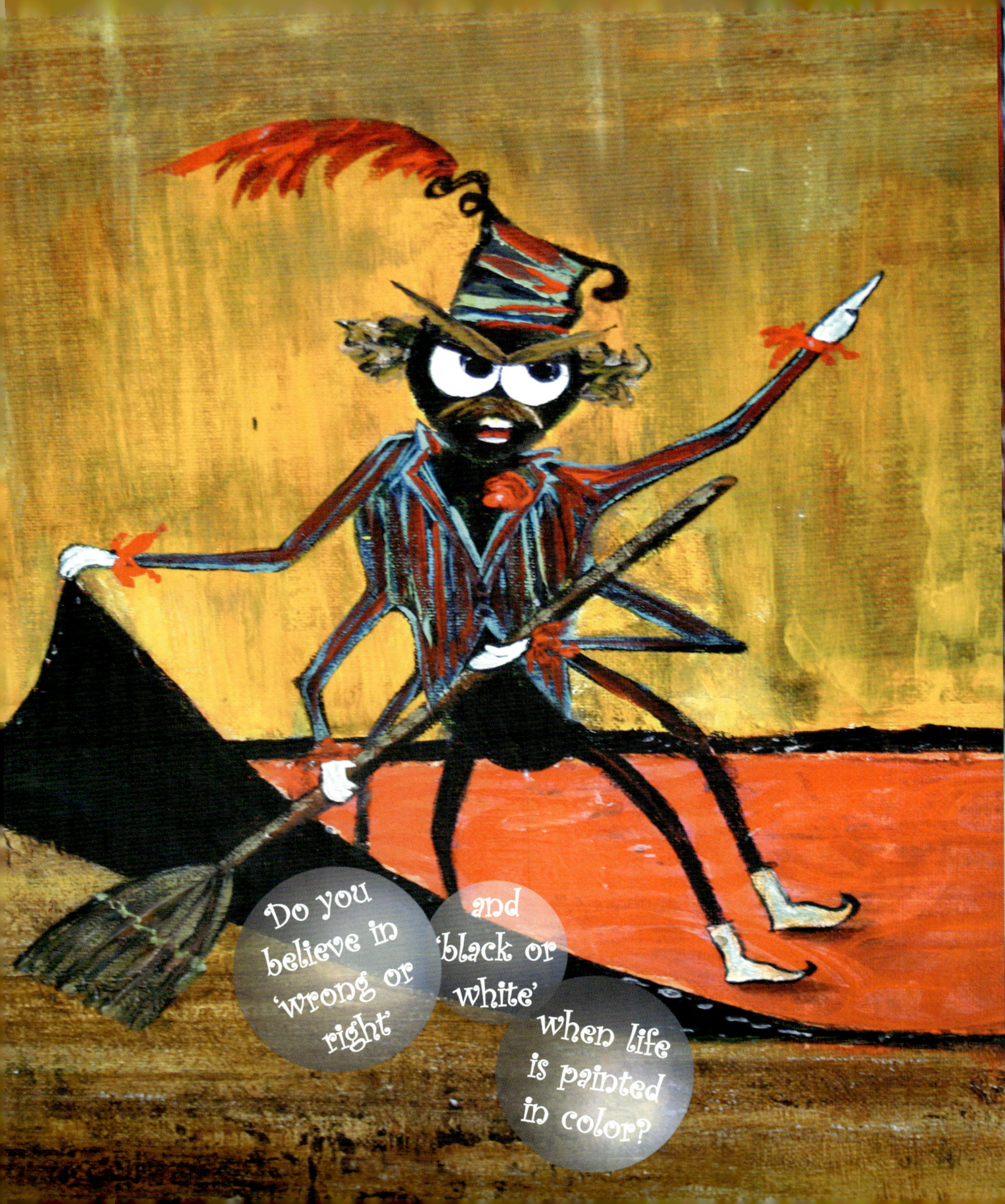
Do you believe in 'wrong or right'
and 'black or white'
when life is painted in color?

Lonely Miss C. was **right**.

Sir Grouchy Spider wasn't really a doll, but a real spider. He was sort of an intrusion on her life, coming around to remind her of the ways she constantly did things **wrong**.

guilt-trip
transitive verb

1. to cause feelings of guilt; *guilt-tripped them into helping.*
2. feeling of guilt or responsibility, esp. one not justified by reality.
3. to play upon the guilt feelings of.

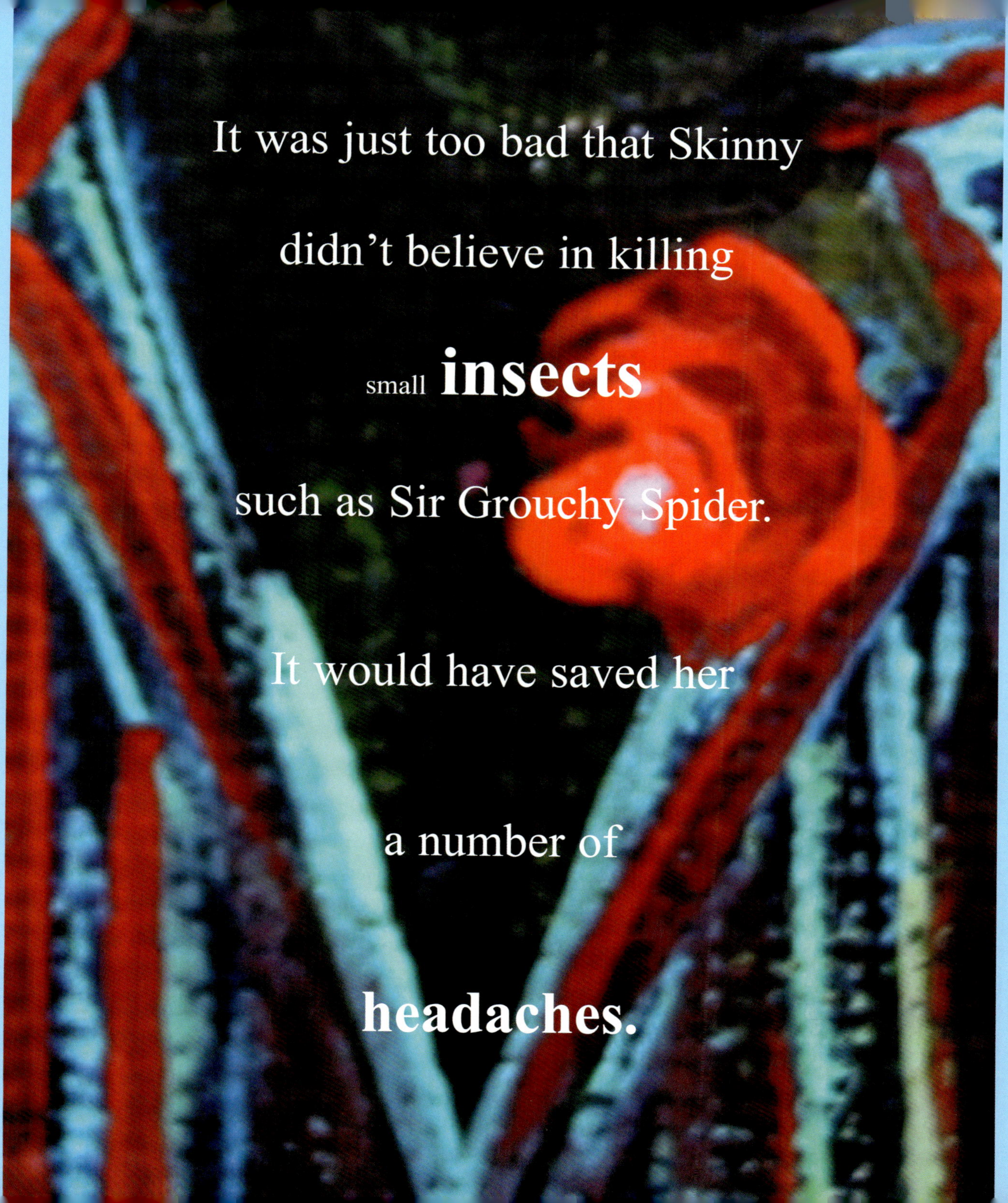

It was just too bad that Skinny

didn't believe in killing

small **insects**

such as Sir Grouchy Spider.

It would have saved her

a number of

headaches.

headache
noun

1. a pain in the head. [or at times in the ass]
2. something, such as a problem, that causes annoyance or trouble.

Dean Doll was her newest doll. He was skinny like her and she liked his flamboyant flavored dry sense of humor. The best part about him was that he was a reversible doll. When you turned him over to his backside, he became a priest doll so she got two dolls in one, and they had each other.

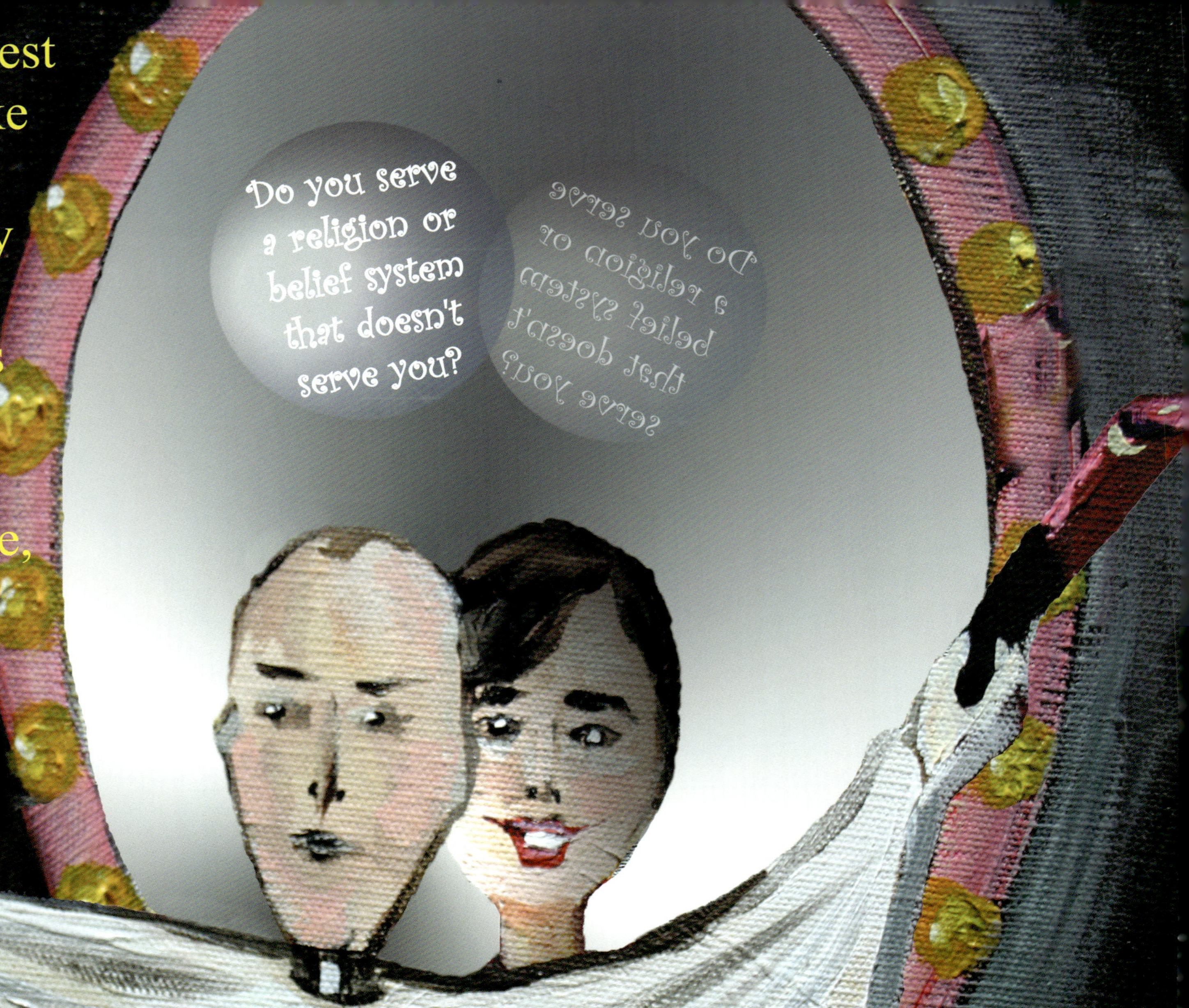
Do you serve a religion or belief system that doesn't serve you?

Skinny named him ***Father Deana Marie***. She thought that was funny, although Skinny didn't like how Father Deana Marie always told Dean Doll to stay hidden behind his back. Father judged Dean Doll ever since the day Skinny brought them out of the closet. **Bad beliefs** can do that.

duplicity

noun

1. deceitfulness in speech or conduct; speaking or acting in two different ways concerning the same matter with intent to deceive [each other in this case] ; double-dealing.

2. a twofold or double state or quality. Two faced. Backstabber.

3. acting in bad faith; deception by pretending to entertain one set of intentions while acting under the influence of another.

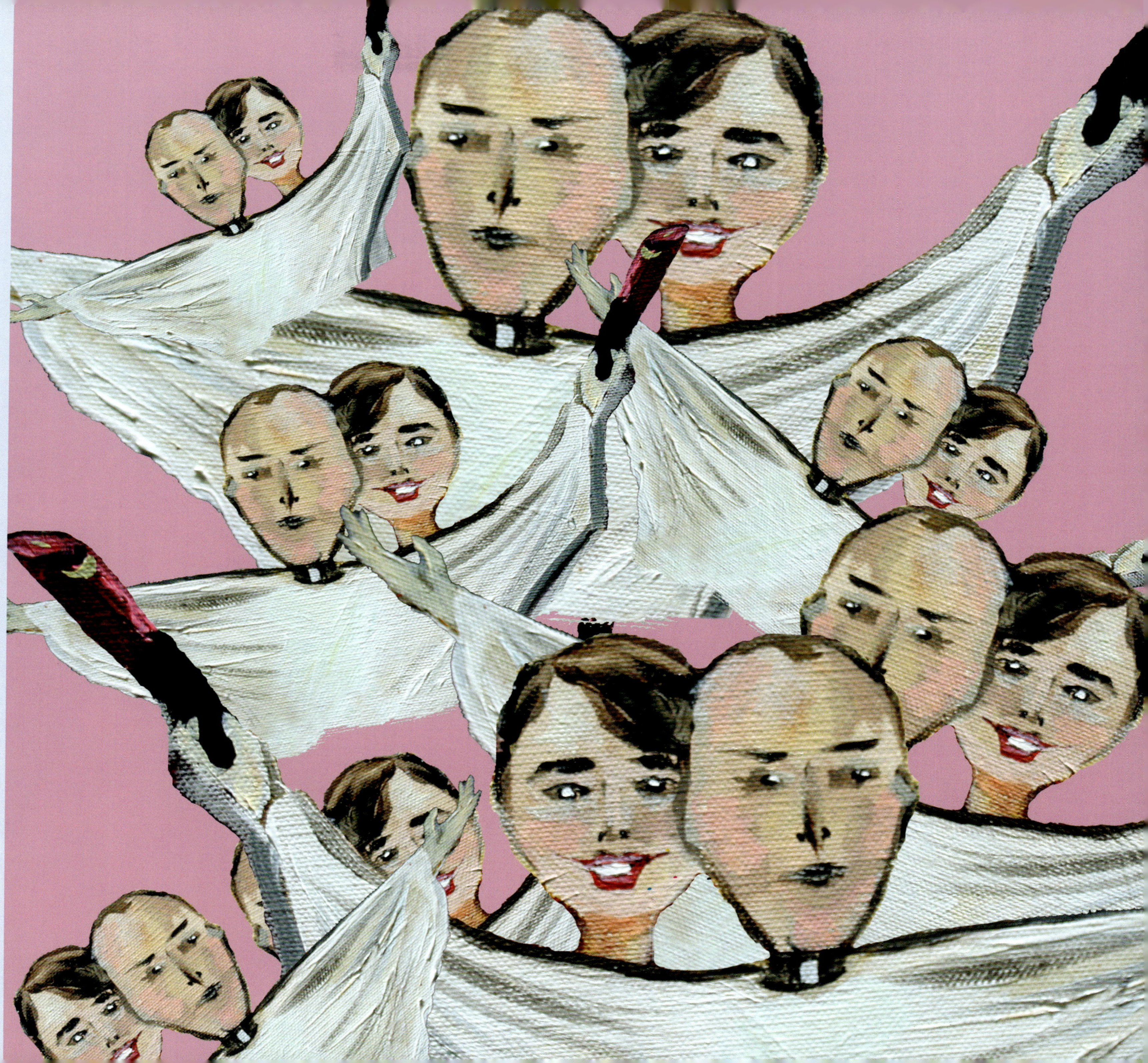

She had other dolls that she hadn't named yet. They were tossed in a box far back in her closet.

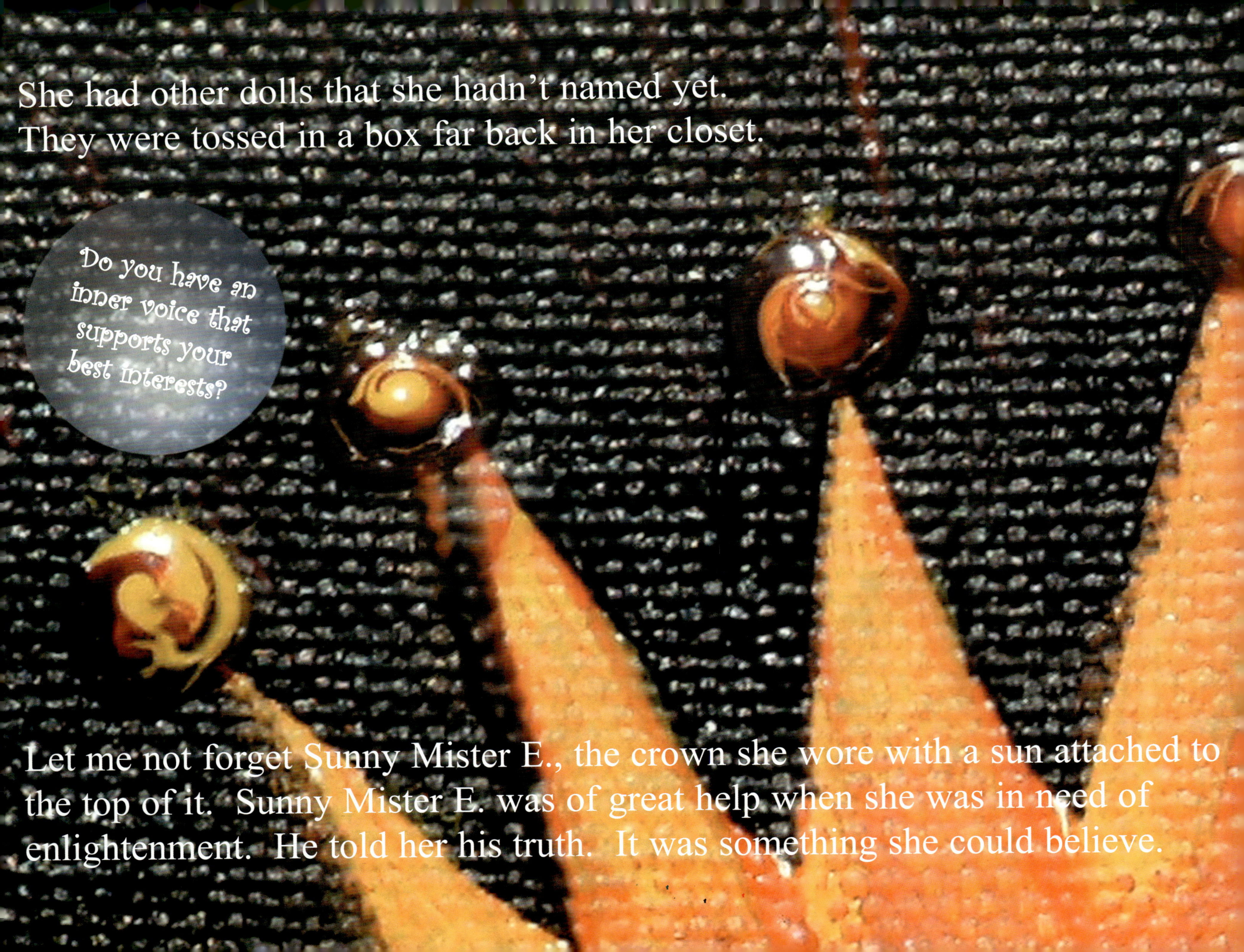

Do you have an inner voice that supports your best interests?

Let me not forget Sunny Mister E., the crown she wore with a sun attached to the top of it. Sunny Mister E. was of great help when she was in need of enlightenment. He told her his truth. It was something she could believe.

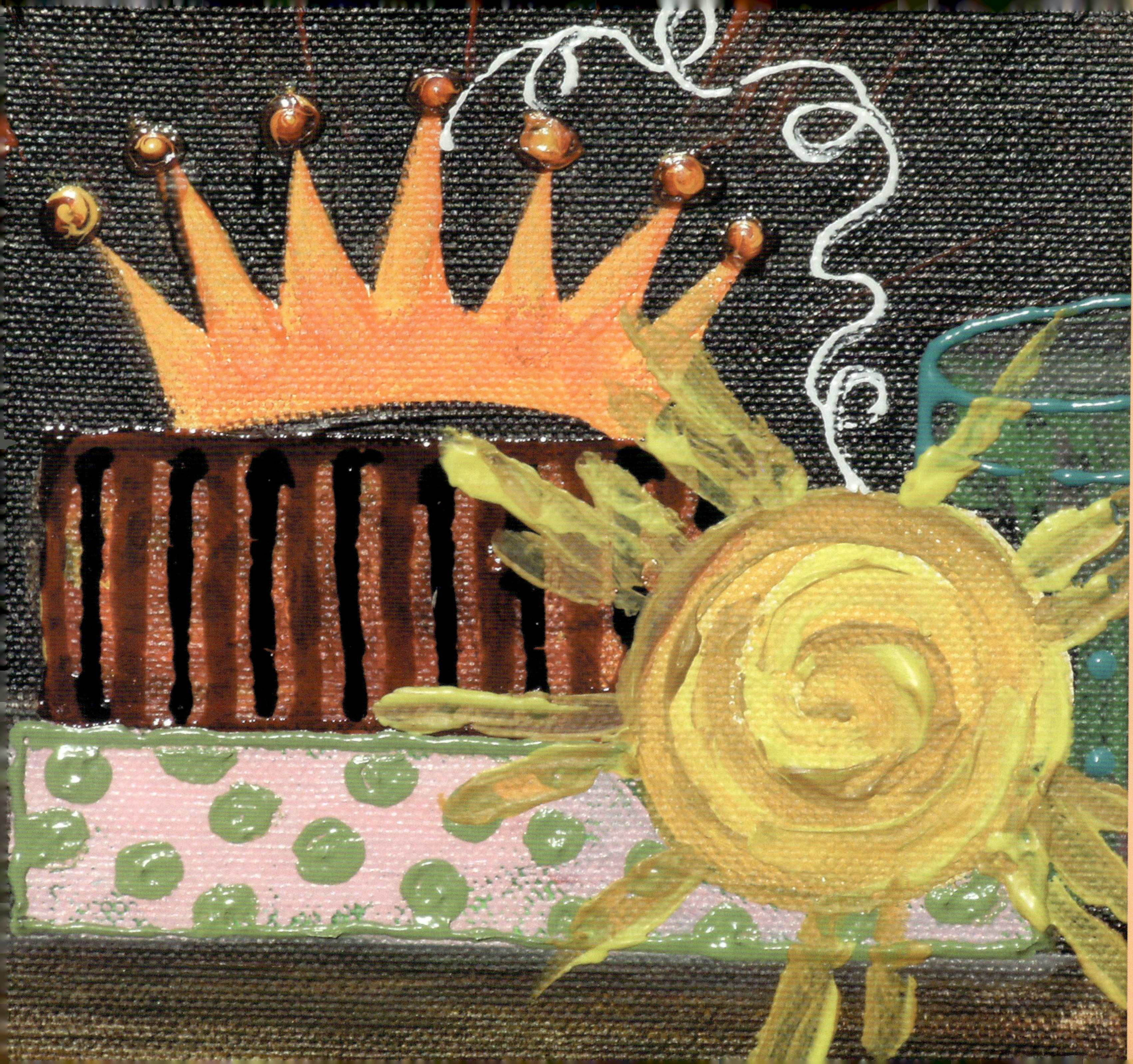

perception
noun

1. the act or faculty of apprehending by means of the senses or of the mind; cognition; understanding.

2. immediate or intuitive recognition or appreciation, as of moral, psychological, or aesthetic qualities; insight; intuition; discernment; *an artist of rare perception.*

Then of course there was me, her stuffed owl who sat high above her
I was there just to watch and that's what made her feel alive. She lived

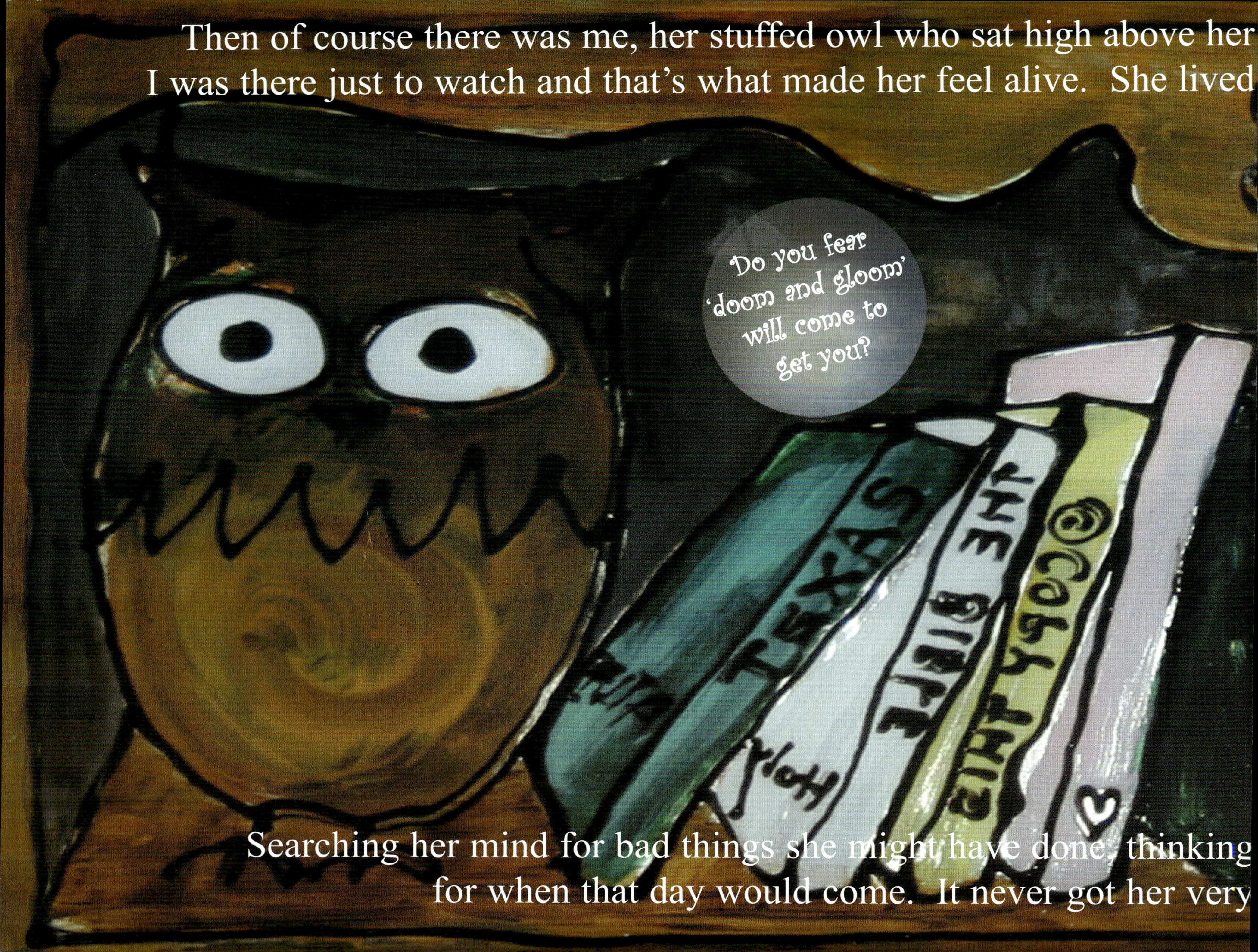
Do you fear 'doom and gloom' will come to get you?

Searching her mind for bad things she might have done, thinking
for when that day would come. It never got her very

room on the tallest of shelves. I never moved or said a word. She knew with the fear of judgment day's arrival in her every waking moment.

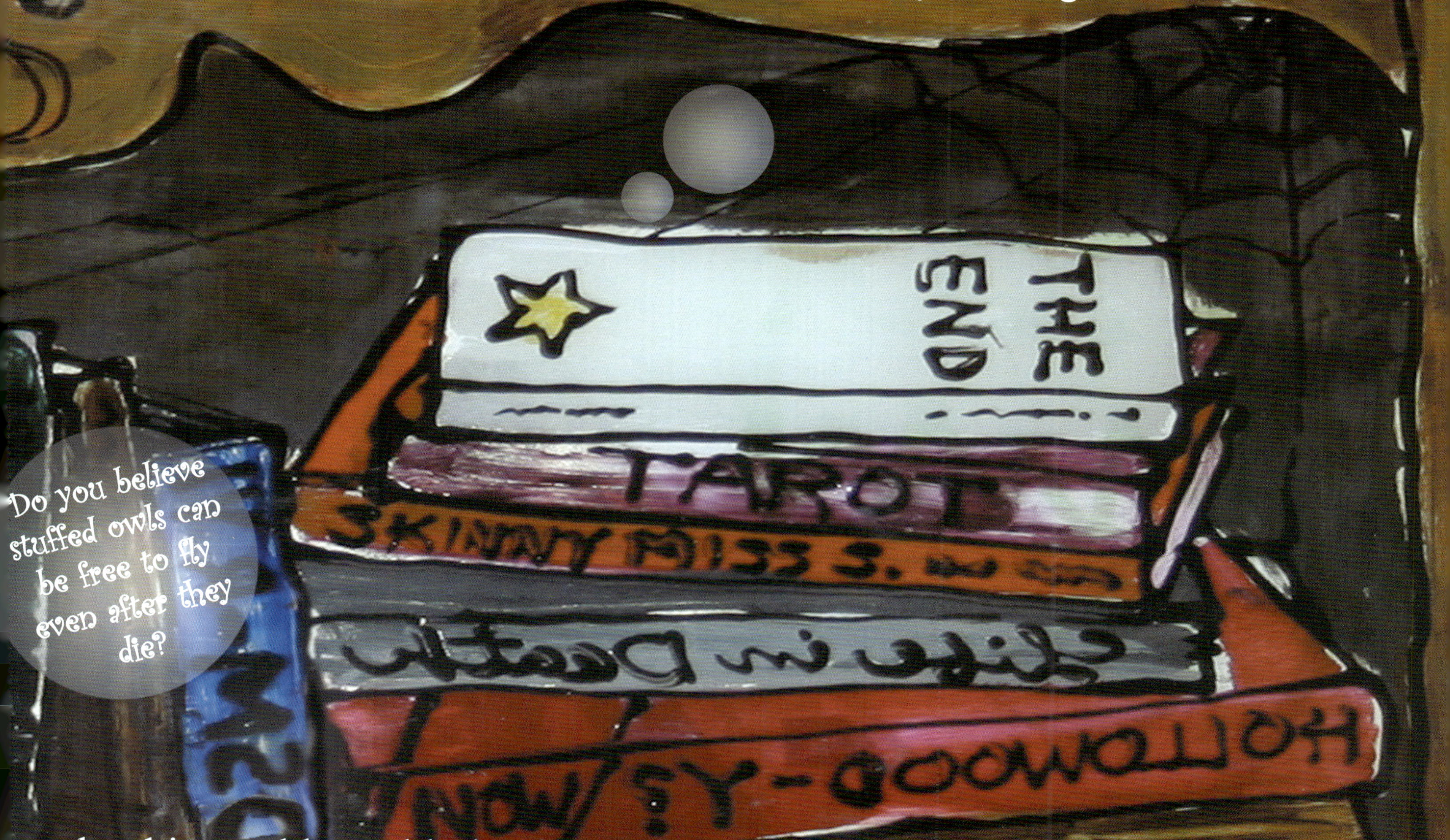
THE END
TAROT
Do you believe stuffed owls can be free to fly even after they die?

naybe this world would give her a clue to what she would be judged ·ar since her sins were all just self-serving shame.

DIAGNOSTIC CRITERIA FOR:

Generalized A n x i e t y Disorder

A. Unrealistic or excessive anxiety or worry (apprehensive expectation) about two or more life circumstances, e.g., worry about possible misfortune to one's child (who is in no danger) and worry about finances (for no good reason),for a period of six months or longer, during which the person has been bothered more days than not by these concerns. In children and adolescents, this may take the form of anxiety and worry about academic, athletic, and social performance.

B. If another Axis I disorder is present, the focus of the anxiety and worry in A is unrelated to it, e.g., the anxiety or worry is not about having panic attack (as in Panic Disorder), being embarrassed in public (as in Social Phobia), being contaminated (as in Obsessive Compulsive Disorder), or gaining weight (as in Anorexia Nervosa).

C. The disturbance does not occur only during the course of a Mood Disorder or a psychotic disorder.

D. At least 6 of the following 18 symptoms are often present when anxious: Motor tension, autonomic hyperactivity, vigilance and scanning.

Anxiety Disorder Not Otherwise Specified:
1. Mixed anxiety-depressive disorder: clinically significant symptoms of anxiety and depression, but the criteria are not met for either a specific Mood Disorder or a specific Anxiety Disorder.[4]

I mean really…who was going to care about the geraniums

in the flower-pots she let accidentally die and rot because she forgot the

watering part?

Do you always think you are doing something wrong?

She would only question herself,
"Did I purposely **forget** or in not **remembering**
did I mean to do it?

I'm such a mess!

Do you dress for depression too?

Do you dress yourself for someone other than you?

It's time I get DRESSED!"

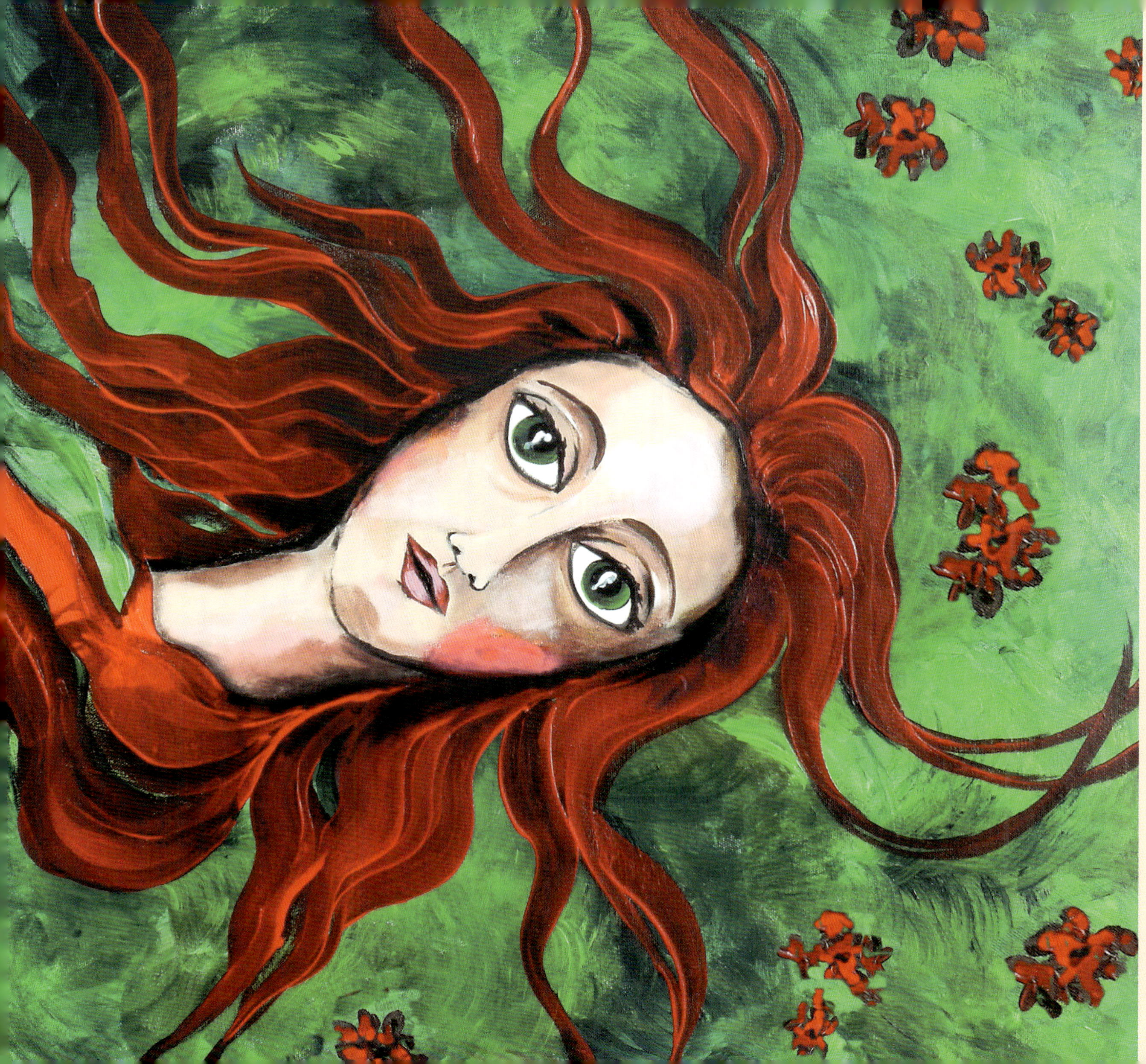

shame

noun, verb

1. the painful feeling arising from the consciousness of something dishonorable, ridiculous, improper, etc., done by oneself or another; *She was overcome with shame.*

2. susceptibility to this feeling; *She could not escape the feelings of shame.*

3. a fact or circumstance bringing disgrace or regret; *The death of the geraniums were a shame.* [It was a shame you couldn't water them.]

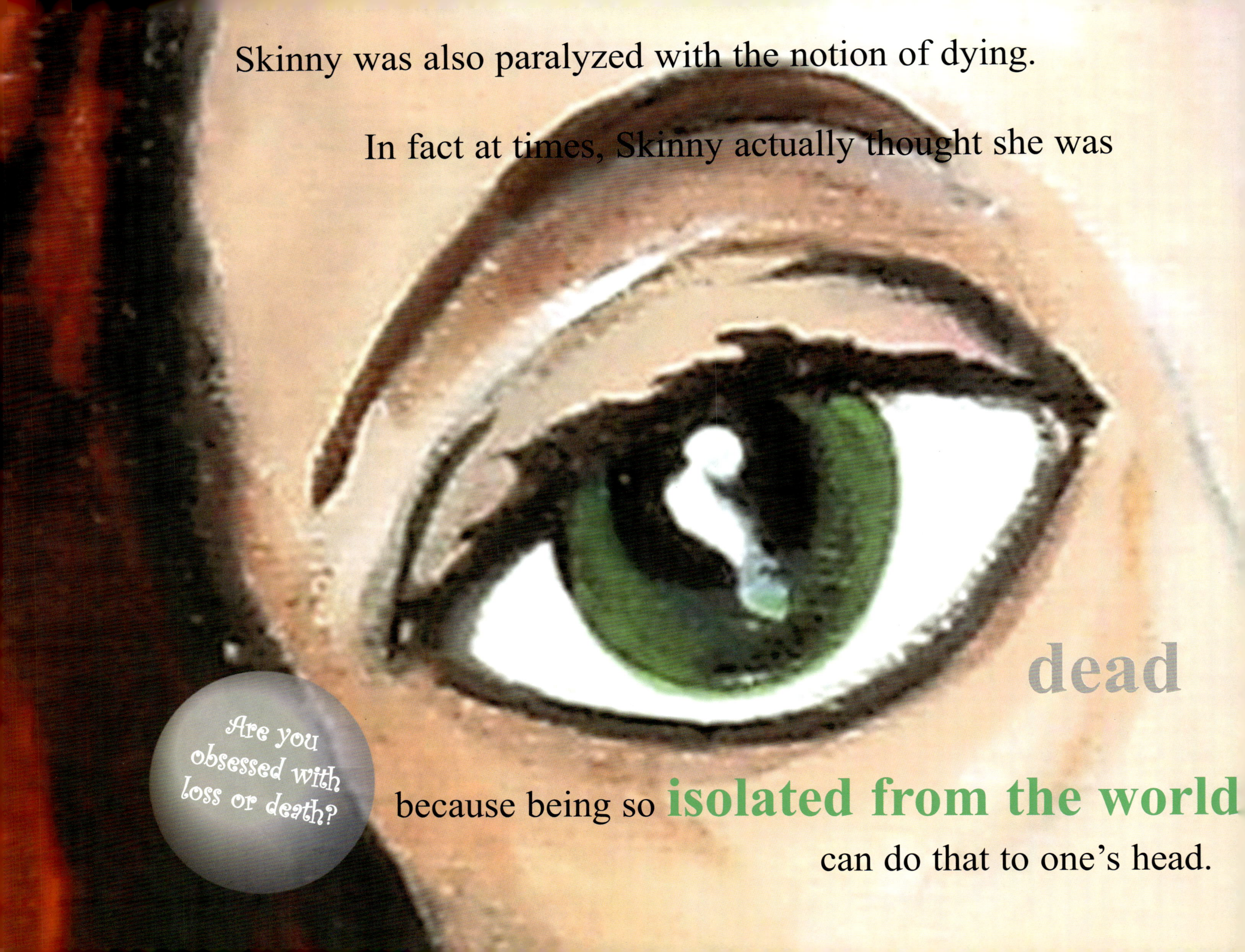

Skinny was also paralyzed with the notion of dying.

In fact at times, Skinny actually thought she was

dead

because being so **isolated from the world**

can do that to one's head.

Are you obsessed with loss or death?

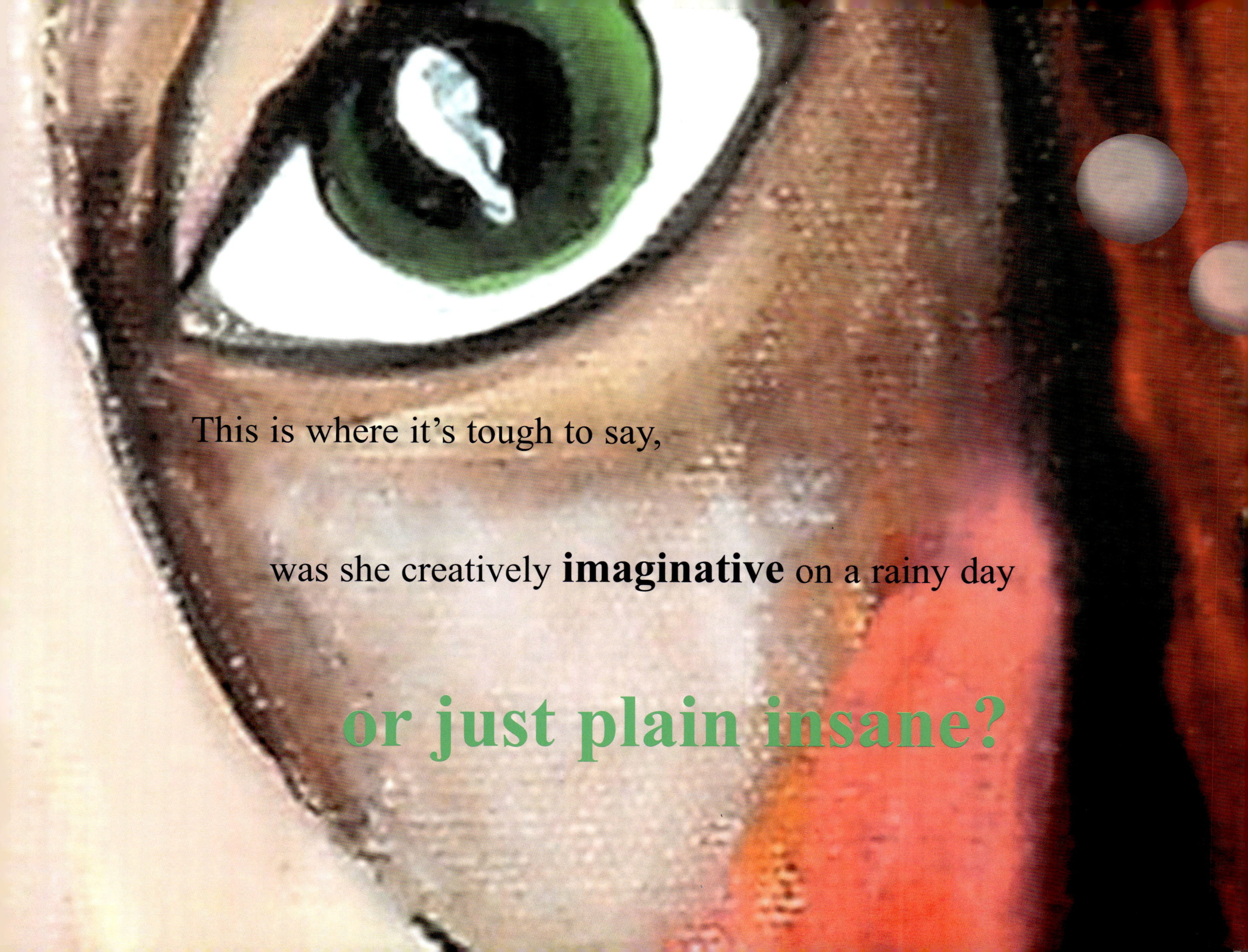

This is where it's tough to say,

was she creatively **imaginative** on a rainy day

or just plain insane?

divination

noun

1. the art or practice that seeks to foresee or foretell future events or discover hidden knowledge usually by the interpretation of omens or by the aid of supernatural powers

2. unusual insight: intuitive perception

Having never seen the world, Skinny had quite an inner world of her own. At times it was more than confusing when she and her voices had different things to say.

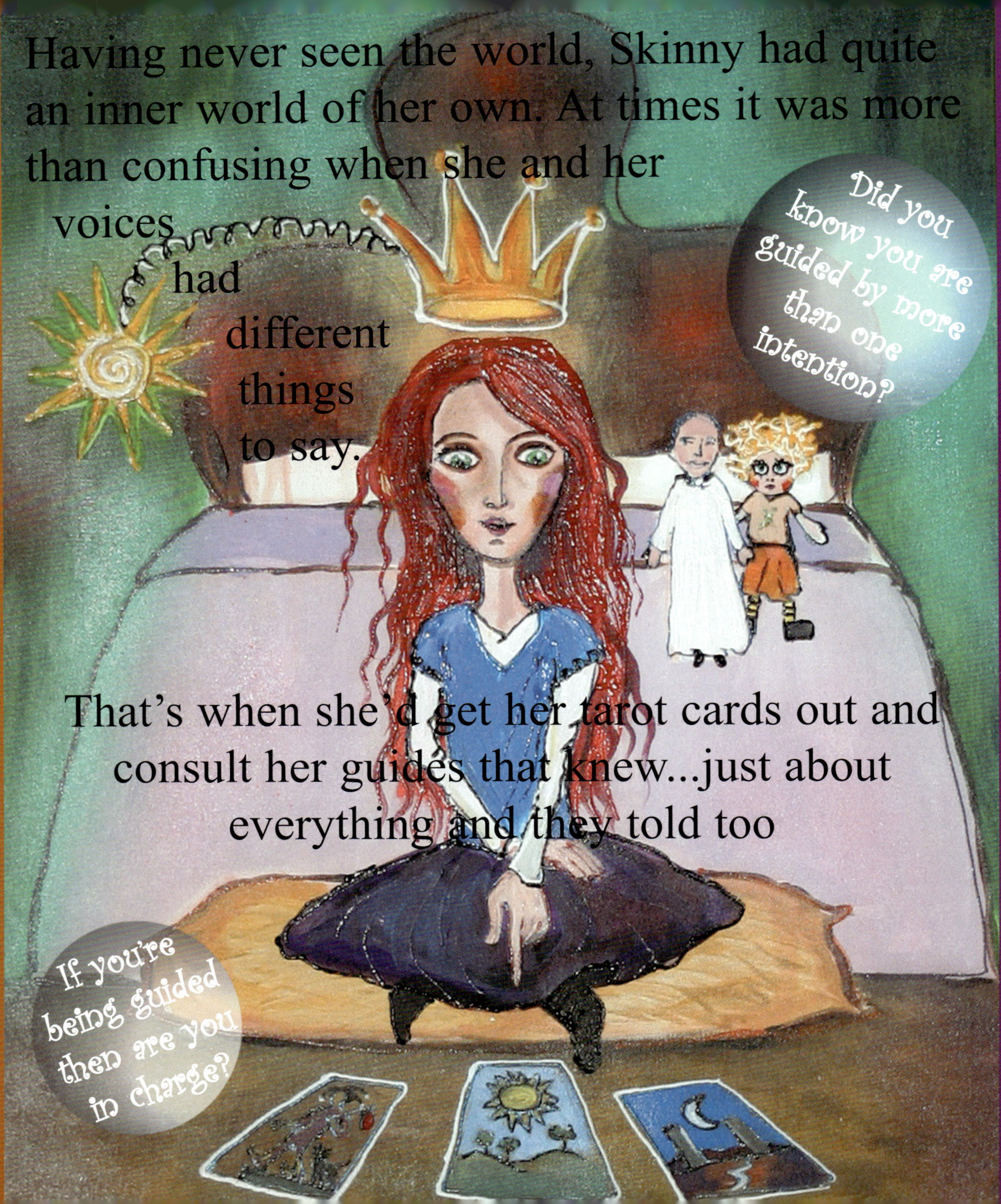
Did you know you are guided by more than one intention?
If you're being guided then are you in charge?

That's when she'd get her tarot cards out and consult her guides that knew...just about everything and they told too

The tarot is typically a set of 78 cards. Tarot cards are utilized primarily for divinatory purposes. The deck is split into the Major Arcana and Minor Arcana which are used in occult tarot and are seldom used by card players. The divinatory meanings of the cards are derived mostly from the Kabbalah of Jewish mysticism and from Medieval Alchemy. Tarot reading revolves around the belief that the cards can be used to gain insight into the current and possible future situations of the subject. Some believe they are guided by a spiritual force, such as Gaia, while others believe the cards help them tap into a collective unconscious or their own creative, brainstorming subconscious.

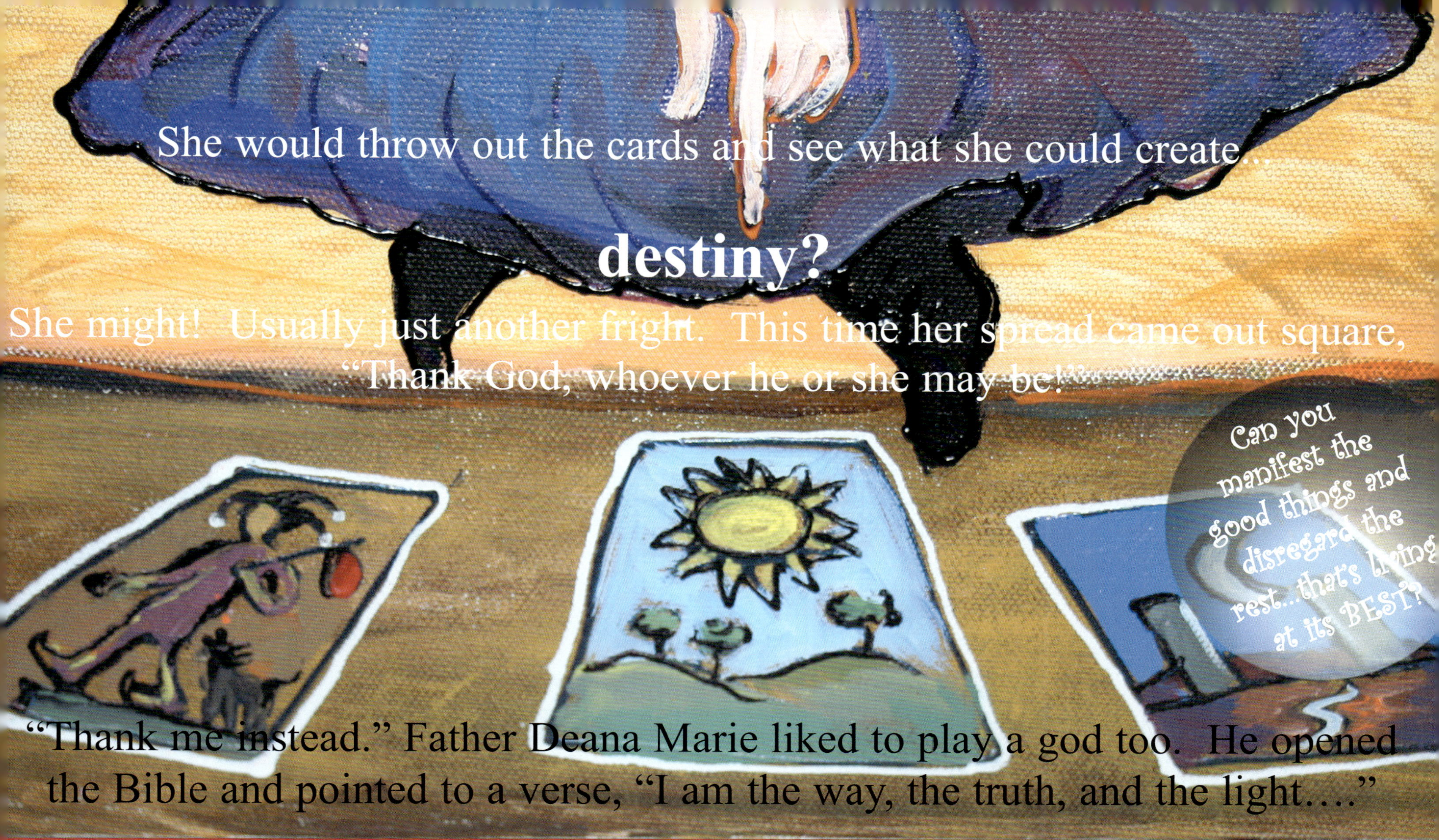

She would throw out the cards and see what she could create...

destiny?

She might! Usually just another fright. This time her spread came out square,
"Thank God, whoever he or she may be!"

Can you manifest the good things and disregard the rest...that's living at its BEST?

"Thank me instead." Father Deana Marie liked to play a god too. He opened the Bible and pointed to a verse, "I am the way, the truth, and the light...."

Bibliomancy is the use of books in divination.

The method of employing sacred books (especially specific words and verses) for 'magical medicine', for removing negative entities, or for divination is universal in all religions of the world. Directions for the method of Bibliomancy: A book is picked that is believed to hold truth. It is balanced on its spine and allowed tc fall open. A passage is picked, with the eyes closed. [It's alot like playing cards.] Among Christians, the Bible is most commonly used. Because book owners frequently have favorite passages that the books open themselves to, some practitioners use dice or another randomiser to choose the page to be opened. This practice was formalized by the use of coins or yarrow stalks in consulting the I Ching. Tarot can also be considered a form of bibliomancy, with the main difference that the cards (pages) are unbound. Another variant requires the selection of a random book from a library before selecting the random passage from that book. This also holds if a book has fallen down from a shelf on its own.[5]

DIAGNOSTIC CRITERIA FOR:

Schizotypal Personality Disorder

A. A pervasive pattern of social and interpersonal deficits marked by acute discomfort with, and reduced capacity for, close relationships as well as by cognitive or perceptual distortions and eccentricities of behavior, beginning early adulthood and present in a variety of contexts, as indicated by five (or more) of the following:

(1) ideas of reference (excluding delusions of reference)
(2) odd beliefs or magical thinking that influences behavior and is inconsistent with subcultural norms (e.g., superstitiousness, belief in clairvoyance, telepathy, or "sixth sense"; in children and adolescents, bizarre fantasies or preoccupations)
(3) unusual perceptual experiences, including bodily illusions
(4) odd thinking and speech (e.g., vague, circumstantial, metaphorical, overelaborate, or stereotyped)
(5) suspiciousness or paranoid ideation
(6) inappropriate or constricted affect
(7) behavior or appearance that is odd, eccentric, or peculiar
(8) lack of close friends or confidants other than first-degree relatives
(9) excessive social anxiety that does not diminish with familiarity and tends to be associated with paranoid fears rather than negative judgments about self

B. Does not occur exclusively during the course of Schizophrenia, a Mood Disorder With Psychotic Features, another Psychotic Disorder, or a Pervasive Developmental Disorder. Note: If criteria are met prior to the onset of Schizophrenia, add "Premorbid," e.g., "Schizotypal Personality Disorder (Premorbid)."[6]

DIAGNOSTIC CRITERIA FOR:

Religious or Spiritual Problem

This category can be used when the focus of clinical attention is a religious or spiritual problem. Examples include distressing experiences that involve loss or questioning of faith, problems associated with conversion to a new faith, or questioning of spiritual values that may not necessarily be related to an organized church or religious institution.[7]

“Oh, have I fed **#9** today? I can never remember...I probably did.” Skinny

That cat is going to be the death of me! Remembering him means he’s like

Her black cat she called **#9** was never seen. She and the dolls knew it was

feed it he was sure to die. **#9** would sneak out late, late at night when

He’s probably scared of me. As if I could really do anything to him in the

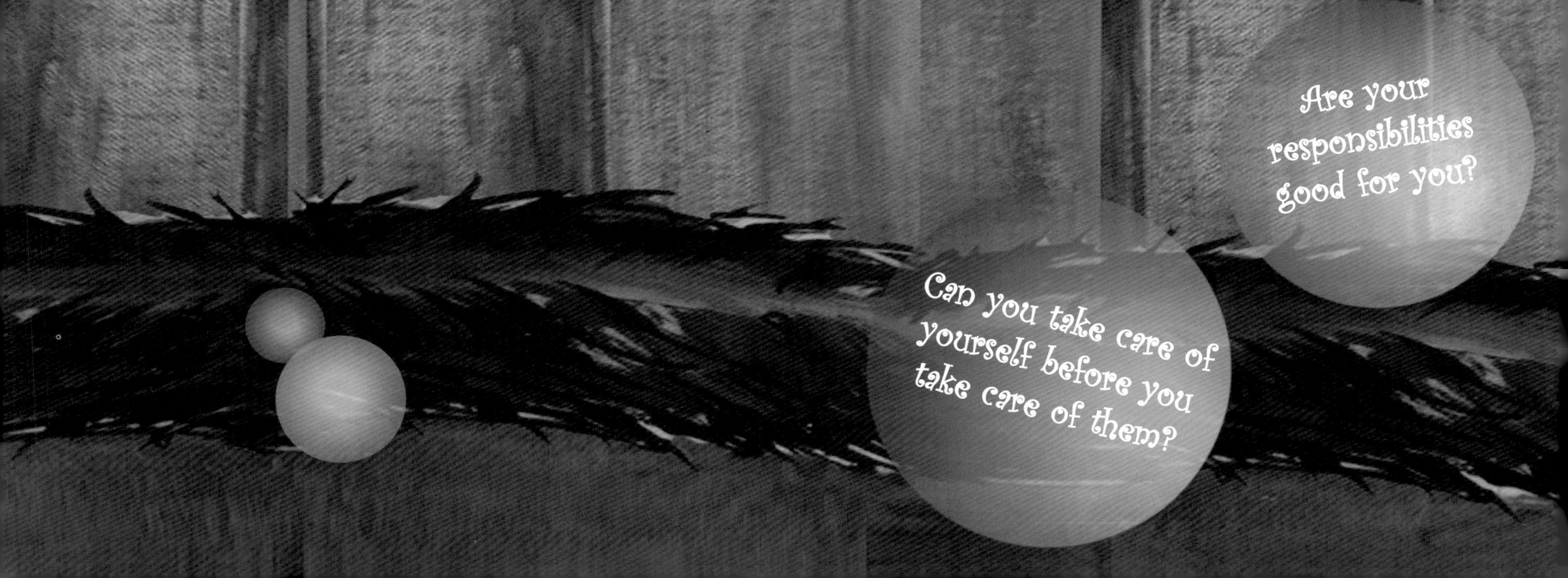
Are your responsibilities good for you?
Can you take care of yourself before you take care of them?

was troubled and nervous inside. "I must have, thank God! Yes, I did!

another memory." Skinny Miss S. avoided most of her black memories.

alive because it ate all of his food each night. She worried if she didn't

Skinny was finally asleep. I've seen his shadow a couple of times.

condition I'm in. Cats are weird though, they're ***rarely never spooked…***

thus begins the amazing adventures of

Skinny Miss S.

Do you escape only to find yourself in darkness?

Skinny Miss S. was very **depressed.**

When she tried to eat a little something,

it made her **sick with anxiety.**

Skinny said, "I don't feel like eating. It's much more fun to pretend."

Lonely replied, "But you'll die if you don't want to thrive.

Is that what you intend?"

anxiety

noun

1. painful or apprehensive uneasiness of mind usually over an impending or anticipated ill.

2. fearful concern or interest

3. an abnormal and overwhelming sense of fear often marked by physiological signs (as sweating, tension, and increased pulse), by doubt concerning the reality and nature of the threat, and by self-doubt about one's capacity to cope with it

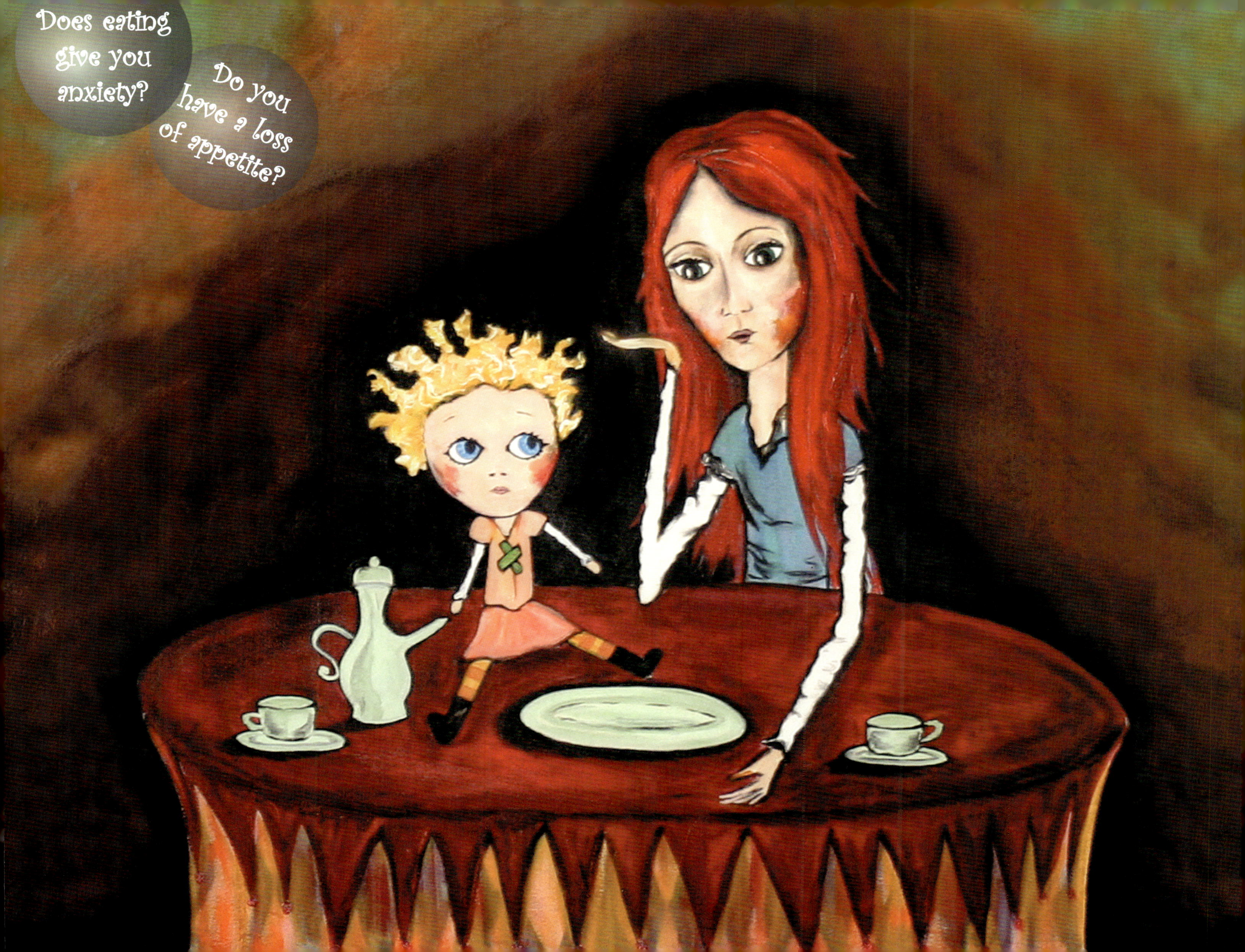
Does eating give you anxiety?
Do you have a loss of appetite?

DIAGNOSTIC CRITERIA FOR:

Anorexia Nervosa

A. Refusal to maintain body weight at or above a minimally normal weight for age and height (e.g., weight loss leading to maintenance of body weight less than 85% of that expected; or failure to make expected weight gain during period of growth, leading to body weight less than 85% of that expected).

B. Intense fear of gaining weight or becoming fat, even though underweight.

C. Disturbance in the way in which one's body weight or shape is experienced, undue influence of body weight or shape on self-evaluation, or denial of the seriousness of the current low body weight.

D. In postmenarcheal females, amenorrhea, i.e., the absence of at least three consecutive menstrual cycles. (A woman is considered to have amenorrhea if her periods occur only following hormone, e.g., estrogen, administration).

Specify type:

Restricting Type: during the current episode of Anorexia Nervosa, the person has not regularly engaged in binge-eating or purging behavior (i.e., self-induced vomiting or the misuse of laxatives, diuretics, or enemas).

Binge-Eating/Purging Type: during the current episode of Anorexia Nervosa, the person has regularly engaged in binge-eating or purging behavior (i.e., self-induced vomiting or the misuse of laxatives, diuretics, or enemas).[8]

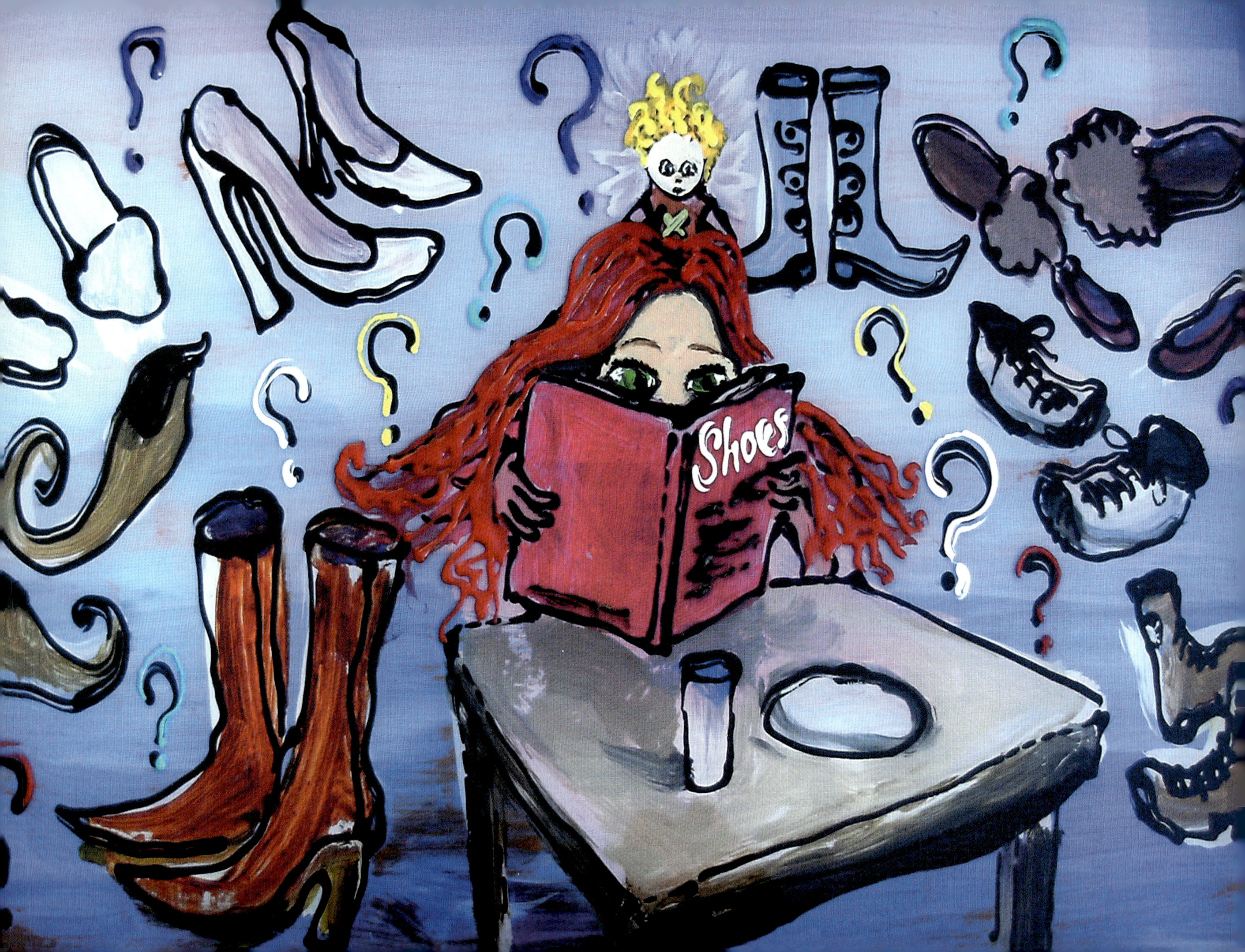
Shoes

When she would try to make a simple decision, she decided she could not, so she thought and thought and tought... until she forgot. Sometimes she would count how many times the thought stepped back in. It usually came in two's, like the pairs of her shoes.

"Which ones should I choose?!" Skinny really couldn't decide, "I need shoes to go outside and check the mail. I just can't seem to decide on which pair!"

Lonely could, but didn't dare share, "It shouldn't be that hard to figure out what shoes to wear!"

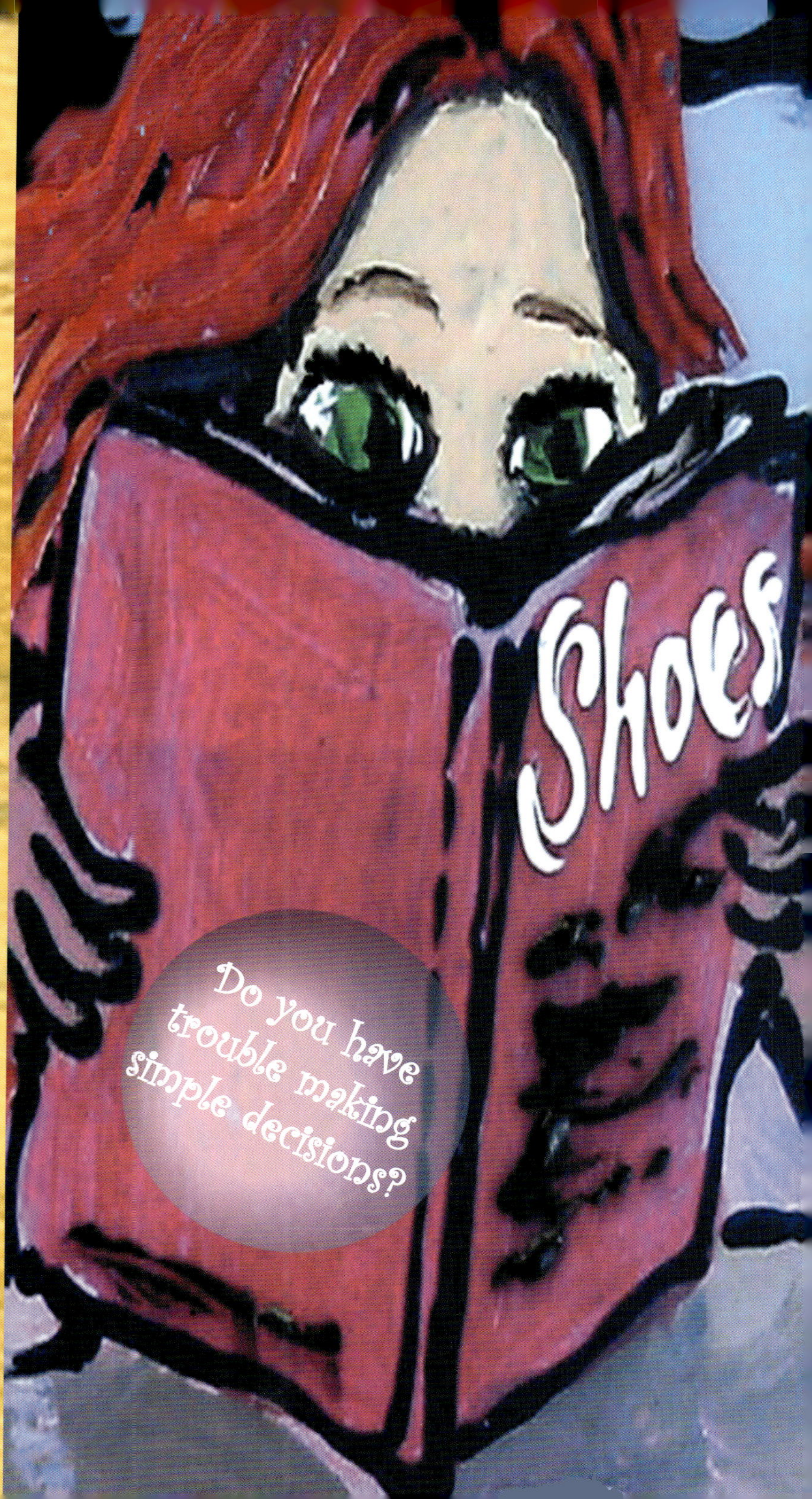

DIAGNOSTIC CRITERIA FOR:

Obsessive-Compulsive Disorder

A. Either obsessions or compulsions: Obsessions as defined by (1), (2), (3), and (4):

(1) recurrent and persistent thoughts, impulses, or images that are experienced, at some time during the disturbance, as intrusiv and inappropriate and that cause marked anxiety or distress

(2) the thoughts, impulses, or images are not simply excessive worries about real-life problems

(3) the person attempts to ignore or suppress such thoughts, impules, or images, or to neutralize them with some other thought or action

(4) the person recognizes that the obsessional thoughts, impulses, or images are a product of his or her own mind (not imposed from without as in thought insertion)

Compulsions as defined by (1) and (2):

(1) repetitive behaviors (e.g., hand washing, ordering, checking) or mental acts (e.g., praying, counting, repeating words silently) that the person feels driven to perform in response to an obsession, or according to rules that must be applied rigidly

(2) the behaviors or mental acts are aimed at preventing or reducing distress or preventing some dreaded event or situation; however, these behaviors or mental acts either are not connected in a realistic way with what they are designed to neutralize or prevent or are clearly excessive.

B. At some point during the course of the disorder, the person has recognized that the obsessions or compulsions are excessive or unreasonable. Note: This does not apply to children.

C. The obsessions or compulsions cause marked distress, are time consuming (take more than 1 hour a day), or significantly interfere with the person's normal routine, occupational (or academic) functioning, or usual social activities or relationships.

D. If another Axis I disorder is present, the content of the obsessions or compulsions is not restricted to it (e.g., preoccupation with food in the presence of an Eating Disorder; hair pulling in the presence of Trichotillomania; concern with appearance in the presence of Body Dysmorphic Disorder; preoccupation with drugs in the presence of a Substance Use Disorder; preoccupation with having a serious illness in the presence of Hypochondriasis; preoccupation with sexual urges or fantasies in the presence of a Paraphilia; or guilty ruminations in the presence of Major Depressive Disorder).

E. The disturbance is not due to the direct physiological effects of a substance (e.g., a drug of abuse, a medication) or a general medical condition.

Specify if:

With Poor Insight: if, for most of the time during the current episode, the person does not recognize that the obsessions and compulsions are excessive or unreasonable.[9]

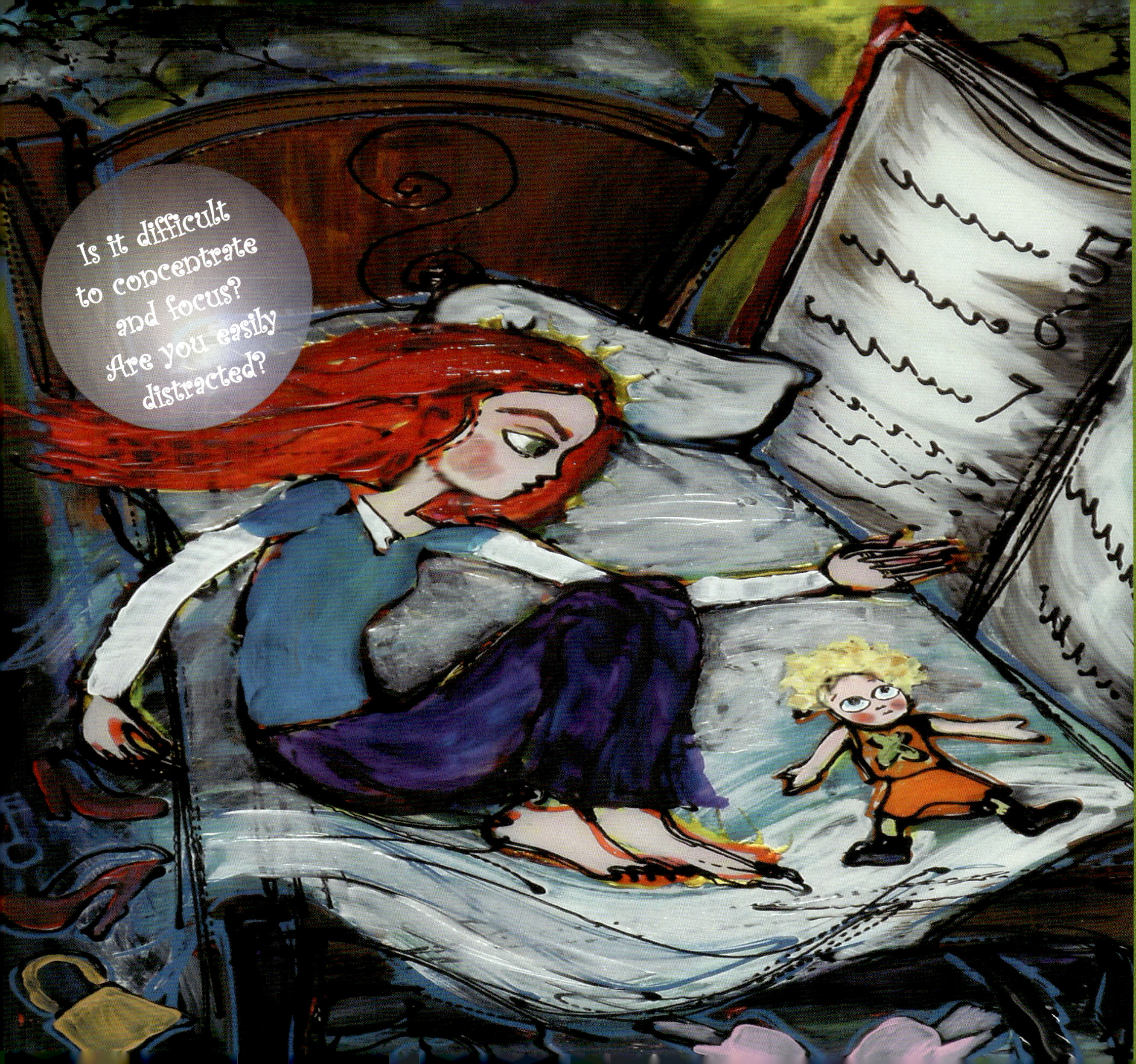
Is it difficult to concentrate and focus? Are you easily distracted?

concentration

noun

1. the act or process of concentrating
2. the state of being concentrated; *esp:* direction of attention to a single object.
3. an academic major or area of focus within a major.
4. a concentrated mass or thing.
5. the amount of a component in a given area or volume.

When she tried to read a little something, the words blurred into a lot of something else. Skinny laid in bed with a book open to the page,

"Seven Ways to Celebrate Yourself:"

She was driven to distraction when concentrating between the words in her mind and the words on the page. She read out loud to herself as she thought of all she had to do.

"**Number 1.** Draw your family tree and honor your roots. [*I haven't taken the trash out in weeks!*]
Number 2. Find your favorite childhood picture and have a conversation with it. [*The dishes are piling up.*]
Number 3. Make a collage from magazine clippings which best represents you. [*How am I going to pay my bills today?*]
Number 4. Go on a date with guess who, YOU! [*Oh yes, and I can't forget there are clothes all over the floor.*]
Number 5. Sit in silence in a warm bath and think about nothing. [*I haven't taken a shower in days. I should think about taking one.*]
Number 7. Just because you want a hug…buy yourself a teddy!
[*Haven't I read that line already? Oh no, I skipped* ***Number 6.*** *That one's about making a wish.* ***This book is full of it.***]"

DIAGNOSTIC CRITERIA FOR:

Attention-Deficit/Hyperactivity Disorder

A. Either (1) or (2):

(1) six (or more) of the following symptoms of inattention have persisted for at least 6 months to a degree that is maladaptive and inconsistent with developmental level:

Inattention

(a) often fails to give close attention to details or makes careless mistakes in schoolwork, work, or other activities

(b) often has difficulty sustaining attention in tasks or play activities

(c) often does not seem to listen when spoken to directly

(d) often does not follow through on instructions and fails to finish schoolwork, chores, or duties in the workplace (not due to oppositional behavior or failure to understand instructions)

(e) often has difficulty organizing tasks and activities

(f) often avoids, dislikes, or is reluctant to engage in tasks that require sustained mental effort (such as schoolwork or homework)

(g) often loses things necessary for tasks or activities (e.g., toys, school assignments, pencils, books, or tools)

(h) is often easily distracted by extraneous stimuli

(i) is often forgetful in daily activities

(2) six (or more) of the following symptoms of hyperactivity-impulsivity have persisted for at least 6 months to a degree that is maladaptive and inconsistent with developmental level: Hyperactivity

(a) often fidgets with hands or feet or squirms in seat
(b) often leaves seat in classroom or in other situations in which remaining seated is expected
(c) often runs about or climbs excessively in situations in which it is inappropriate (in adolescents or adults, may be limited to subjective feelings of restlessness)
(d) often has difficulty playing or engaging in leisure activities quietly
(e) is often "on the go" or often acts as if "driven by a motor"
(f) often talks excessively Impulsivity
(g) often blurts out answers before questions have been completed
(h) often has difficulty awaiting turn
(i) often interrupts or intrudes on others (e.g., butts into conversations or games)

B. Some hyperactive-impulsive or inattentive symptoms that caused impairment were present before age 7 years.

C. Some impairment from the symptoms is present in two or more settings (e.g., at school [or work] and at home).

D. There must be clear evidence of clinically significant impairment in social, academic, or occupational functioning.

E. The symptoms do not occur exclusively during the course of a Pervasive Developmental Disorder, Schizophrenia, or other Psychotic Disorder and are not better accounted for by another mental disorder (e.g., Mood Disorder, Anxiety Disorder, Dissociative Disorder, or a Personality Disorder).[10]

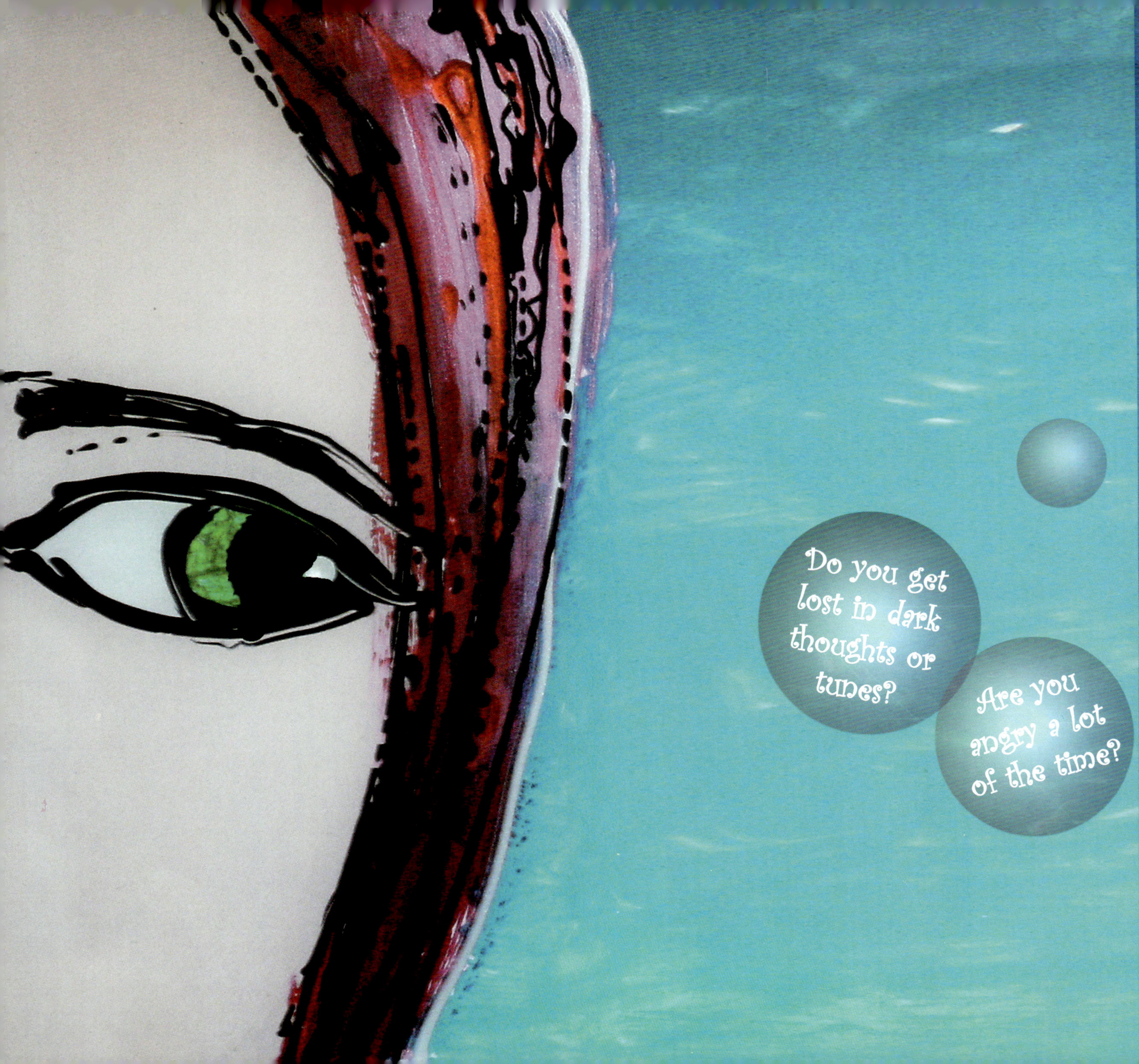
Do you get lost in dark thoughts or tunes?
Are you angry a lot of the time?

sabotage

noun

1. destruction of an employer's property or the hindering of manufacturing by discontented workers.

2. destructive or obstructive action carried on by a civilian or enemy agent to hinder a nation's war effort.

3. an act or process tending to hamper or hurt deliberate subversion.

spacey

adjective

1. dazed or stupefied by or as if by a narcotic substance.

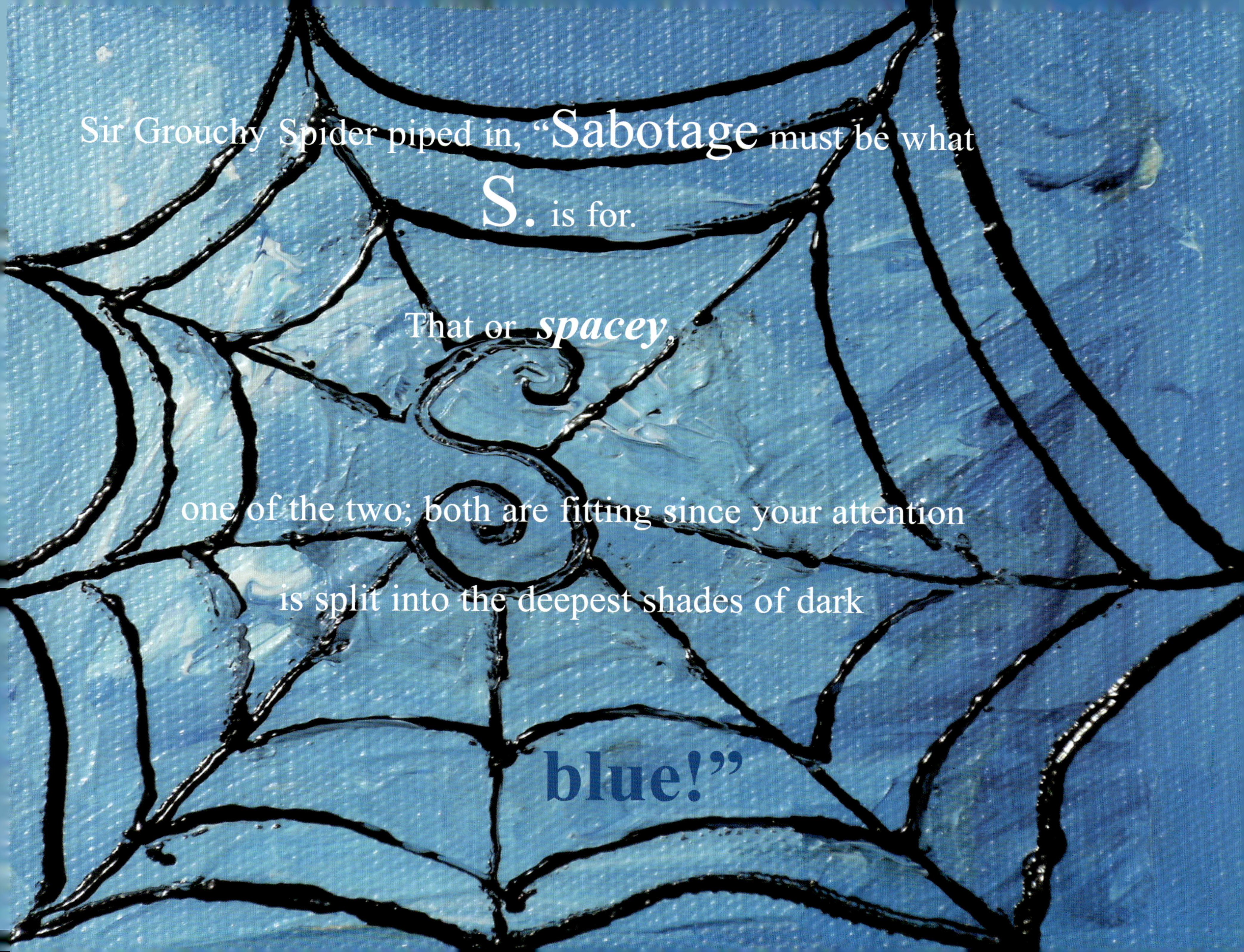

Sir Grouchy Spider piped in, "**Sabotage** must be what **S.** is for.

That or ***spacey***,

one of the two; both are fitting since your attention is split into the deepest shades of dark

blue!"

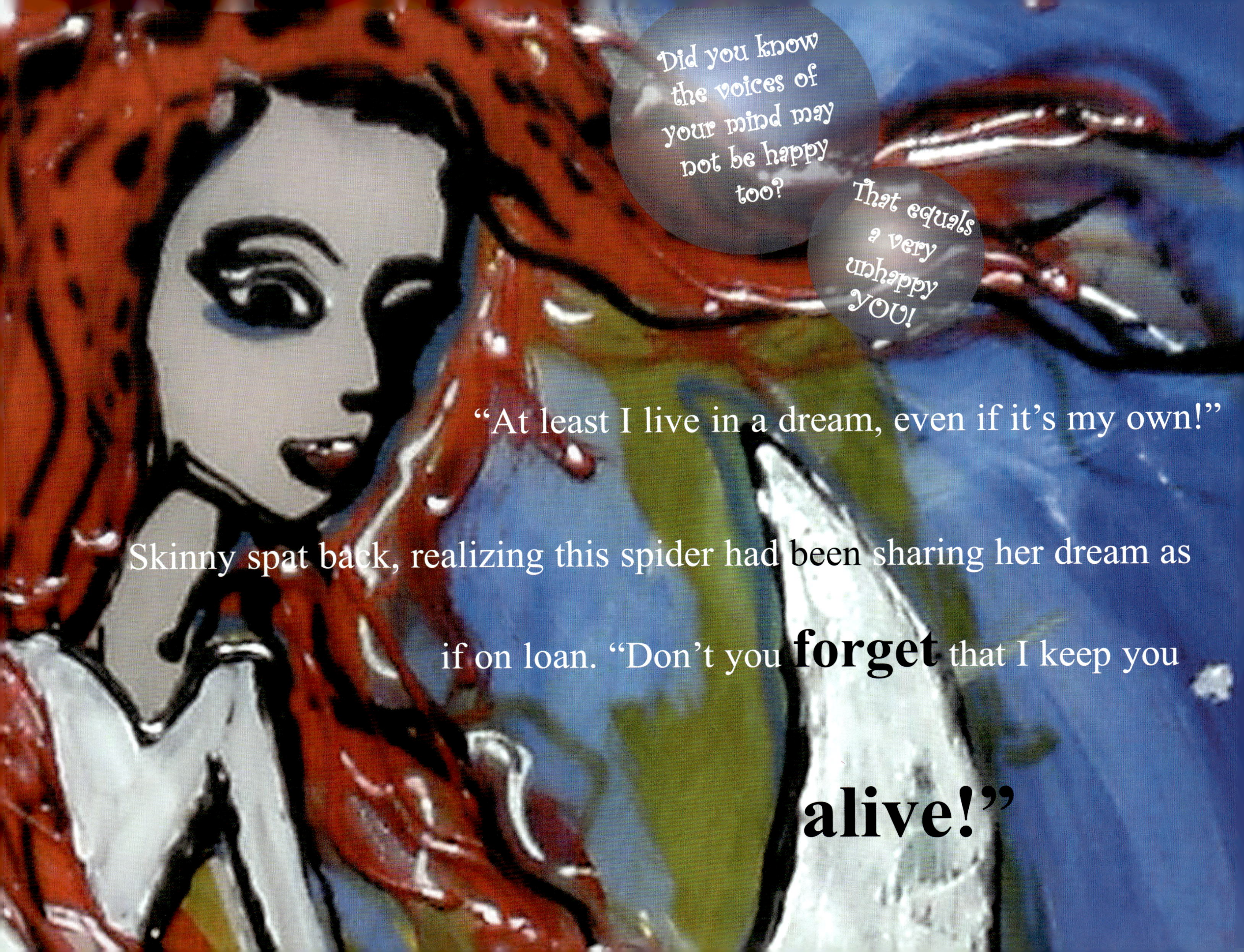
Did you know the voices of your mind may not be happy too?
That equals a very unhappy YOU!

"At least I live in a dream, even if it's my own!"

Skinny spat back, realizing this spider had been sharing her dream as if on loan. "Don't you **forget** that I keep you **alive!**"

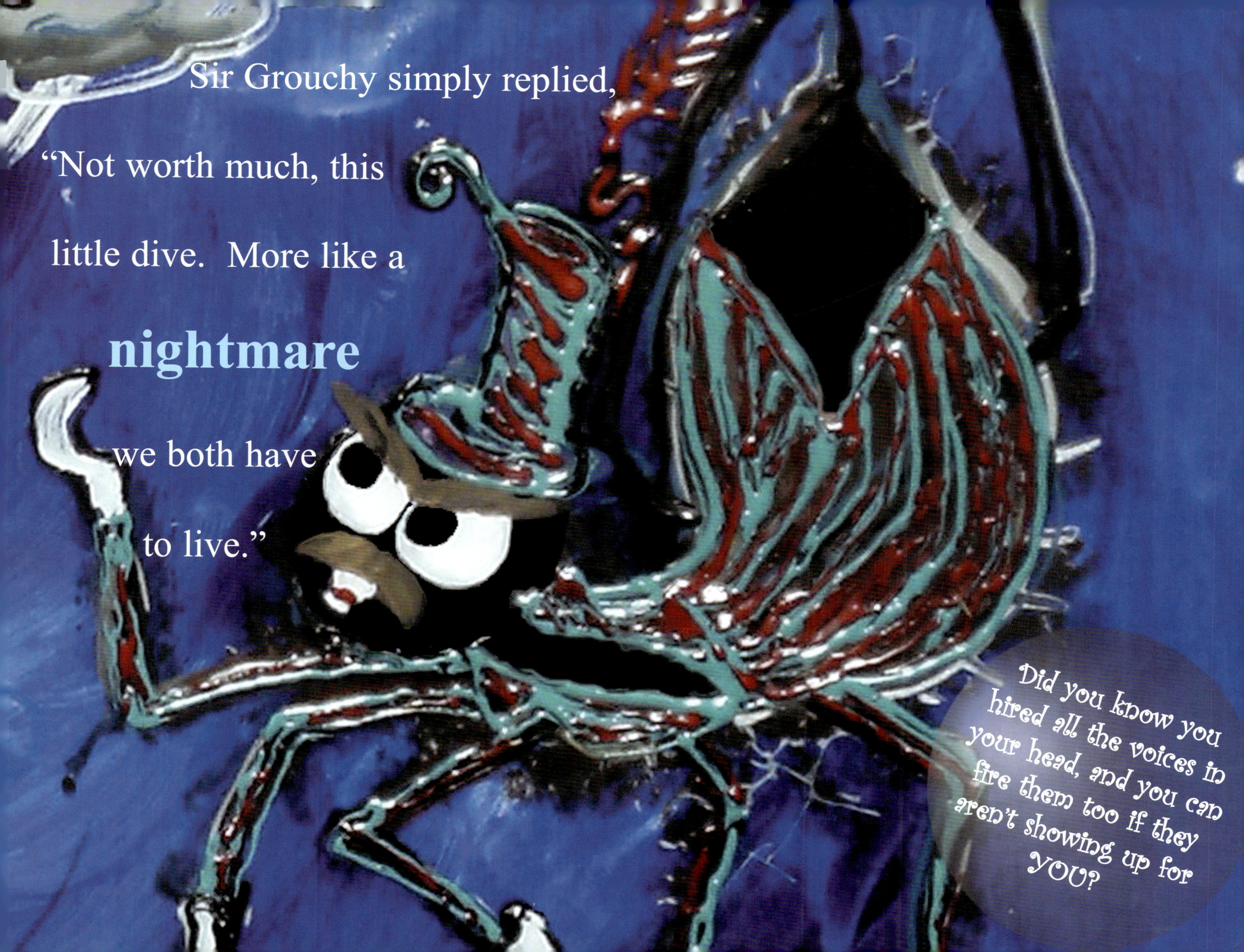

Sir Grouchy simply replied,

"Not worth much, this little dive. More like a **nightmare** we both have to live."

Did you know you hired all the voices in your head, and you can fire them too if they aren't showing up for YOU?

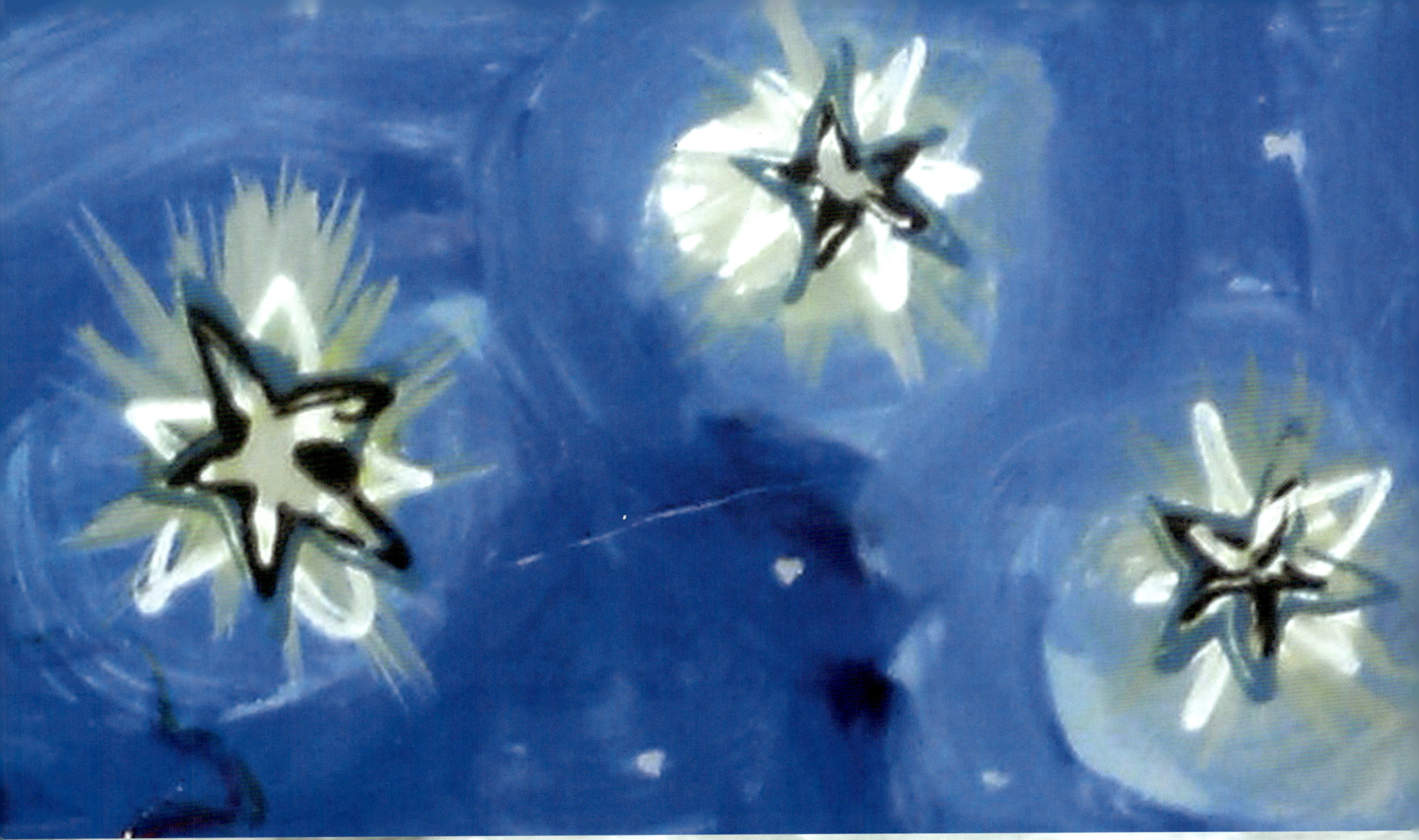

nightmare

noun

1. an evil spirit formerly thought to oppress people during sleep.

2. a frightening dream that usually awakens the sleeper.

3. something (as an experience, situation, or object) having the monstrous character of a nightmare or producing a feeling of anxiety or terror.

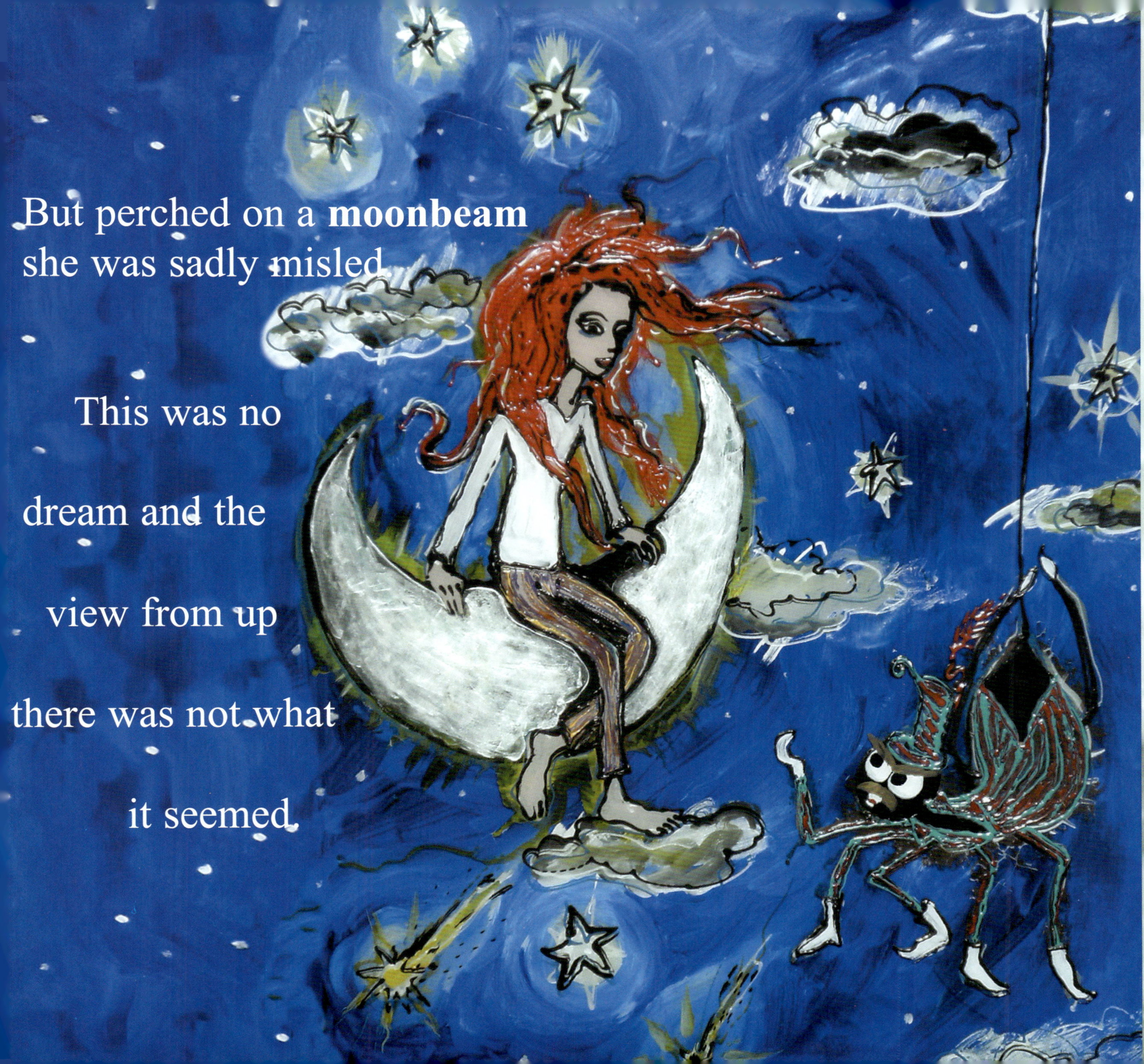

But perched on a **moonbeam**
she was sadly misled.

This was no
dream and the
view from up
there was not what
it seemed.

fantasy
noun

1. the free play of creative imagination.
2. a creation of the imaginative faculty whether expressed or conceived as a fantastic notion.
3. the process of creating especially unrealistic mental images in response to psychological needs; also a series of mental images *(as a daydream); sexual fantasies of adolescence*

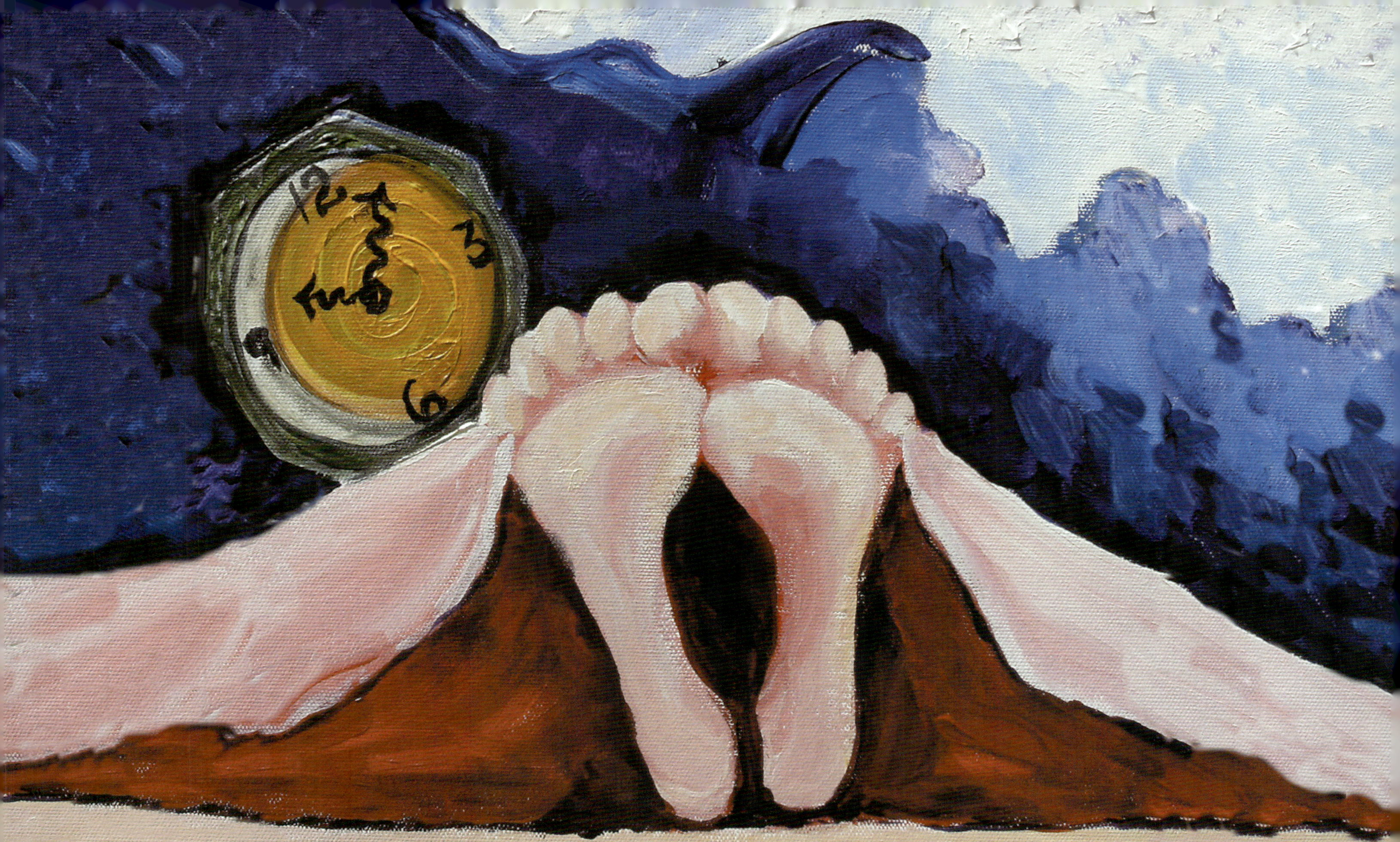

Skinny Miss S. was very depressed.

When she tried to stay awake, she fell asleep and when she tried to sleep, she was nothing but awake.

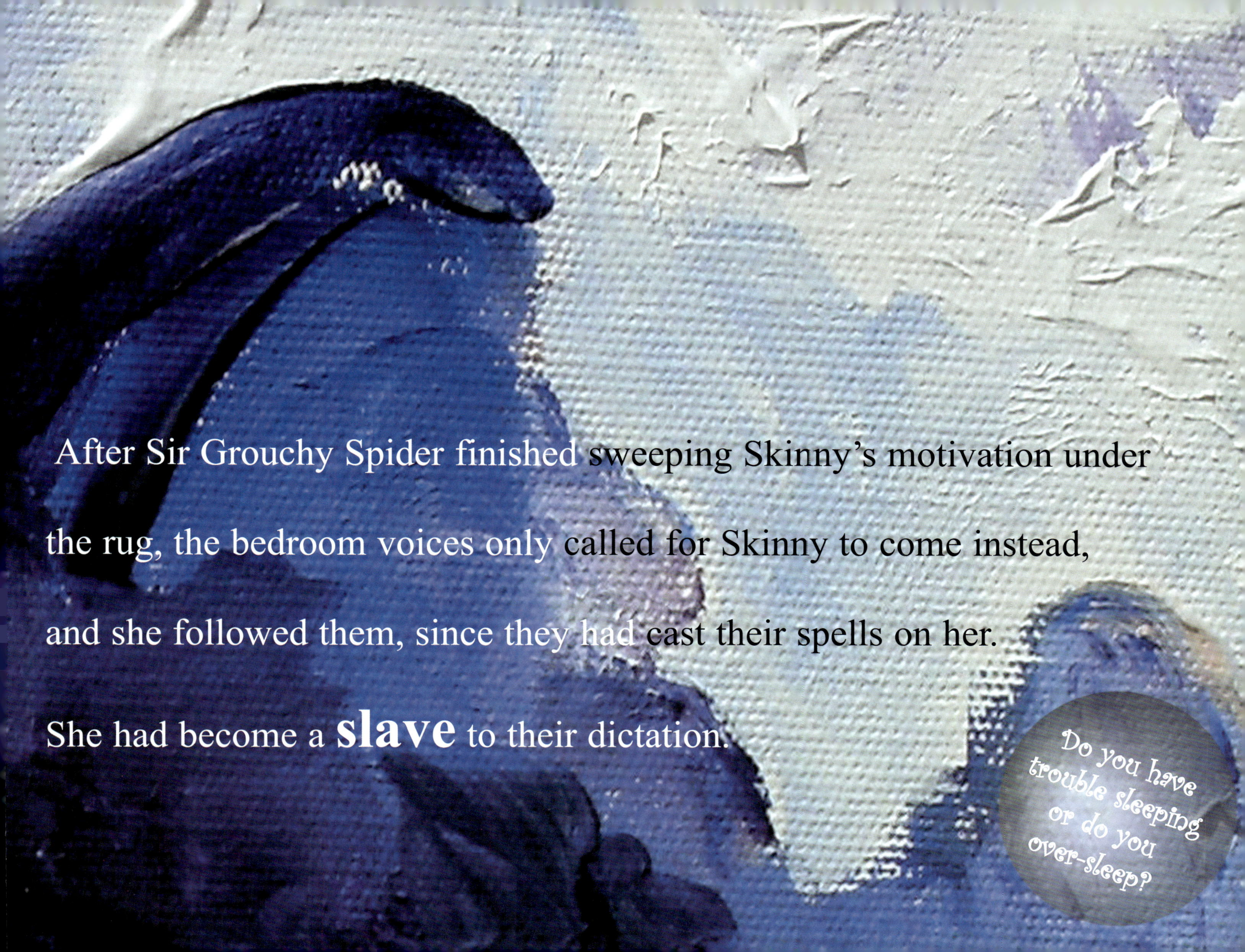

After Sir Grouchy Spider finished sweeping Skinny's motivation under the rug, the bedroom voices only called for Skinny to come instead, and she followed them, since they had cast their spells on her. She had become a **slave** to their dictation.

Do you have trouble sleeping or do you over-sleep?

DIAGNOSTIC CRITERIA FOR:

Primary Insomnia

A. The predominant complaint is difficulty initiating or maintaining sleep, or nonrestorative sleep, for at least 1 month.

B. The sleep disturbance (or associated daytime fatigue) causes clinically significant distress or impairment in social, occupational, or other important areas of functioning.

C. The sleep disturbance does not occur exclusively during the course of Narcolepsy, Breathing-Related Sleep Disorder, Circadian Rhythm Sleep Disorder, or a Parasomnia.

D. The disturbance does not occur exclusively during the course of another mental disorder (e.g., Major Depressive Disorder, Generalized Anxiety Disorder, a delirium).

E. The disturbance is not due to the direct physiological effects of a substance (e.g., a drug of abuse, a medication) or a general medical condition.[11]

"Come to bed, Skinny, for just one more hour, who wants to listen to all the unnecessary chatter?

Firm is your bed and soft are its feathers, we'd be glad to wrap you in chains and leather.

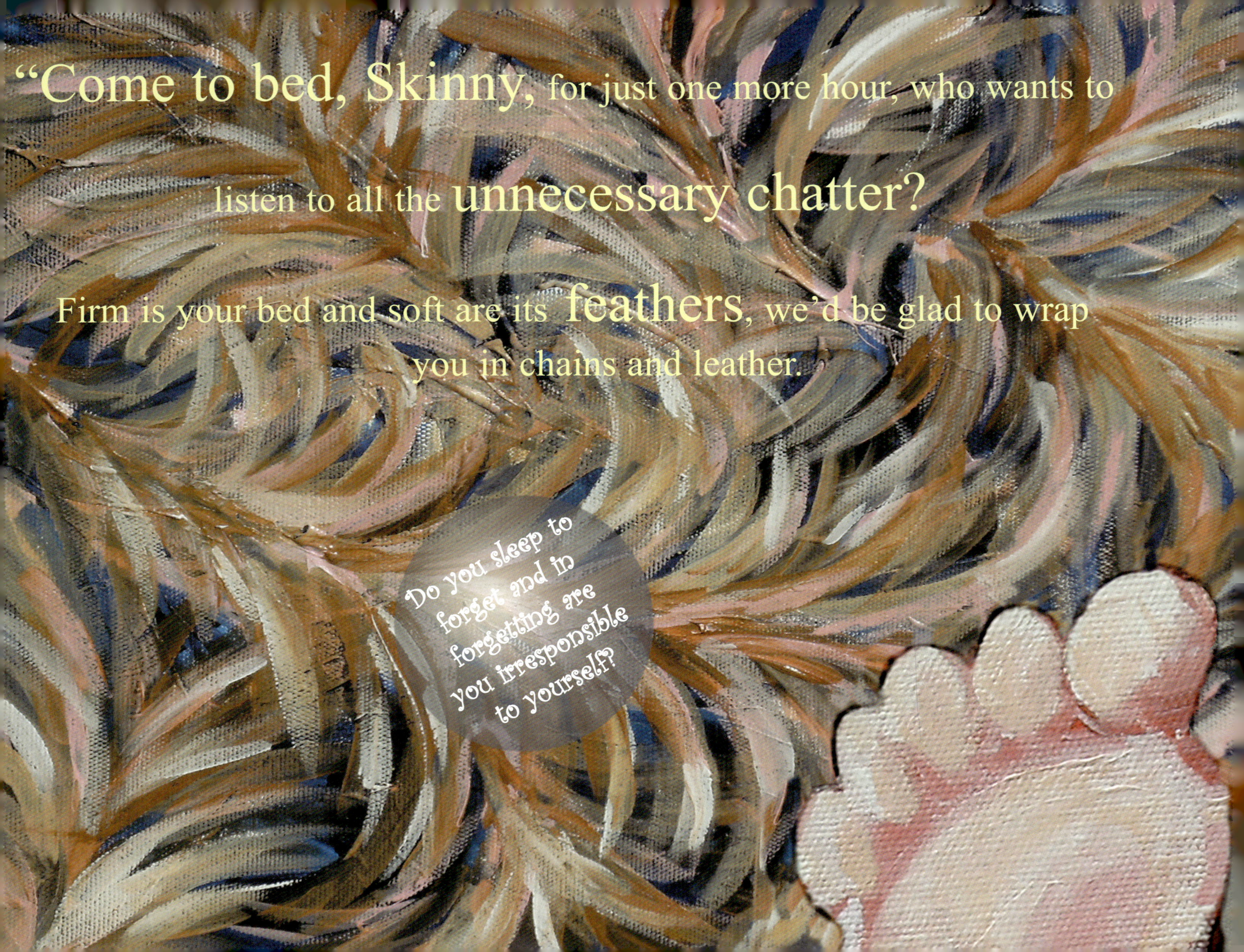

Do you sleep to forget and in forgetting are you irresponsible to yourself?

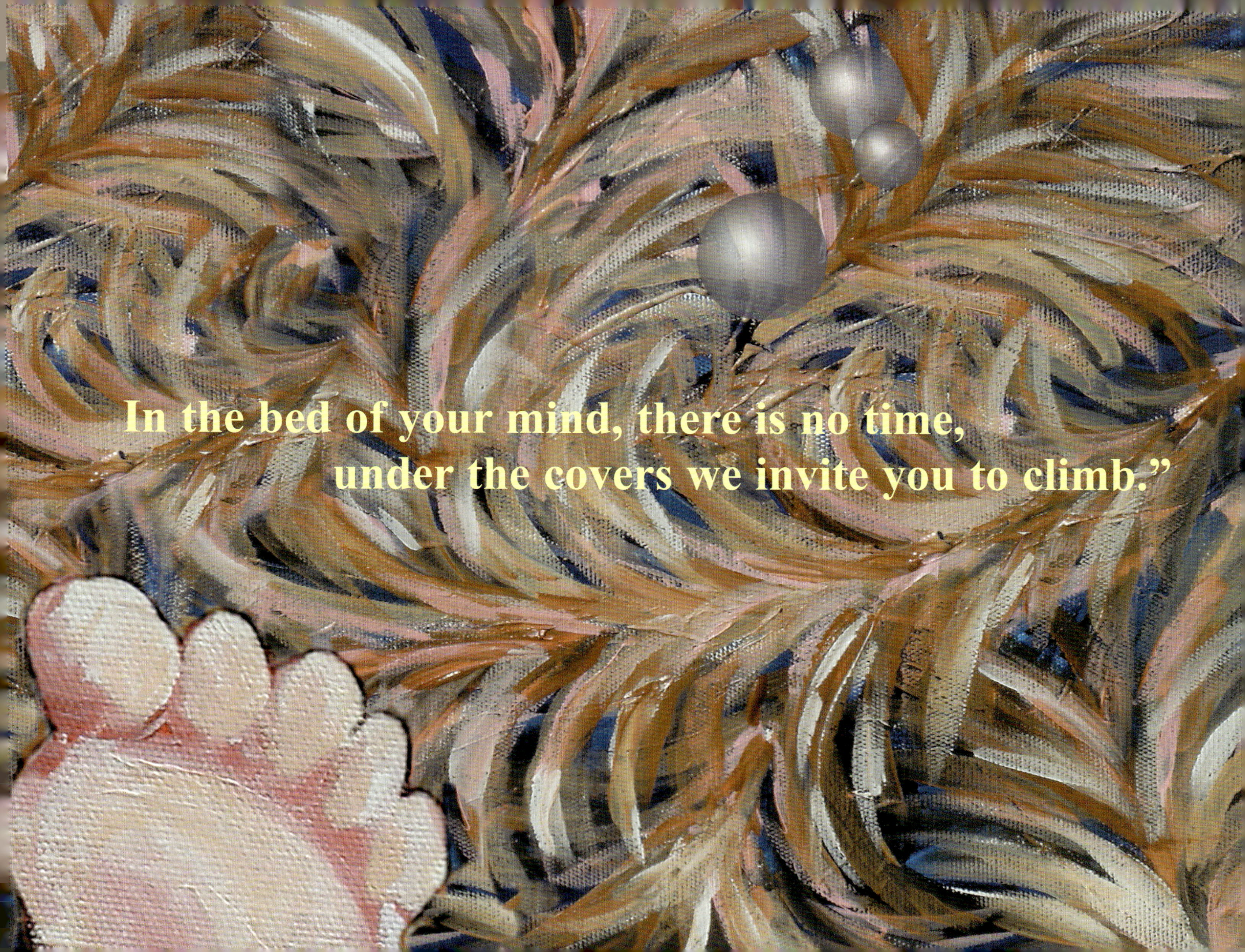

In the bed of your mind, there is no time,
under the covers we invite you to climb."

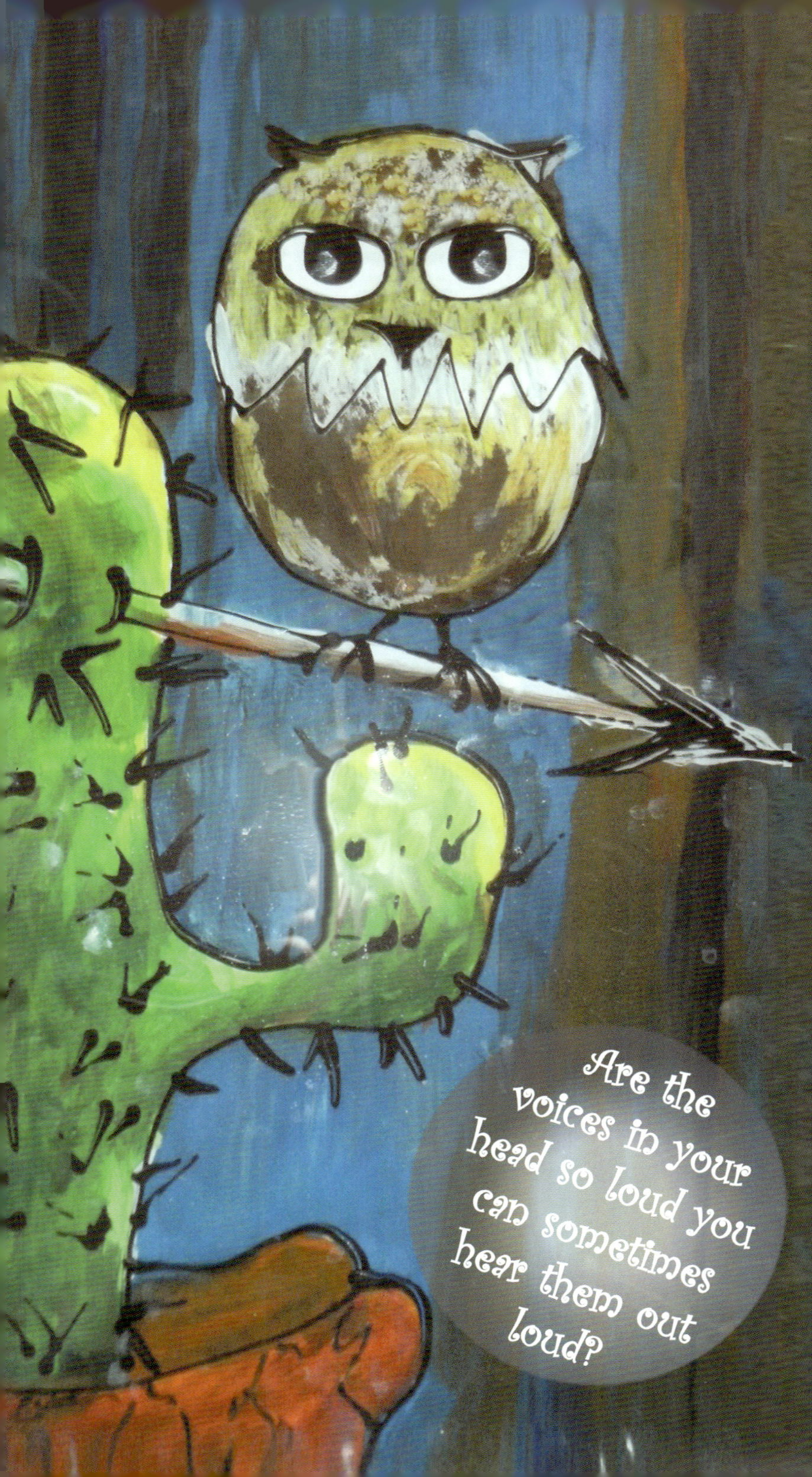
Do you feel like God or ghosts talk to you?
Do they question who you are or just plain say, "boo!"?
Are the voices in your head so loud you can sometimes hear them out loud?

"You take me for a walking zombie don't you?" asked Skinny to no one in particularly.

"WHO ME!?"

I slipped out accidentally.

"Who-ooo, who was that?" asked Skinny Miss S. "My god, I can hear God's voice too! I must be blessed! Is this an inner broadcasting test?"

She eyed me nervously and asked me if it were judgment day. There was nothing I could say. Then she moved me down from high above and placed me on the only house plant she could keep alive.

I suppose now I wasn't just watching her.

Her bed was the only place where she felt relieved and she believed the bedroom voices were the only companions who truly understood, but those voices were really me. Imagine that! An owl taming down an over imaginary girl to get some peace and quiet! After all, I am dead and stuffed now and I deserve a little silence. I knew she had found comfort in becoming invisible to the world, so I gave that to her. Her mind was brilliant to have learned to listen to me. How else would she have survived? I only led her to bed because that was where her subconscious lived. A conscious life would be too much for her head. Besides there I could visit her in her dreams and watch all of the things she use to do before she turned blue and delusional too. I kept an **eye** on her because it worried me how much my voices caused her to rest. Yes, she truly ***worried*** me, and maybe that's why I slipped out a "who...me?", thinking maybe this time I would come clean.

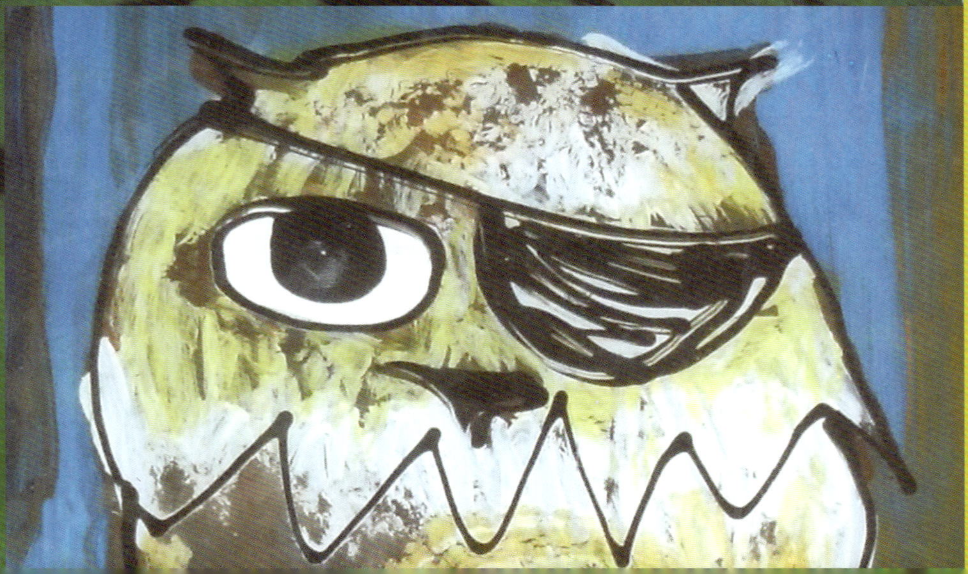

worry
verb

1. to subject to persistent or nagging attention or effort.
2. to afflict with mental distress or agitation; make anxious; torment.
3. to experience concern or anxiety; *Worrying about his healthy eye made him a hypochondriac.*

DIAGNOSTIC CRITERIA FOR:

Delusional Disorder

A. Nonbizarre delusions (i.e., involving situations that occur in real life, such as being followed, poisoned, infected, loved at a distance, or deceived by spouse or lover, or having a disease) of at least 1 month's duration.

B. Criterion A for Schizophrenia has never been met. Note: Tactile and olfactory hallucinations may be present in Delusional Disorder if they are related to the delusional theme.

C. Apart from the impact of the delusion(s) or its ramifications, functioning is not markedly impaired and behavior is not obviously odd or bizarre.

D. If mood episodes have occurred concurrently with delusions, their total duration has been brief relative to the duration of the delusional periods.

E. The disturbance is not due to the direct physiological effects of a substance (e.g., a drug of abuse, a medication) or a general medical condition.

Specify type (the following types are assigned based on the predominant delusional theme):

Erotomanic Type: delusions that another person, usually of higher status, is in love with the individual

Grandiose Type: delusions of inflated worth, power, knowledge, identity, or special relationship to a deity or famous person

Jealous Type: delusions that the individual's sexual partner is unfaithful

Persecutory Type: delusions that the person (or someone to whom the person is close) is being malevolently treated in some way

Somatic Type: delusions that the person has some physical defect or general medical condition

Mixed Type: delusions characteristic of more than one of the above types but no one theme predominates[12]

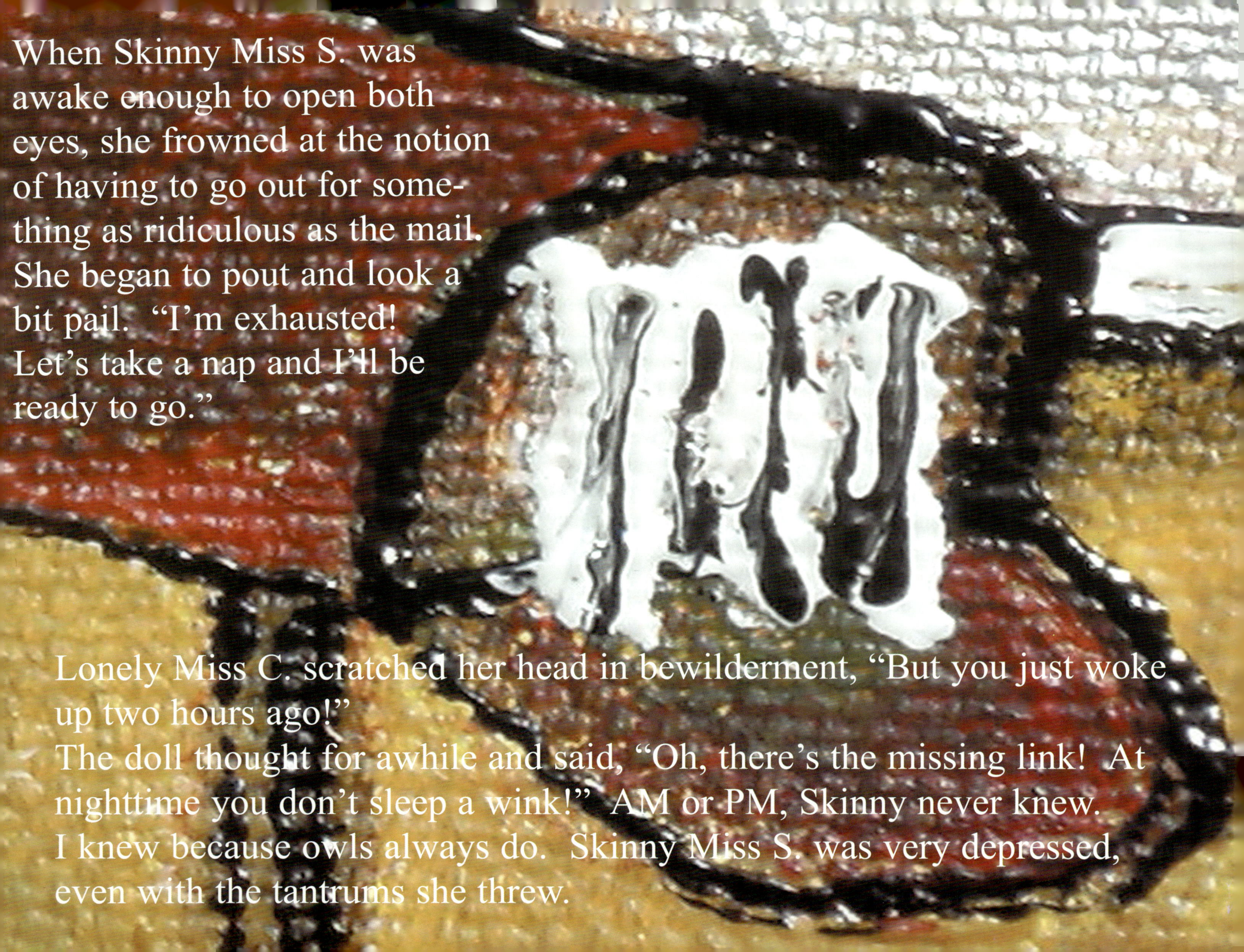

When Skinny Miss S. was awake enough to open both eyes, she frowned at the notion of having to go out for something as ridiculous as the mail. She began to pout and look a bit pail. "I'm exhausted! Let's take a nap and I'll be ready to go."

Lonely Miss C. scratched her head in bewilderment, "But you just woke up two hours ago!"
The doll thought for awhile and said, "Oh, there's the missing link! At nighttime you don't sleep a wink!" AM or PM, Skinny never knew.
I knew because owls always do. Skinny Miss S. was very depressed, even with the tantrums she threw.

tantrum

noun

1. a fit of bad temper: *Her bad tantrums closed the door to any outside connection.*

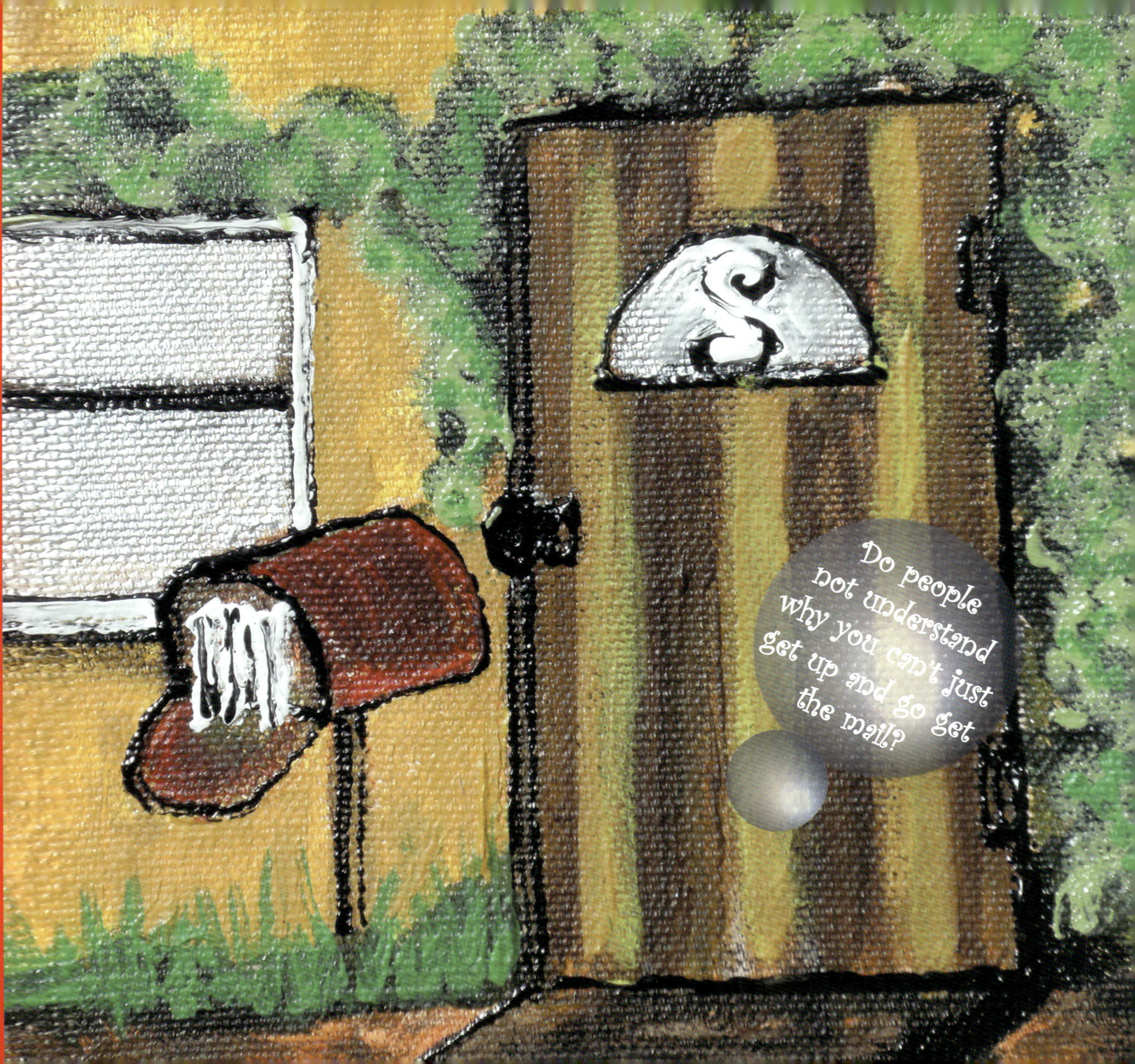
Do people not understand why you can't just get up and go get the mail?

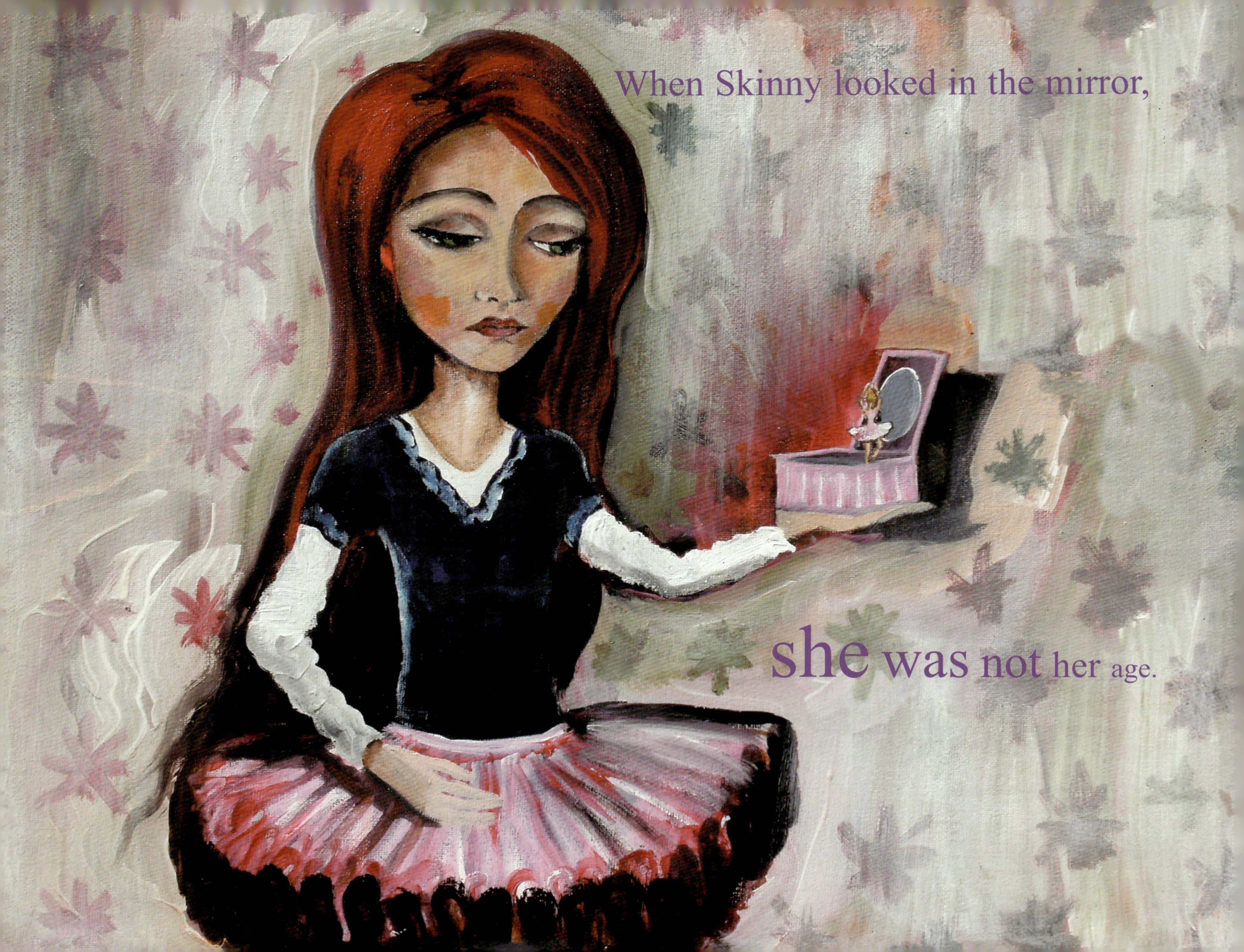

When Skinny looked in the mirror,

she was not her age.

Do you like looking child-like or skinnier than your body wants to naturally be?

reflection

noun

1. an instance of reflecting; especially: the return of light or sound waves from a surface.

2. the production of an image by or as if by a mirror.

3. the action of bending or folding back.

4. something produced by reflecting: as an effect produced by an influence; *Her perception of her image is a reflection of her depression.*

5. obscure or indirect criticism: REPROACH *a reflection on her character*

6. a thought, idea, or opinion formed or a remark made as a result of meditation

7. consideration of some subject matter, idea, or purpose

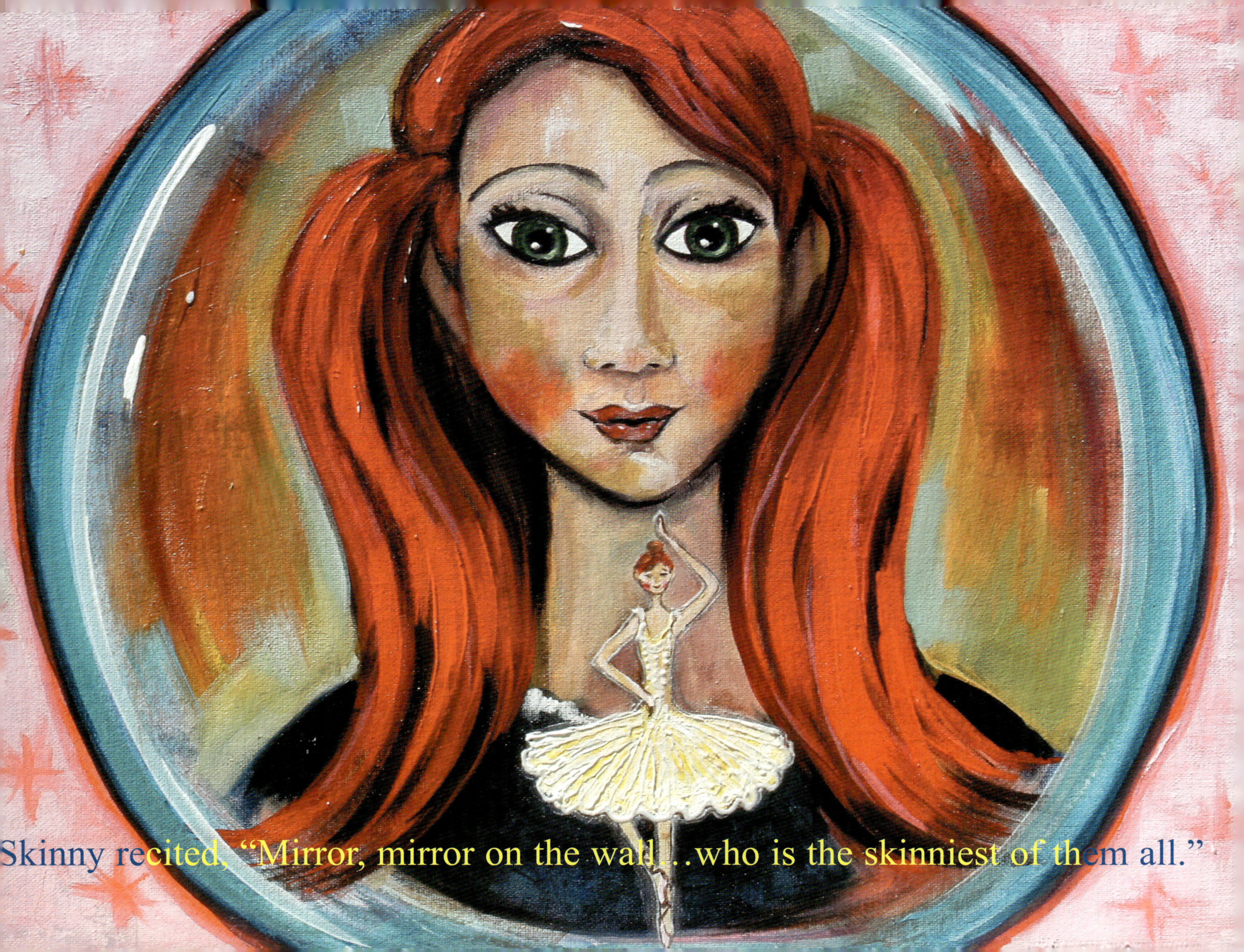

Skinny recited, “Mirror, mirror on the wall…who is the skinniest of them all.”

How do you see yourself today?

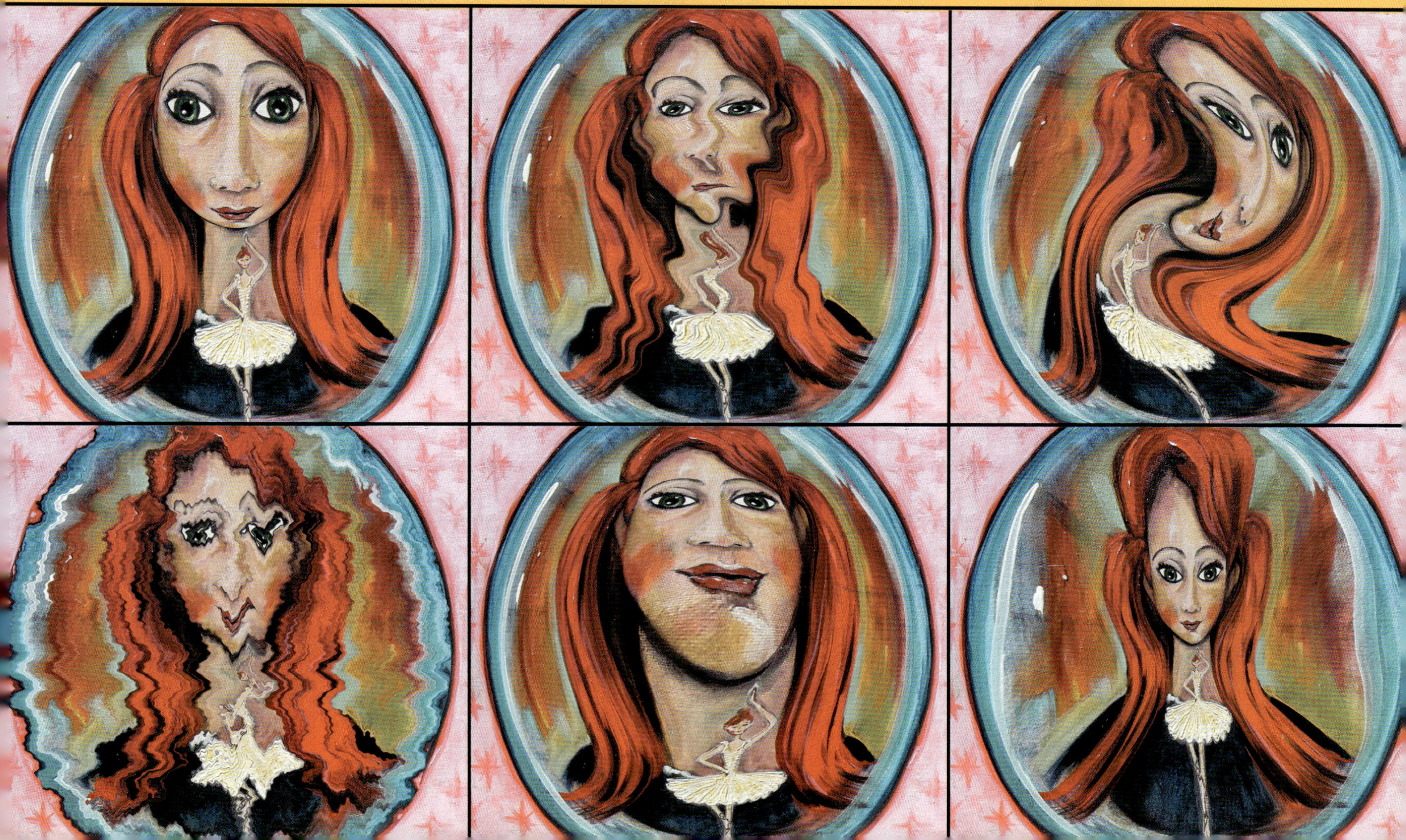

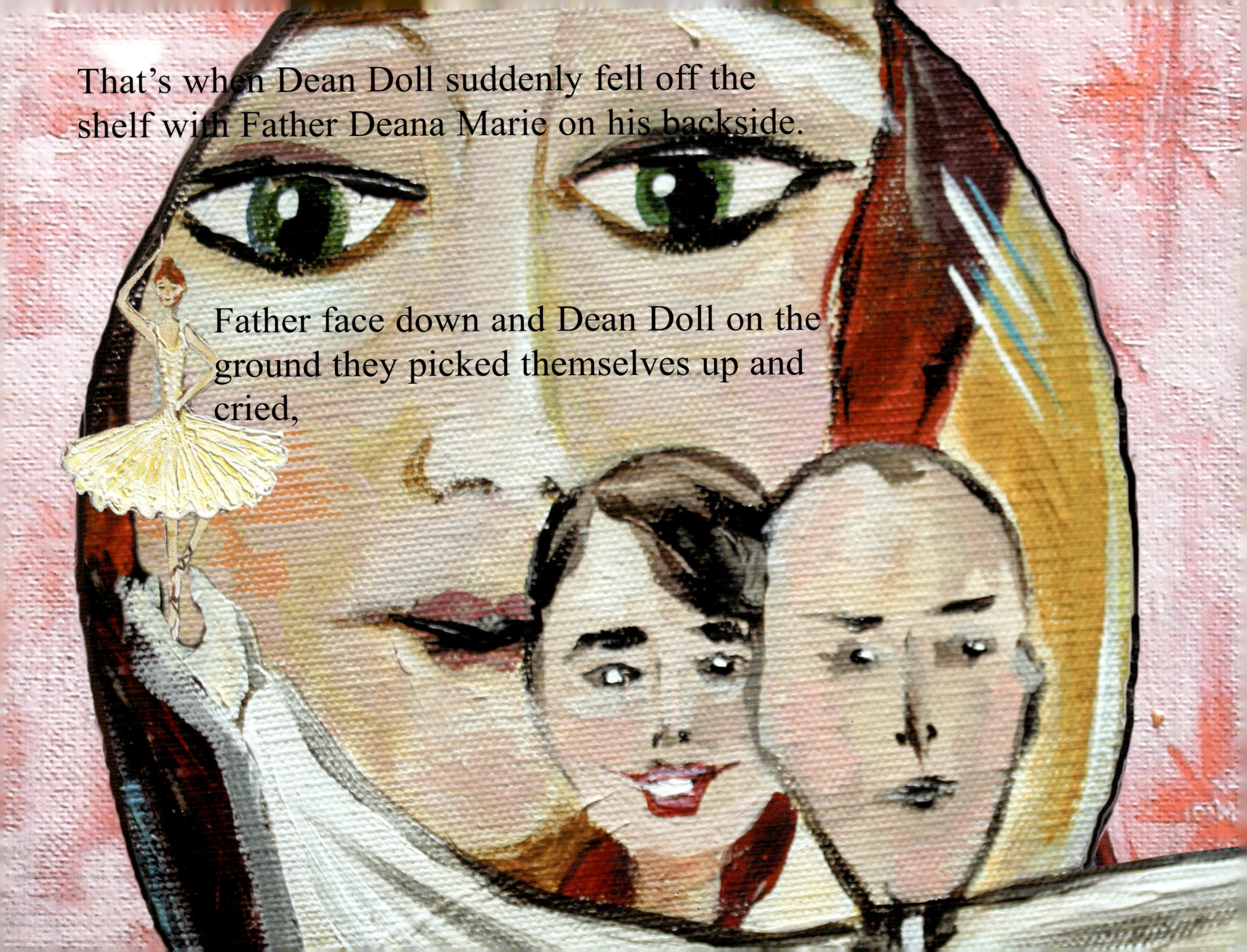

That's when Dean Doll suddenly fell off the shelf with Father Deana Marie on his backside.

Father face down and Dean Doll on the ground they picked themselves up and cried,

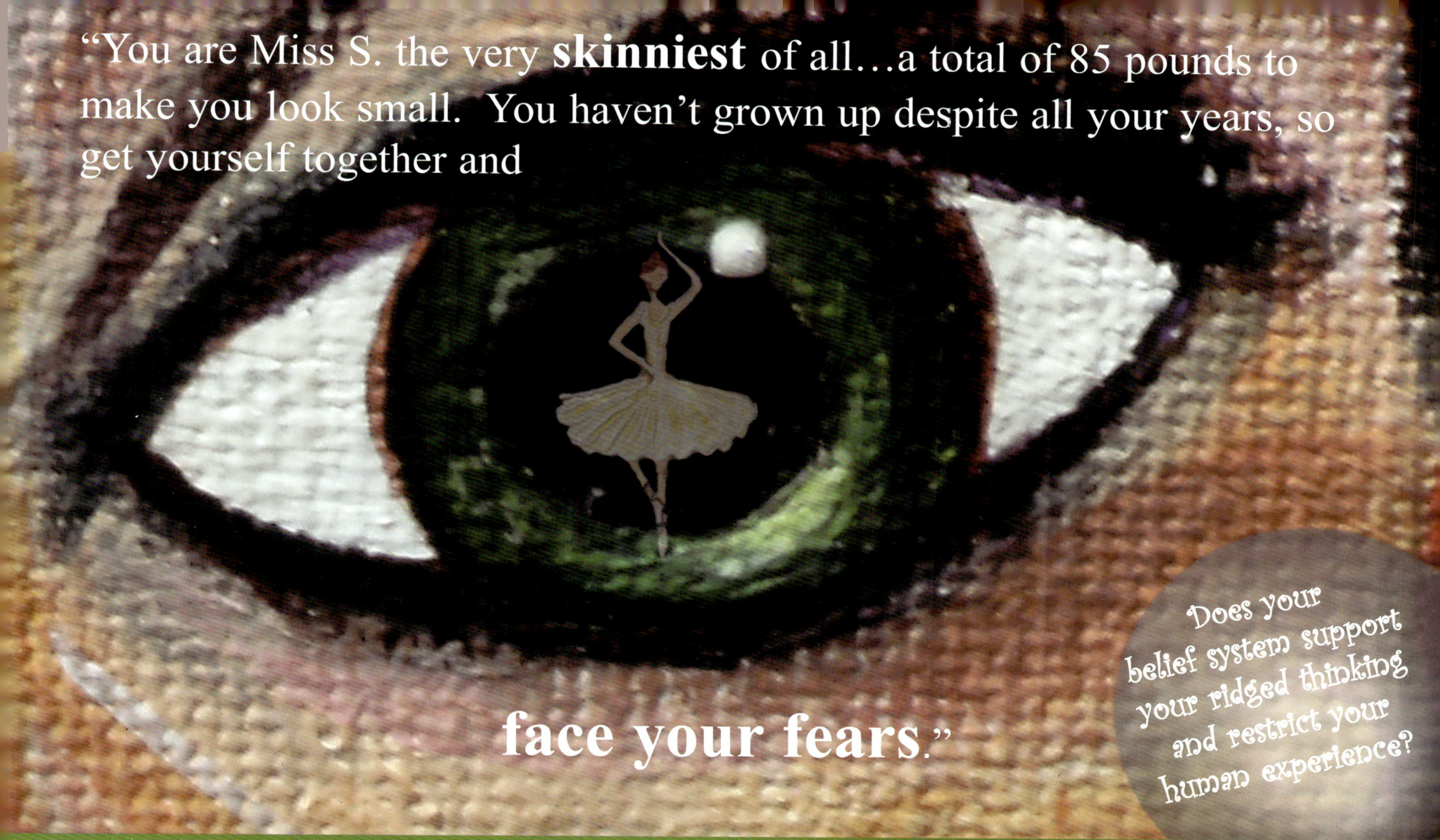
"You are Miss S. the very **skinniest** of all…a total of 85 pounds to make you look small. You haven't grown up despite all your years, so get yourself together and
face your fears."
Does your belief system support your ridged thinking and restrict your human experience?

belief

noun

1. a state or habit of mind in which trust or confidence is placed in some person or thing.

2. something believed; especially: a tenet or body of tenets held by a group.

3. conviction of the truth of some statement or the reality of some being or phenomenon especially when based on examination of evidence. Faith almost always implies certitude even where there is no evidence or proof. *An unshakable faith in God.*

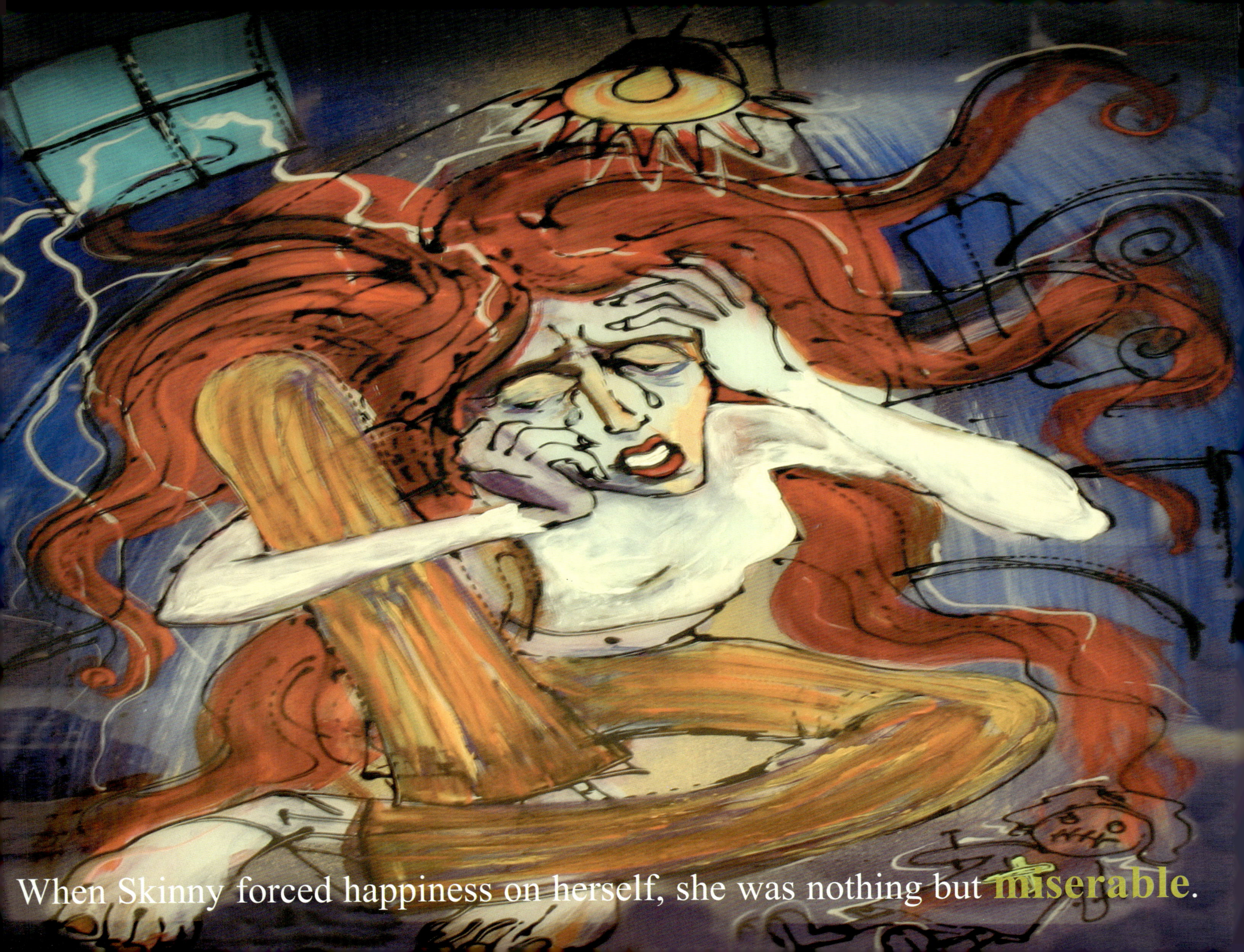

When Skinny forced happiness on herself, she was nothing but miserable.

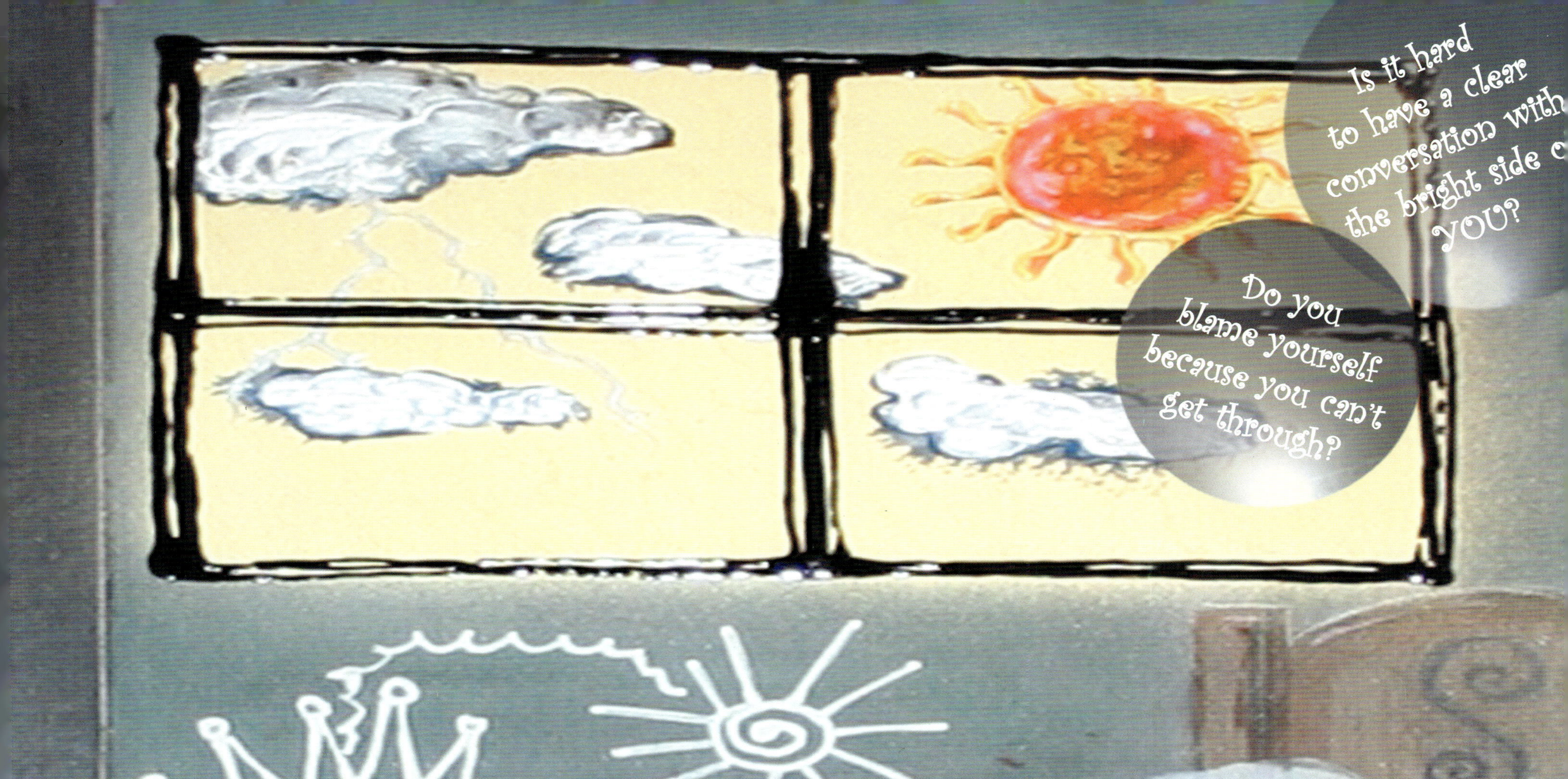
Is it hard
to have a clear
conversation with
the bright side o
YOU?
Do you
blame yourself
because you can't
get through?

"Why doesn't Sunny Mister E. call my name?" Skinny asked.

"Through the thick glass window he asks you the same." Dean Doll replied, although he had voices of his own just the same. They came from the back of his head and filled him with dread. "All the girl needs is to sit nicely in a pew." said Father Deana Marie from the floor, his guilt **WELL** overdue.

DIAGNOSTIC CRITERIA FOR:

A g o r a p h o b i a

A. Anxiety about being in places or situations from which escape might be difficult (or embarrassing) or in which help may not be available in the event of having an unexpected or situationally predisposed Panic Attack or panic-like symptoms. Agoraphobic fears typically involve characteristic clusters of situations that include being outside the home alone; being in a crowd or standing in a line; being on a bridge; and traveling in a bus, train, or automobile. Note: Consider the diagnosis of Specific Phobia if the avoidance is limited to one or only a few specific situations, or Social Phobia if the avoidance is limited to social situations.

B. The situations are avoided (e.g., travel is restricted) or else are endured with marked distress or with anxiety about having a Panic Attack or panic-like symptoms, or require the presence of a companion.

C. The anxiety or phobic avoidance is not better accounted for by another mental disorder, such as Social Phobia (e.g., avoidance limited to social situations because of fear of embarrassment), Specific Phobia (e.g., avoidance limited to a single situation like elevators), Obsessive-Compulsive Disorder (e.g., avoidance of dirt in someone with an obsession about contamination), Posttraumatic Stress Disorder (e.g., avoidance of stimuli associated with a severe stressor), or Separation Anxiety Disorder (e.g., avoidance of leaving home or relatives).[13]

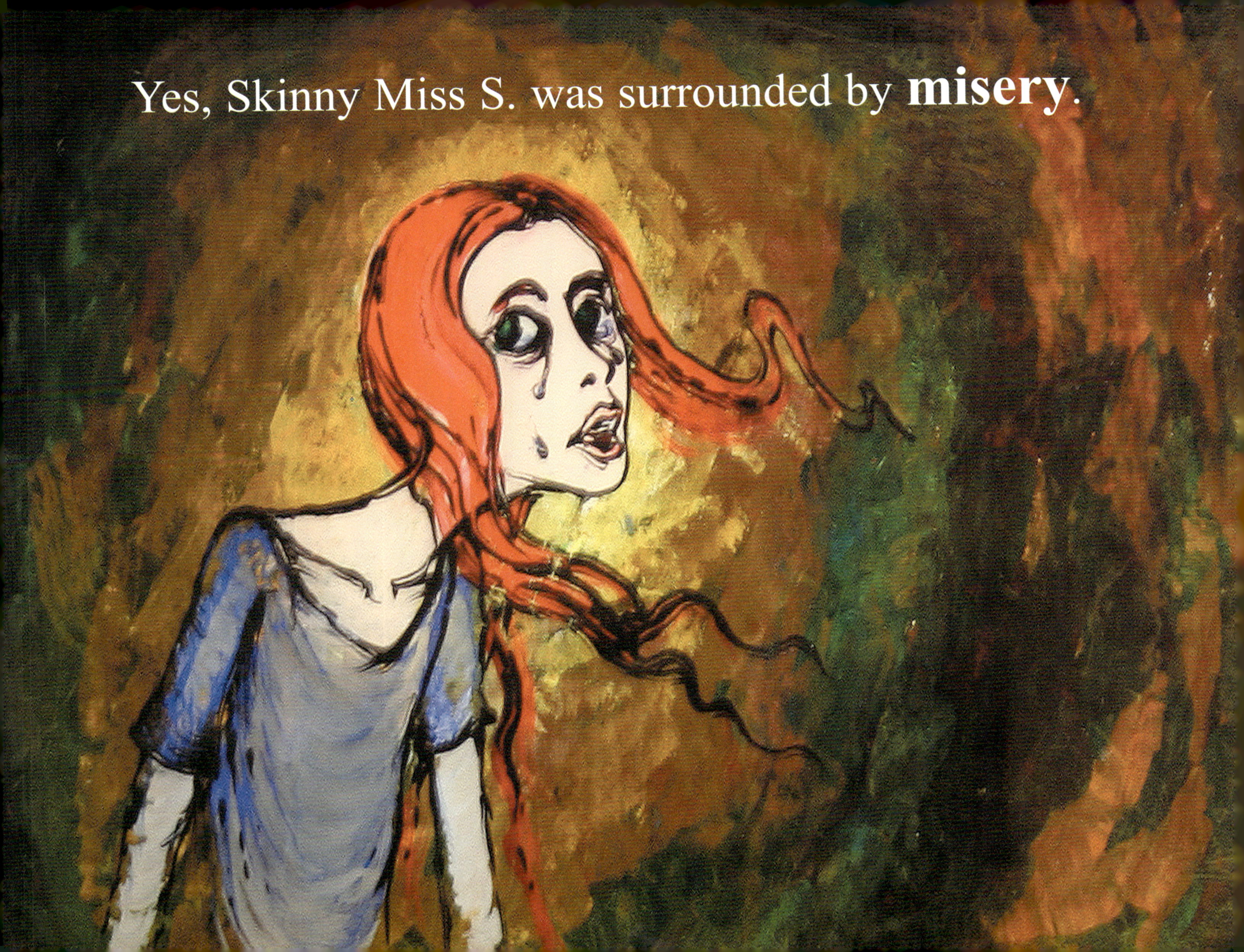
Yes, Skinny Miss S. was surrounded by **misery**.

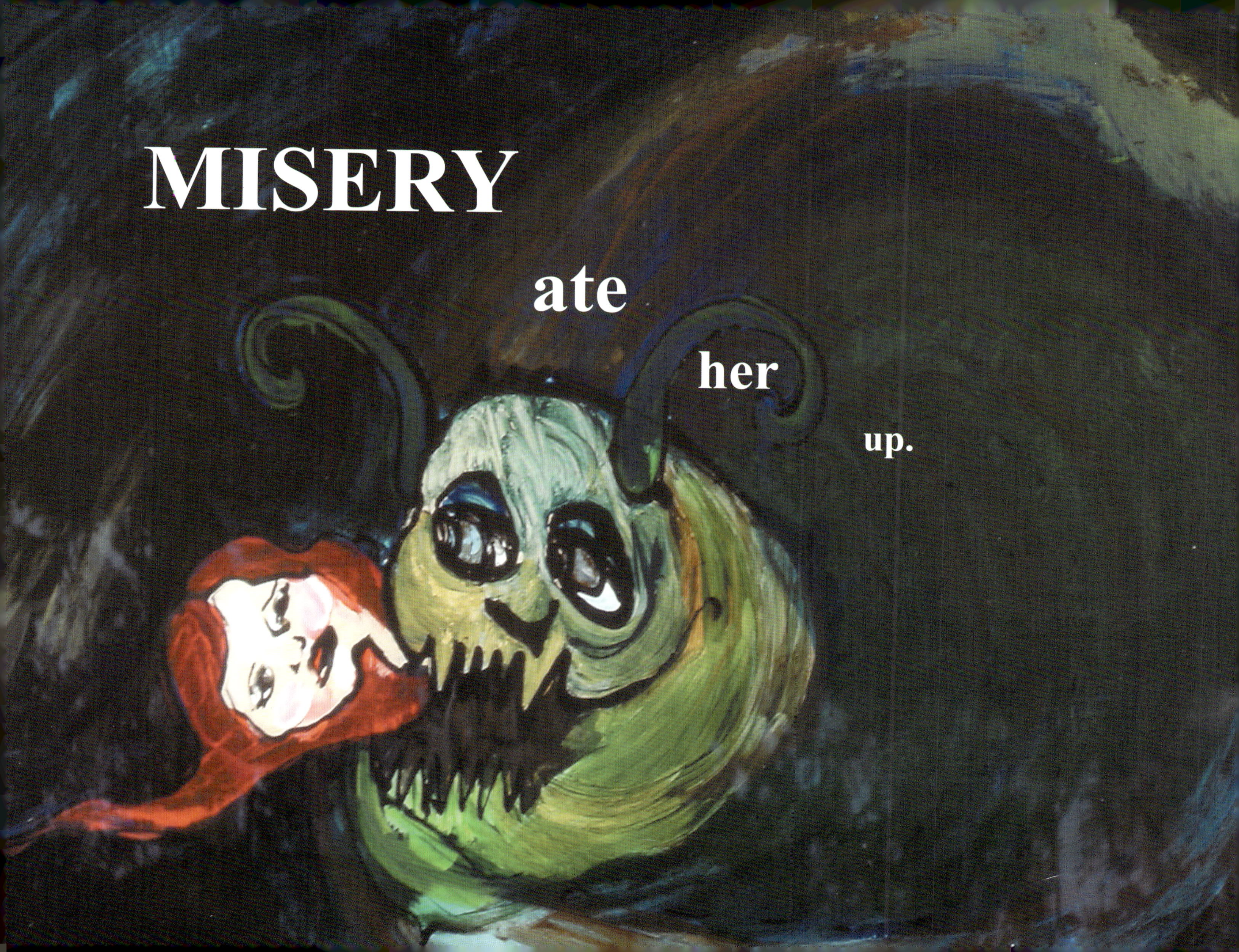
MISERY
ate
her
up.

DIAGNOSTIC CRITERIA FOR:

Major Depressive Episode

A. Five (or more) of the following symptoms have been present during the same 2-week period and represent a change from previous functioning; at least one of the symptoms is either (1) depressed mood or (2) loss of interest or pleasure.

Note: Do not include symptoms that are clearly due to a general medical condition, or mood-incongruent delusions or hallucinations.

(1) depressed mood most of the day, nearly every day, as indicated by either subjective report (e.g., feels sad or empty) or observation made by others (e.g., appears tearful). Note: In children and adolescents, can be irritable mood.

(2) markedly diminished interest or pleasure in all, or almost all, activities most of the day, nearly every day (as indicated by either subjective account or observation made by others)

(3) significant weight loss when not dieting or weight gain or decrease or increase in appetite nearly every day. Note: In children, consider failure to make expected weight gains.

(4) insomnia or hypersomnia nearly every day

(5) psychomotor agitation or retardation nearly every day (observable by others, not merely subjective feelings of restlessness or being slowed down)

(6) fatigue or loss of energy nearly every day

(7) feelings of worthlessness or excessive or inappropriate guilt (which may be delusional) nearly every day (not merely self-reproach or guilt about being sick)

(8) diminished ability to think or concentrate, or indecisiveness, nearly every day (either by subjective account or as observed by others)

(9) recurrent thoughts of death (not just fear of dying), recurrent suicidal ideation without a specific plan, or a suicide attempt or a specific plan for committing suicide

B. The symptoms do not meet criteria for a Mixed Episode.

C. The symptoms cause clinically significant distress or impairment in social, occupational, or other important areas of functioning.

D. The symptoms are not due to the direct physiological effects of a substance (e.g., a drug of abuse, a medication) or a general medical condition (e.g., hypothyroidism).

E. The symptoms are not better accounted for by Bereavement, i.e., after the loss of a loved one, the symptoms persist for longer than 2 months or are characterized by marked functional impairment, morbid preoccupation with worthlessness, suicidal ideation, psychotic symptoms, or psychomotor retardation.[14]

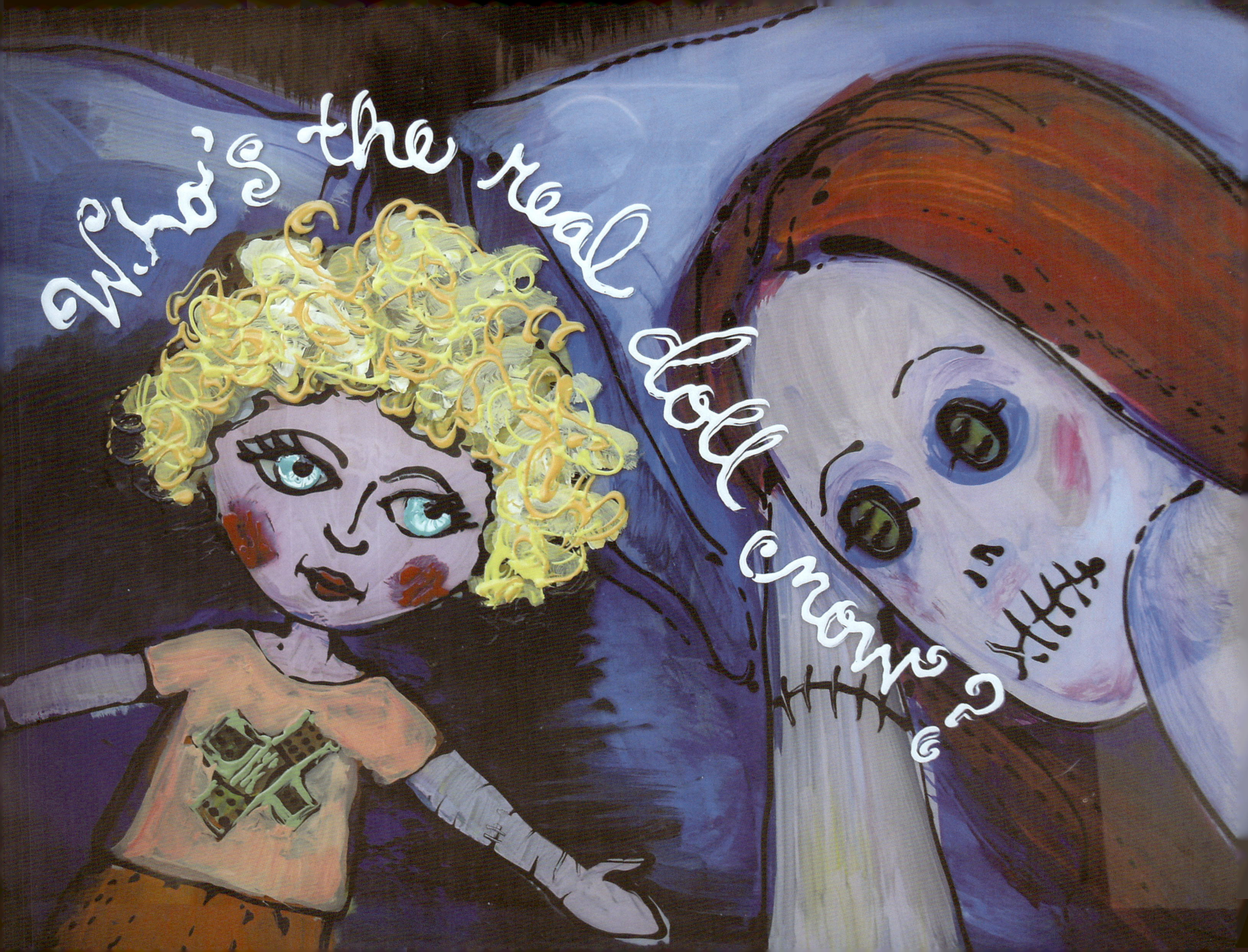
Who's the real doll now?

joy
noun

1. the emotion evoked by well-being, success, or good fortune or by the prospect of possessing what one desires.

2. the expression or exhibition of such emotion.

3. a state of happiness or felicity.

4. a source or cause of delight.

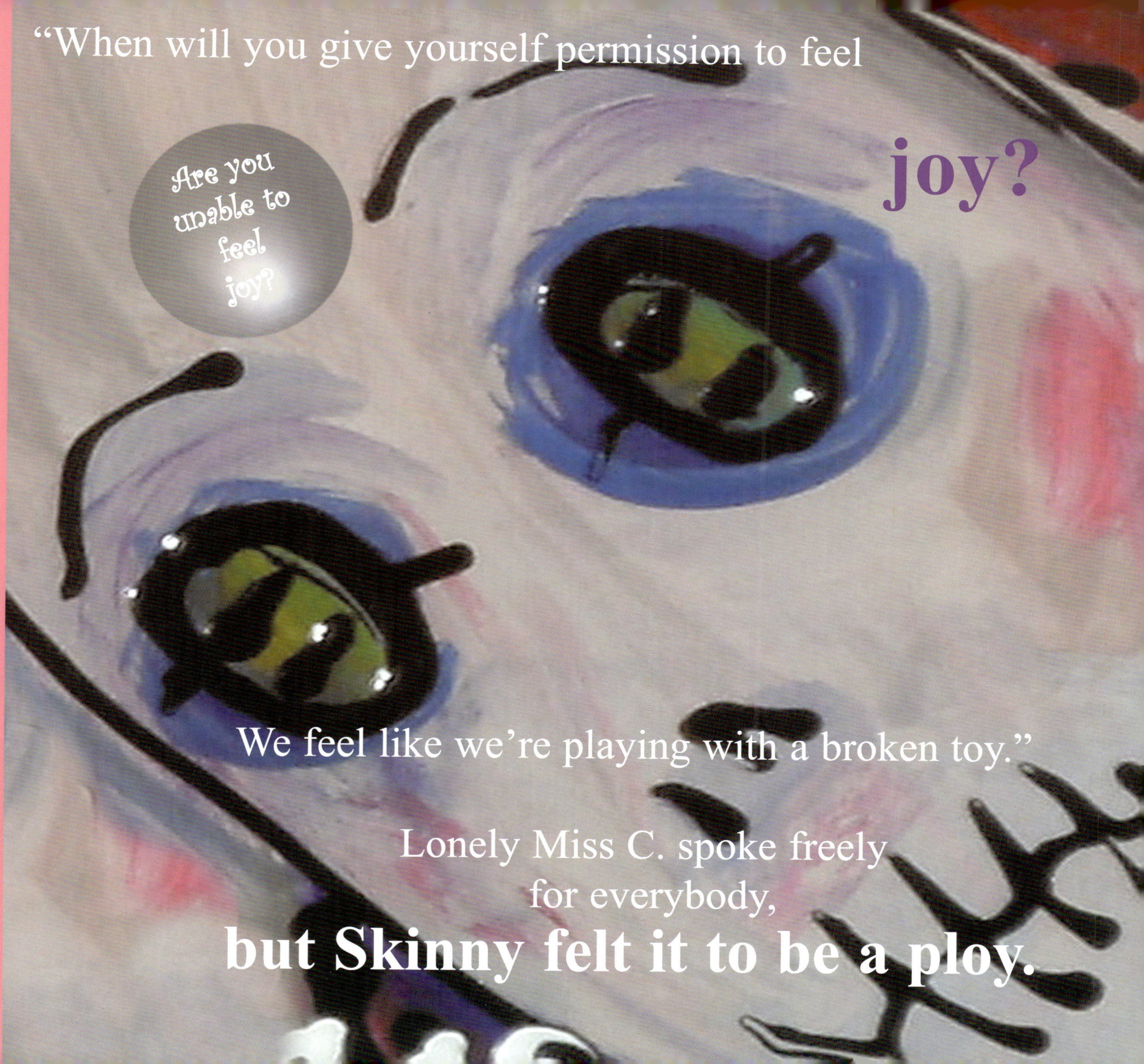

"When will you give yourself permission to feel

Are you unable to feel joy?

joy?

We feel like we're playing with a broken toy."

Lonely Miss C. spoke freely
for everybody,
but Skinny felt it to be a ploy.

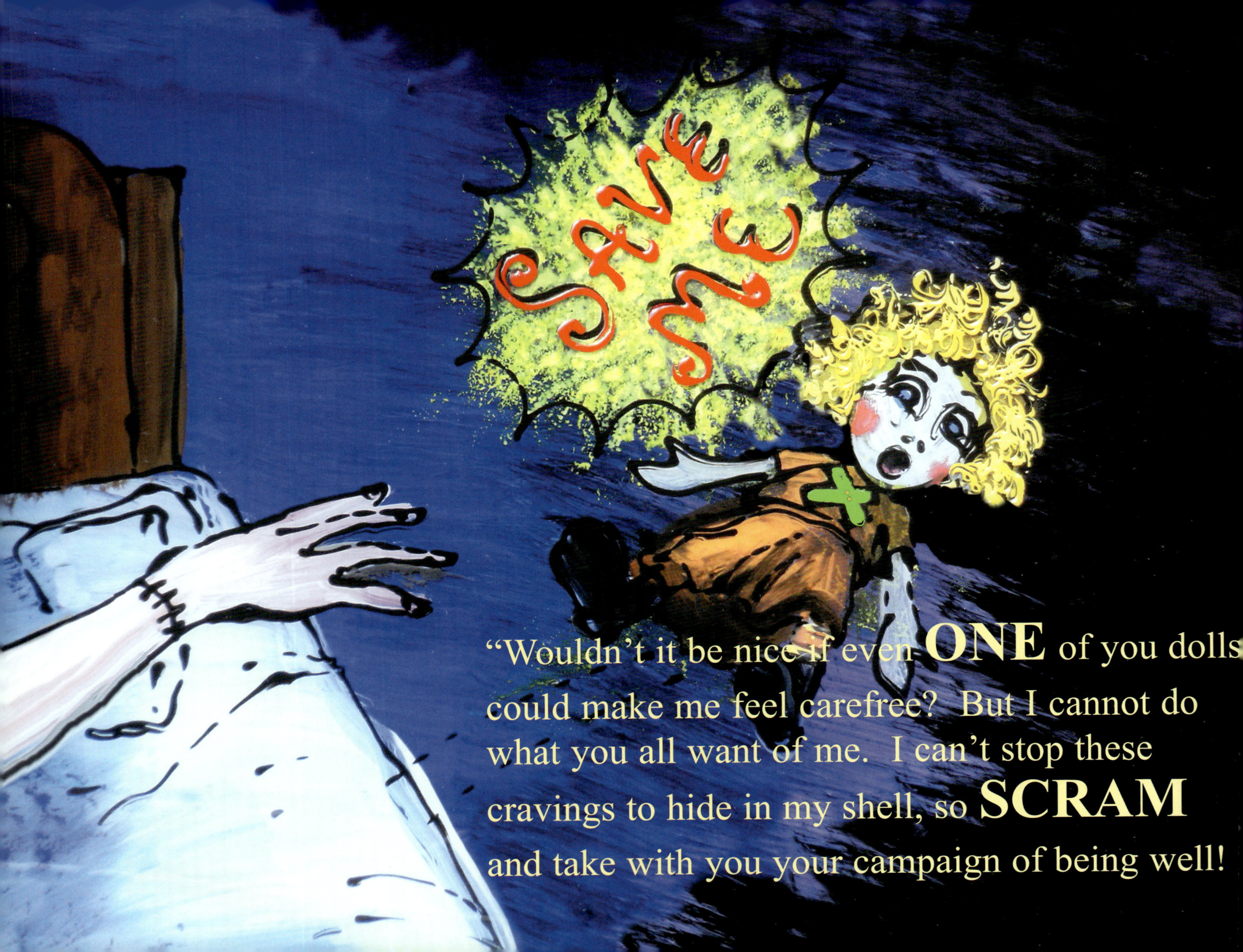

"Wouldn't it be nice if even **ONE** of you dolls could make me feel carefree? But I cannot do what you all want of me. I can't stop these cravings to hide in my shell, so **SCRAM** and take with you your campaign of being well!

You, Miss C., with all your positive notions you sling…might be ‘lonely’ because you ***see*** everything!” With that she threw her in the closet far, far away. Lonely Miss C. was shocked with dismay.

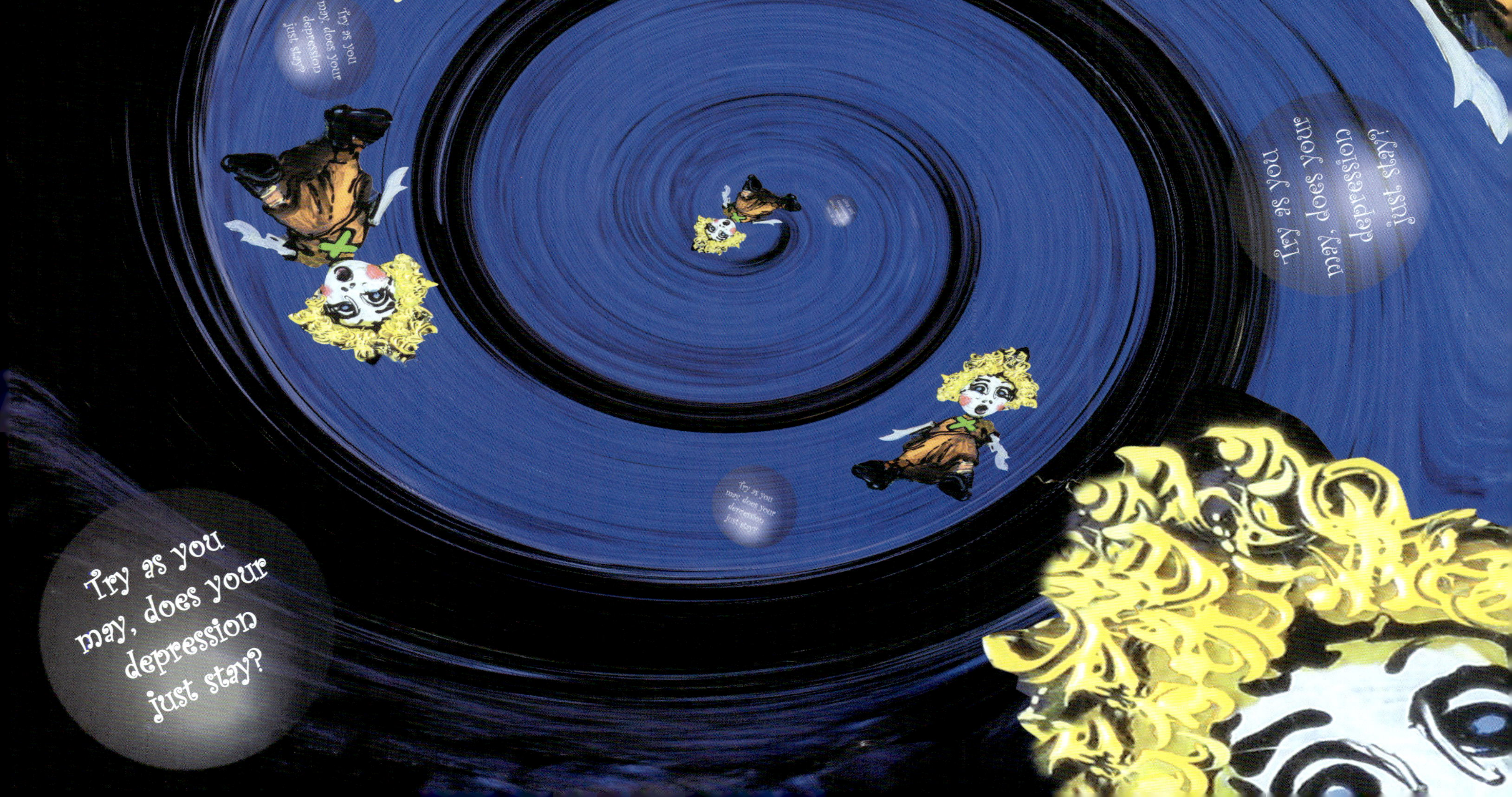

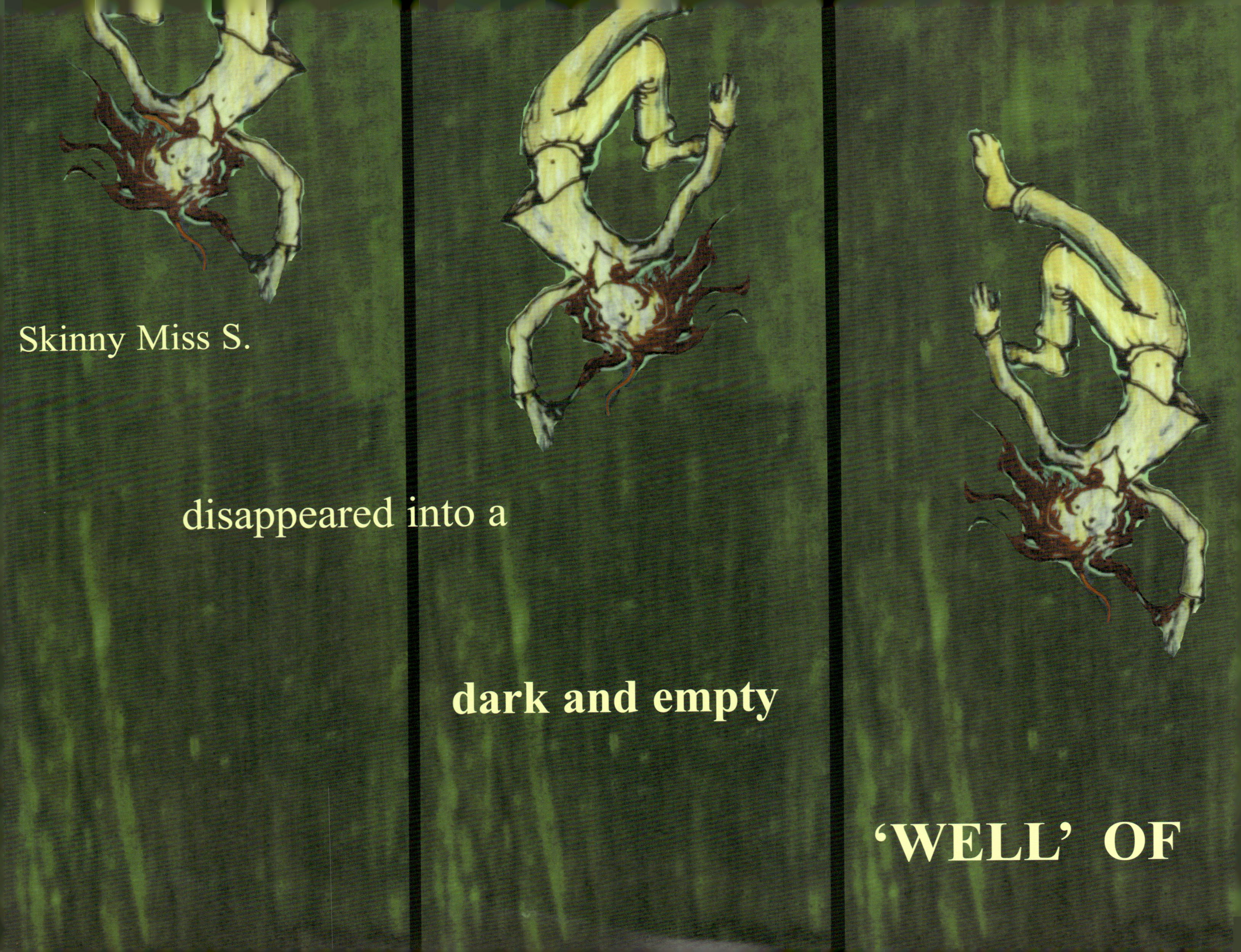

Skinny Miss S.

disappeared into a

dark and empty

'WELL' OF

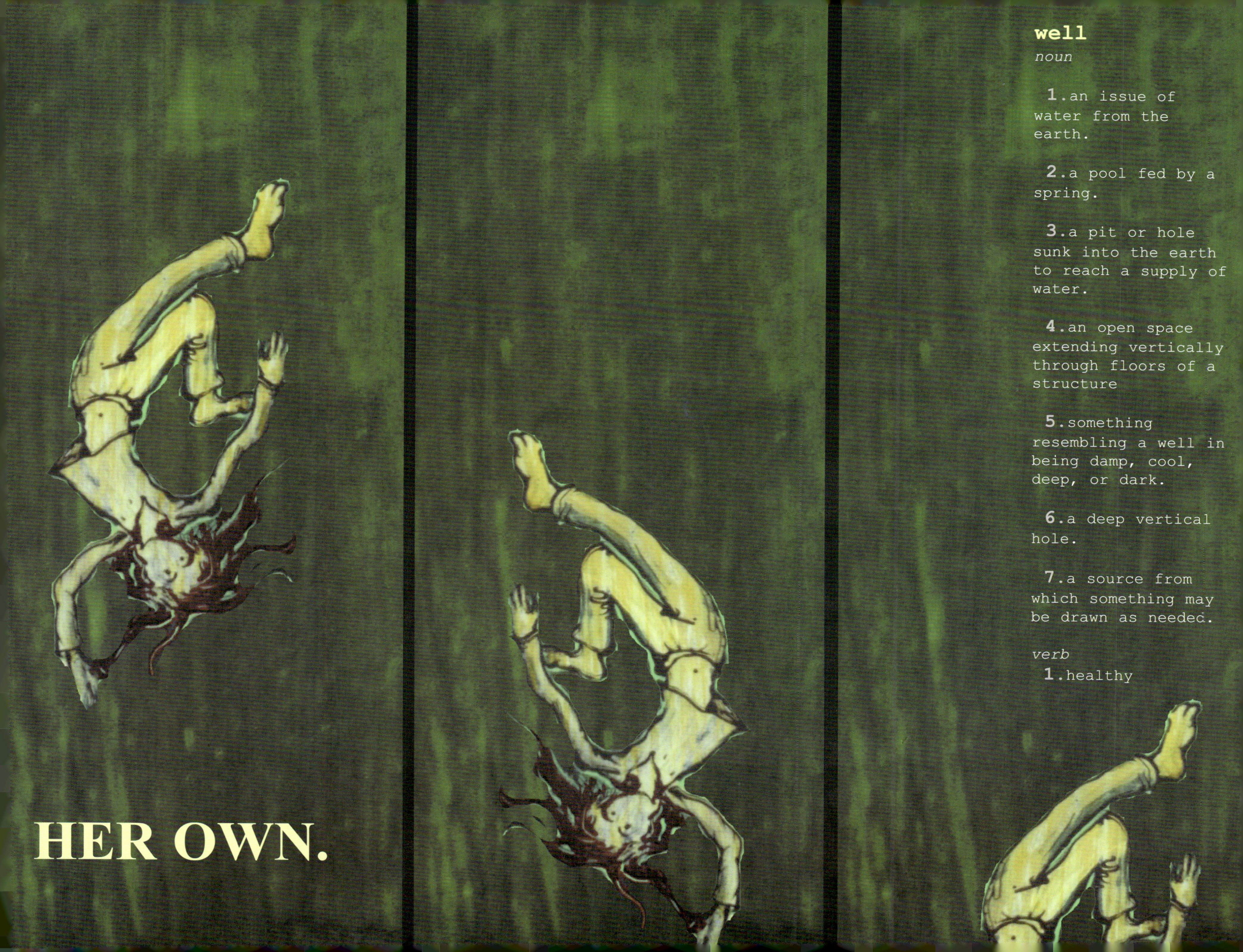
HER OWN.
well
noun
1.an issue of water from the earth.
2.a pool fed by a spring.
3.a pit or hole sunk into the earth to reach a supply of water.
4.an open space extending vertically through floors of a structure
5.something resembling a well in being damp, cool, deep, or dark.
6.a deep vertical hole.
7.a source from which something may be drawn as needed.
verb
1.healthy

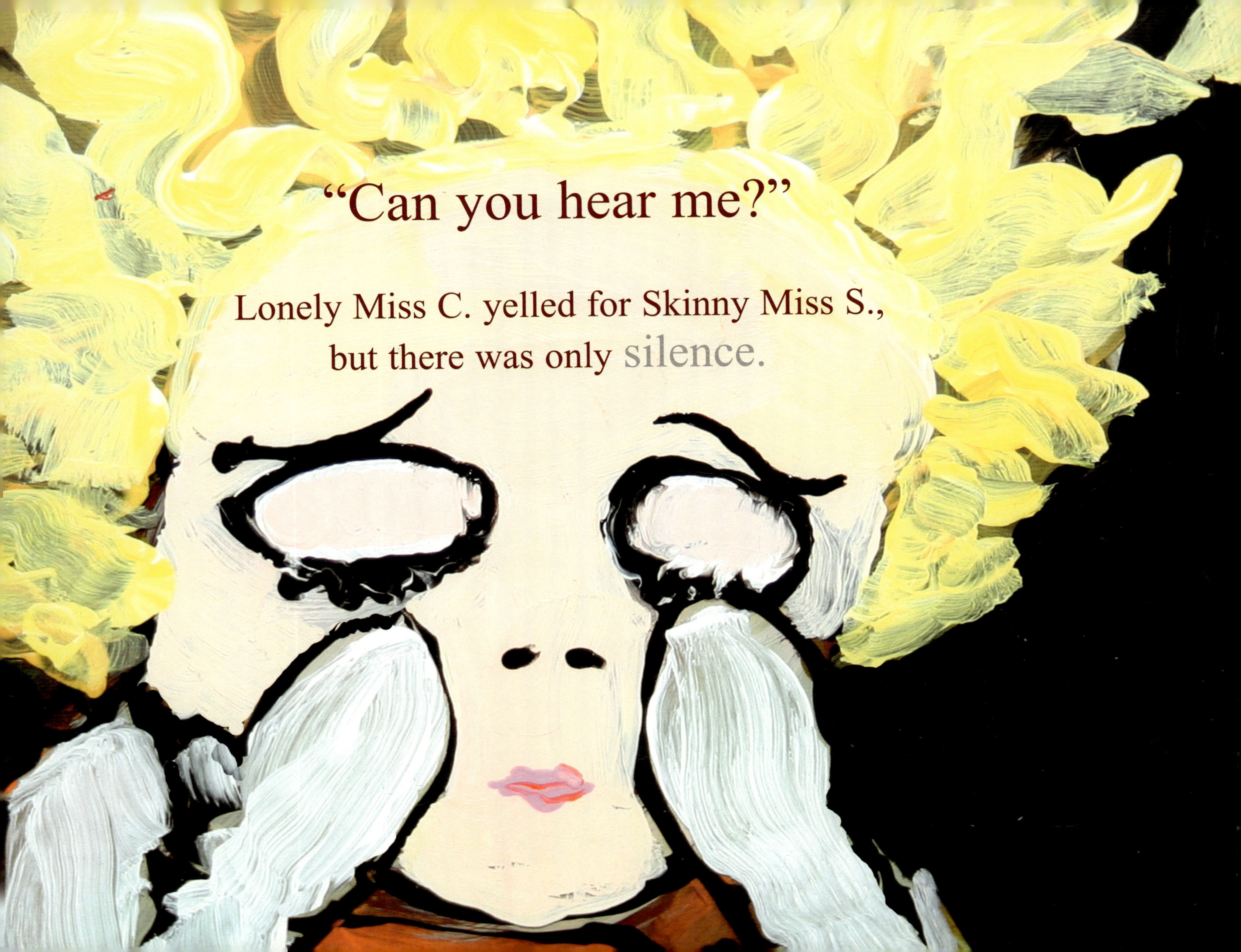

"Can you hear me?"

Lonely Miss C. yelled for Skinny Miss S.,
but there was only silence.

There Skinny Miss S. sat in isolation from her dolls for many days. Finally Skinny's echo came through, "Do you hear me?"

"You can't hear me." they whispered unknowingly, simultaneously.

Do you stay silent to punish others?

Do you 'check out' to make the voices go away?

"Will you ever hear me?" sobbed Lonely Miss C.

"Have you ever heard me?" replied Skinny Miss S.

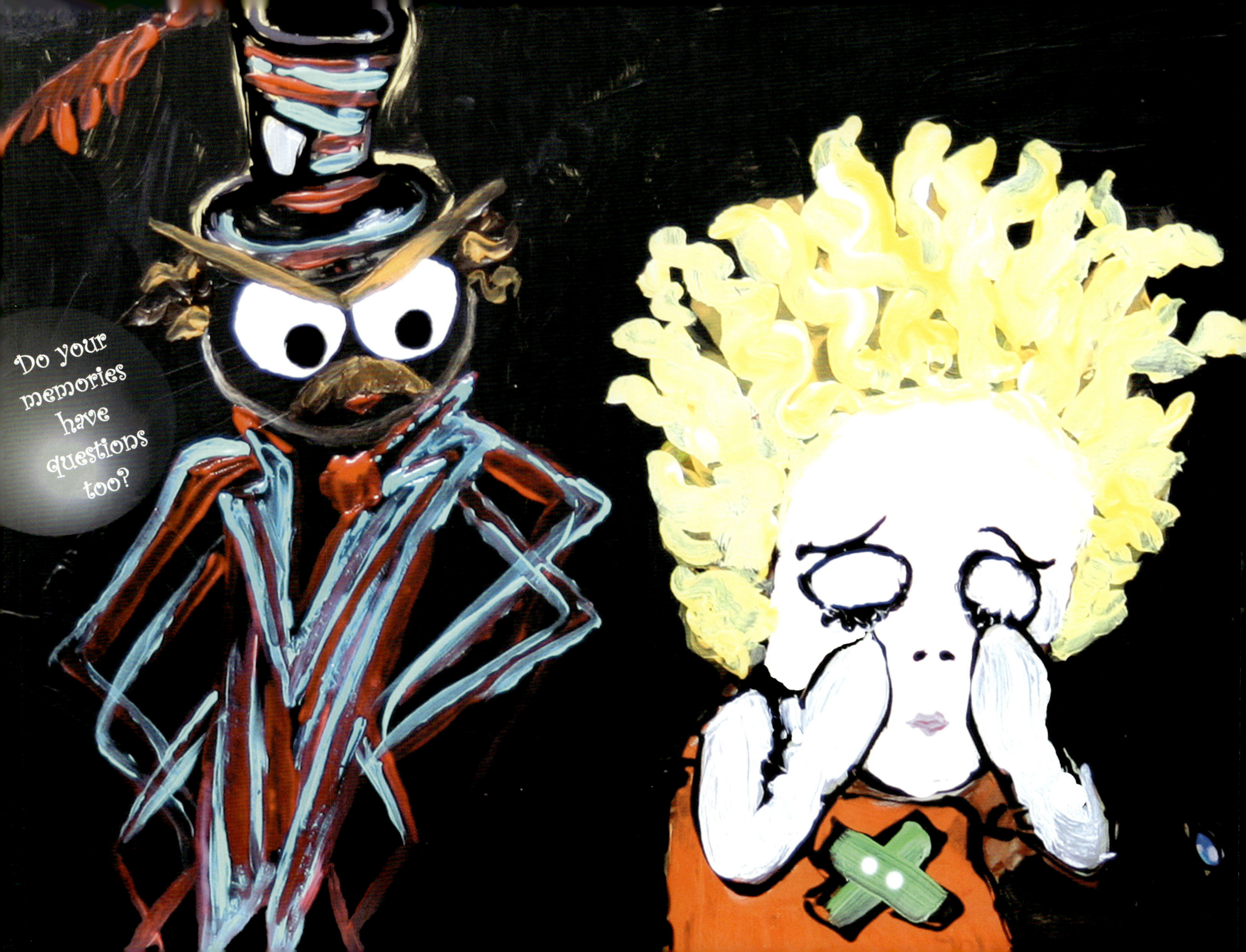
Do your memories have questions too?

Sir Grouchy Spider

spun

down

to Lonely Miss C. and muttered,

Do you have a inner voice that wants to light your way?

Are you as low as you want to go?

"No matter what you do,

she
won't
listen
to
you.

What would it take to reach your bottom?

Look at the poor skinny girl!

I don't see her winning this war!"

pessimism
noun

1. an inclination to emphasize adverse aspects, conditions, and possibilities or to expect the worst possible outcome.
2. the doctrine that reality is essentially evil.
3. the doctrine that evil overbalances happiness in life.

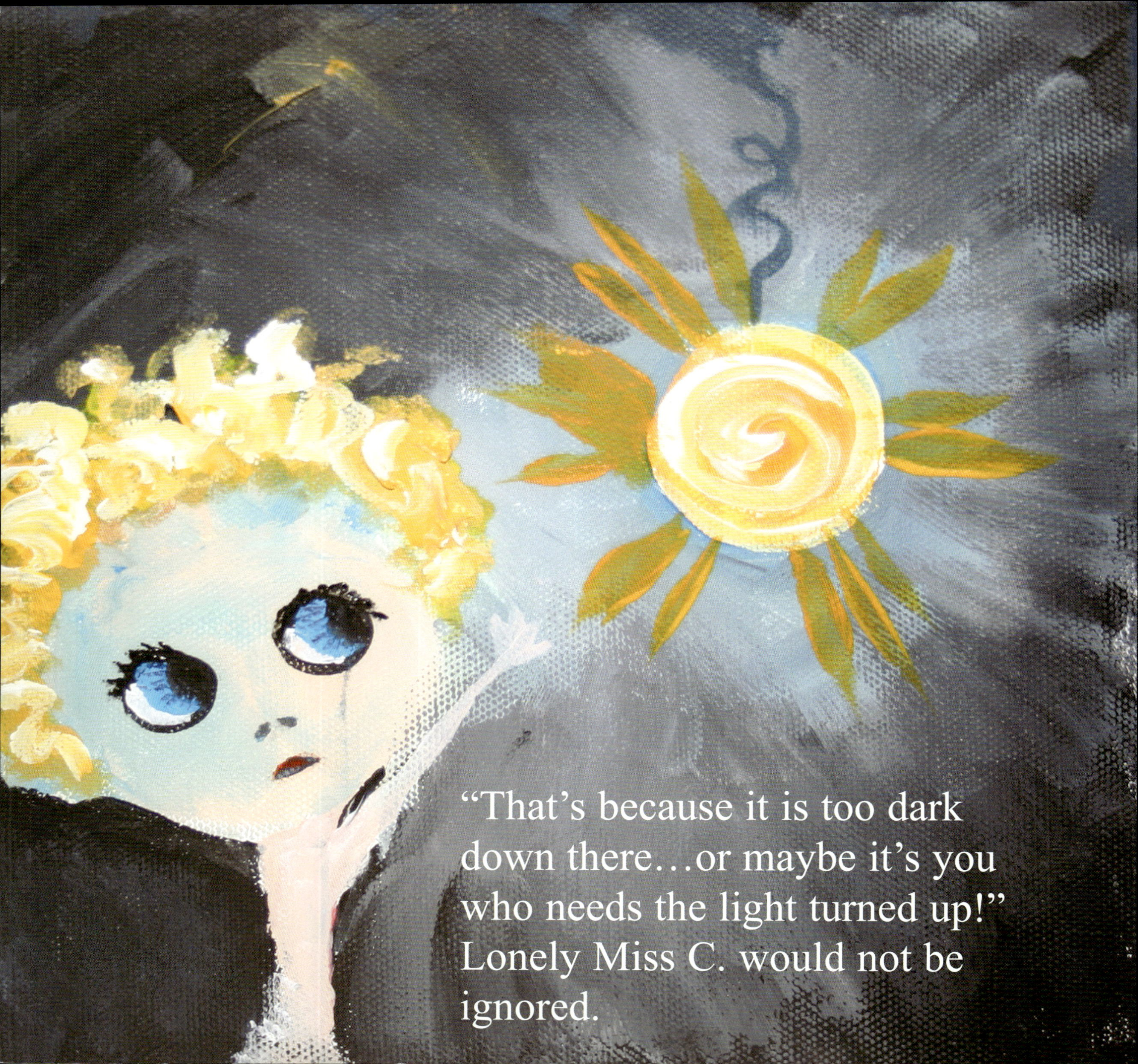

"That's because it is too dark down there…or maybe it's you who needs the light turned up!" Lonely Miss C. would not be ignored.

light
noun

1. something that makes vision possible.

2. electromagnetic radiation of any wavelength and traveling in a vacuum with a speed of about 186,281 miles per second.

3. a source of light: a celestial body

4. illumination; INNER LIGHT, TRUTH, ENLIGHTENMENT.

5. public knowledge; *facts brought to light*, a particular aspect or appearance presented to view; *saw the matter in a different light.*

6. something that enlightens or informs; *shed some light on the problem.*

7. the representation of light in art.

Skinny saw the light that had been turned on coming from afar. She knew someone was searching for her to come home. Skinny suddenly felt so alone since she knew not how to reach back.

"It's okay, Skinny! I'm not going anywhere!" Lonely Miss C. cried down to her.

Did you know sometimes your pain is not your fault, but it's now your responsibility to respond to it?

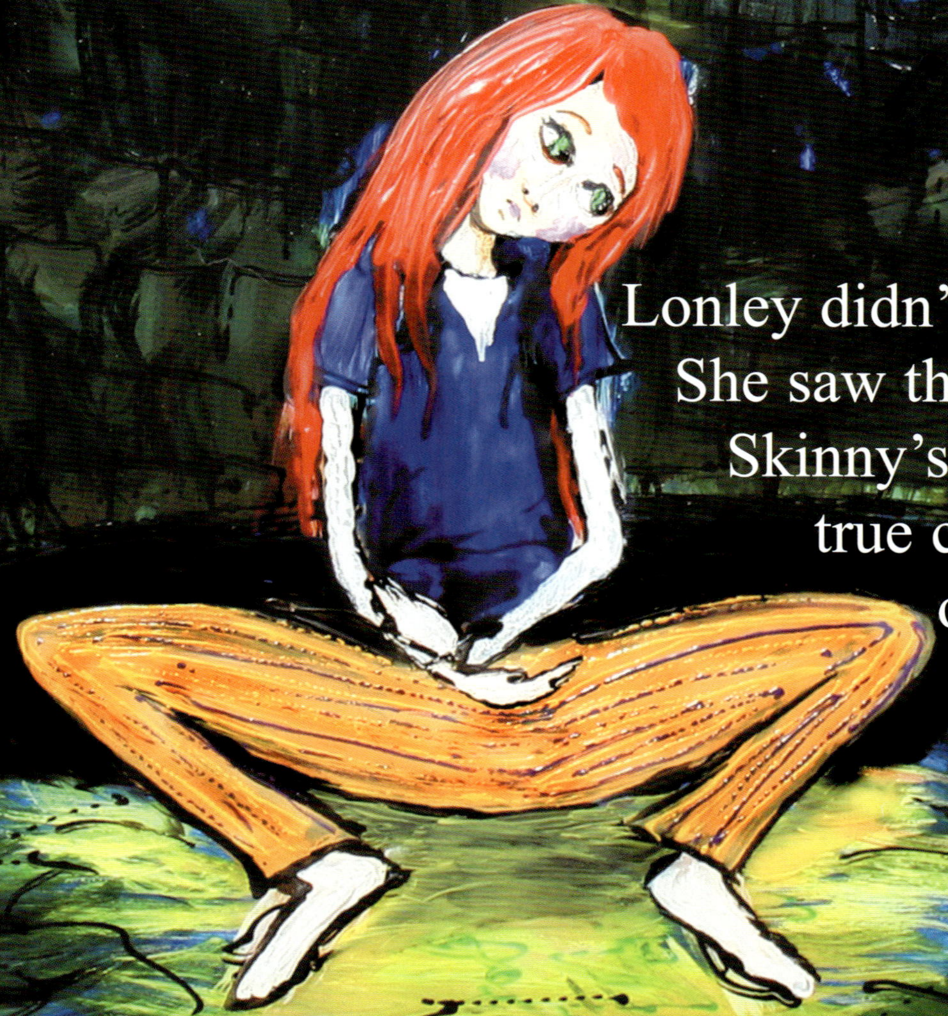

Lonley didn't mind; she saw everything. She saw the pain welled up behind Skinny's denial, coupled with the true confusion behind the origin of her trails.

Do you give yourself time to grieve?

Skinny became angry and screamed toward the light, "I can hear you loud and clear! Now you will hear me my sweet loverly dear!" shouted Skinny Miss S. to her doll who was always there to remind her of what she feared. Skinny Miss S. had indeed something she had forgotten and she had temporarily turned rotten. Skinny told her how Lonely was handcrafted and abandoned by the chrissmas tree when Skinny was three.

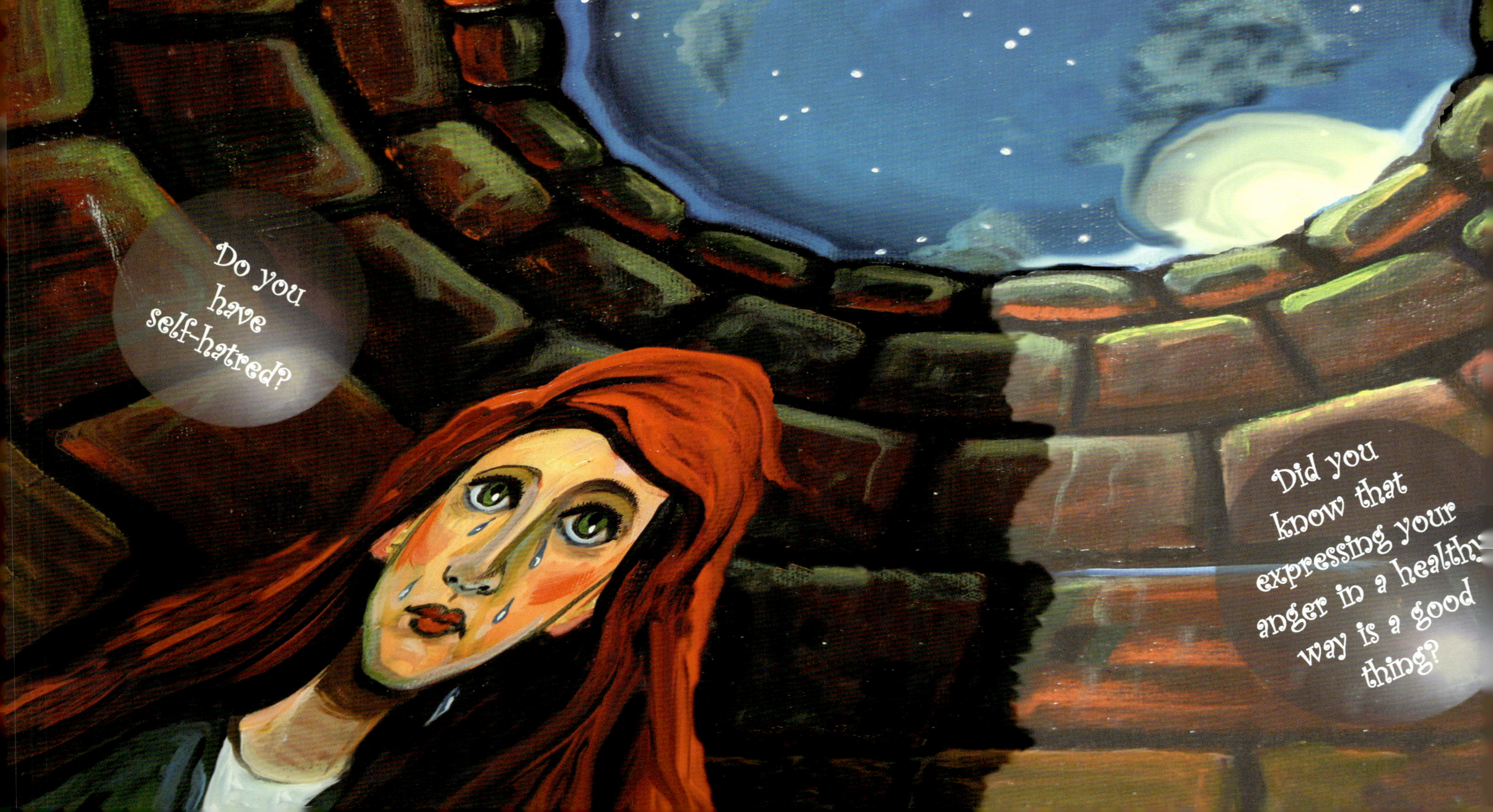

Do you have self-hatred?
Did you know that expressing your anger in a health way is a good thing?

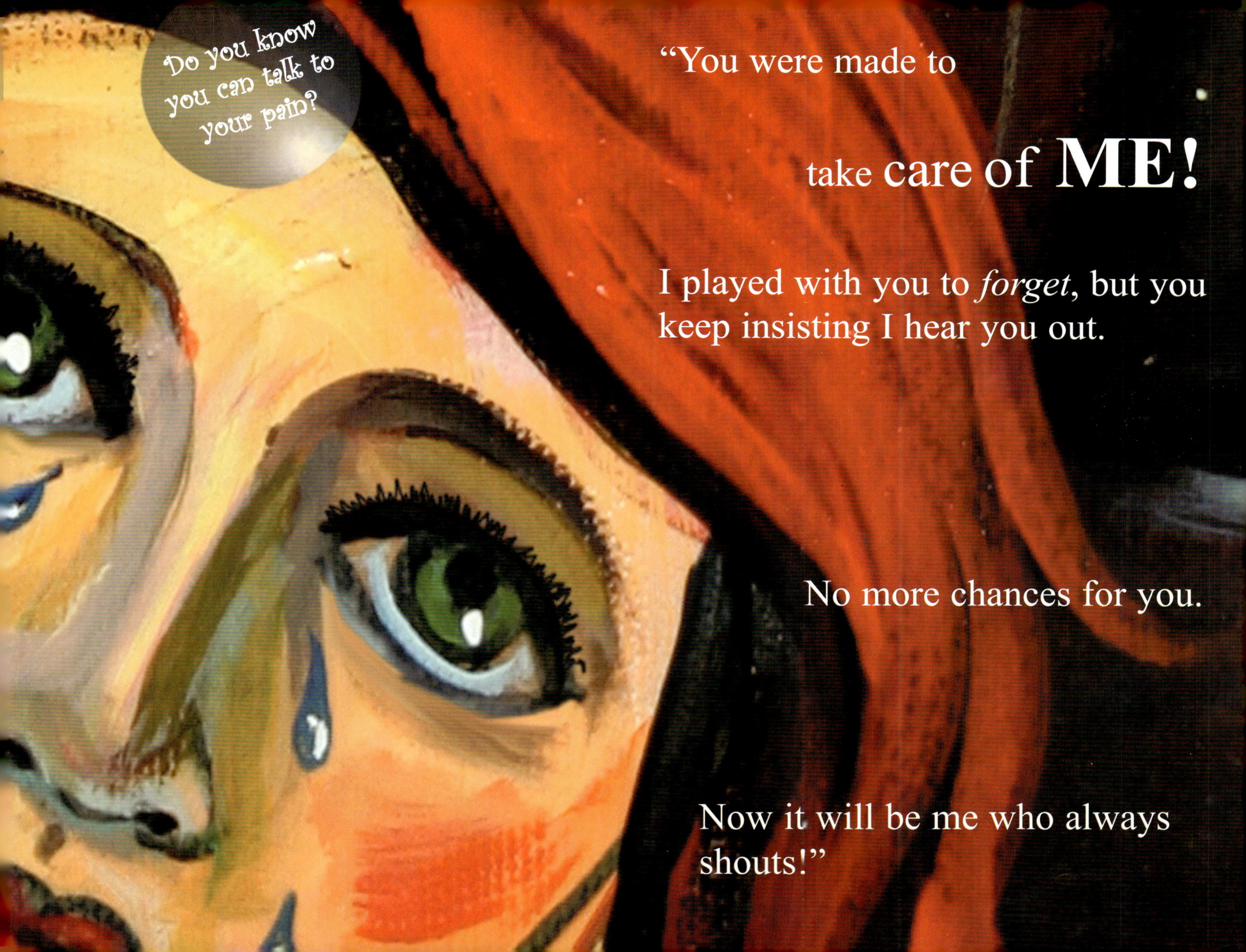

Do you know you can talk to your pain?

“You were made to

take care of **ME!**

I played with you to *forget*, but you keep insisting I hear you out.

No more chances for you.

Now it will be me who always shouts!”

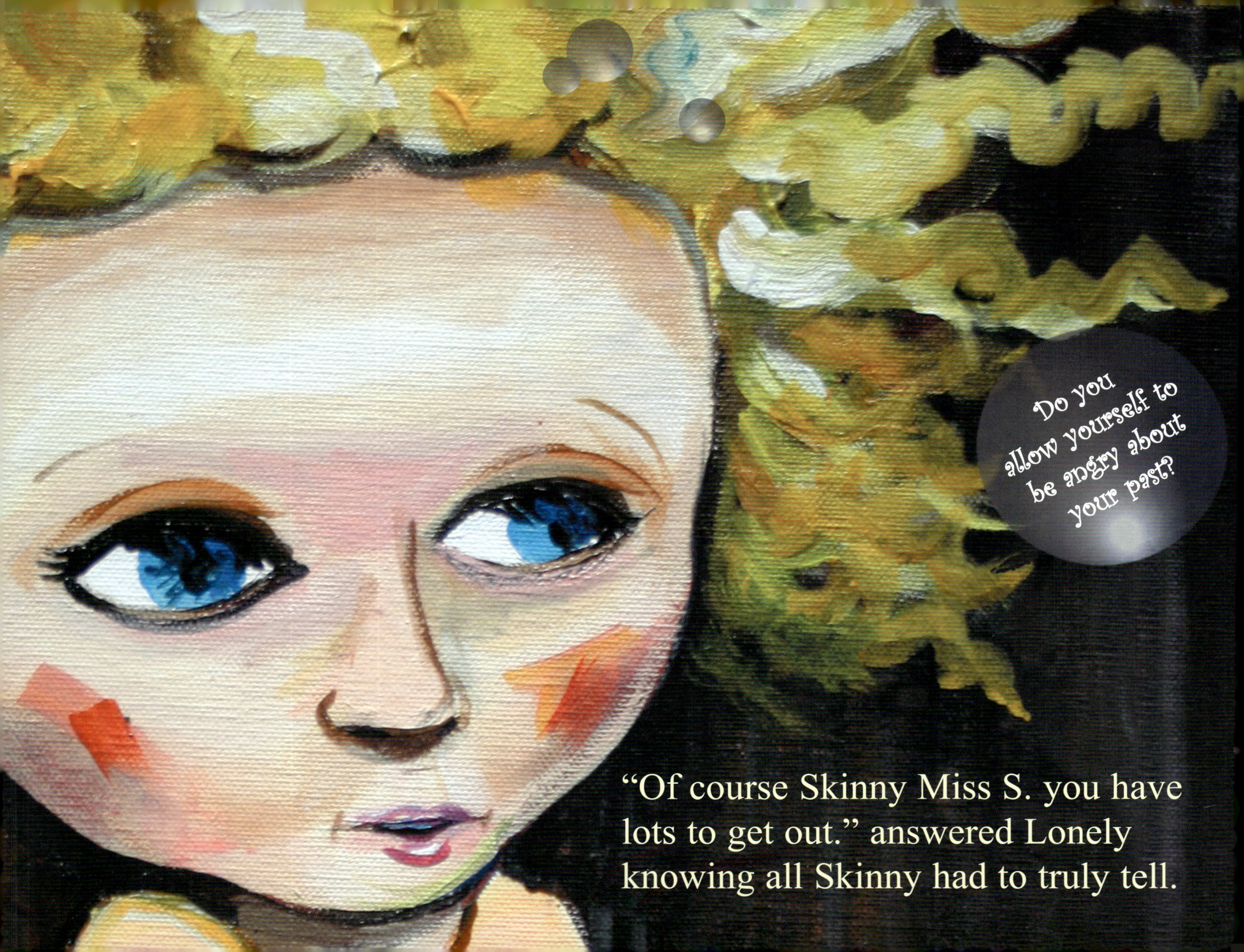
Do you
allow yourself to
be angry about
your past?

"Of course Skinny Miss S. you have lots to get out." answered Lonely knowing all Skinny had to truly tell.

confrontation
noun

1. the act of confronting.

2. the state of being confronted; *as a face-to-face meeting.*

3. forces or ideas: CONFLICT.

4. COMPARISON: *the flashbacks bring into meaningful confrontation present and past, near and far - R. J. Clements.*

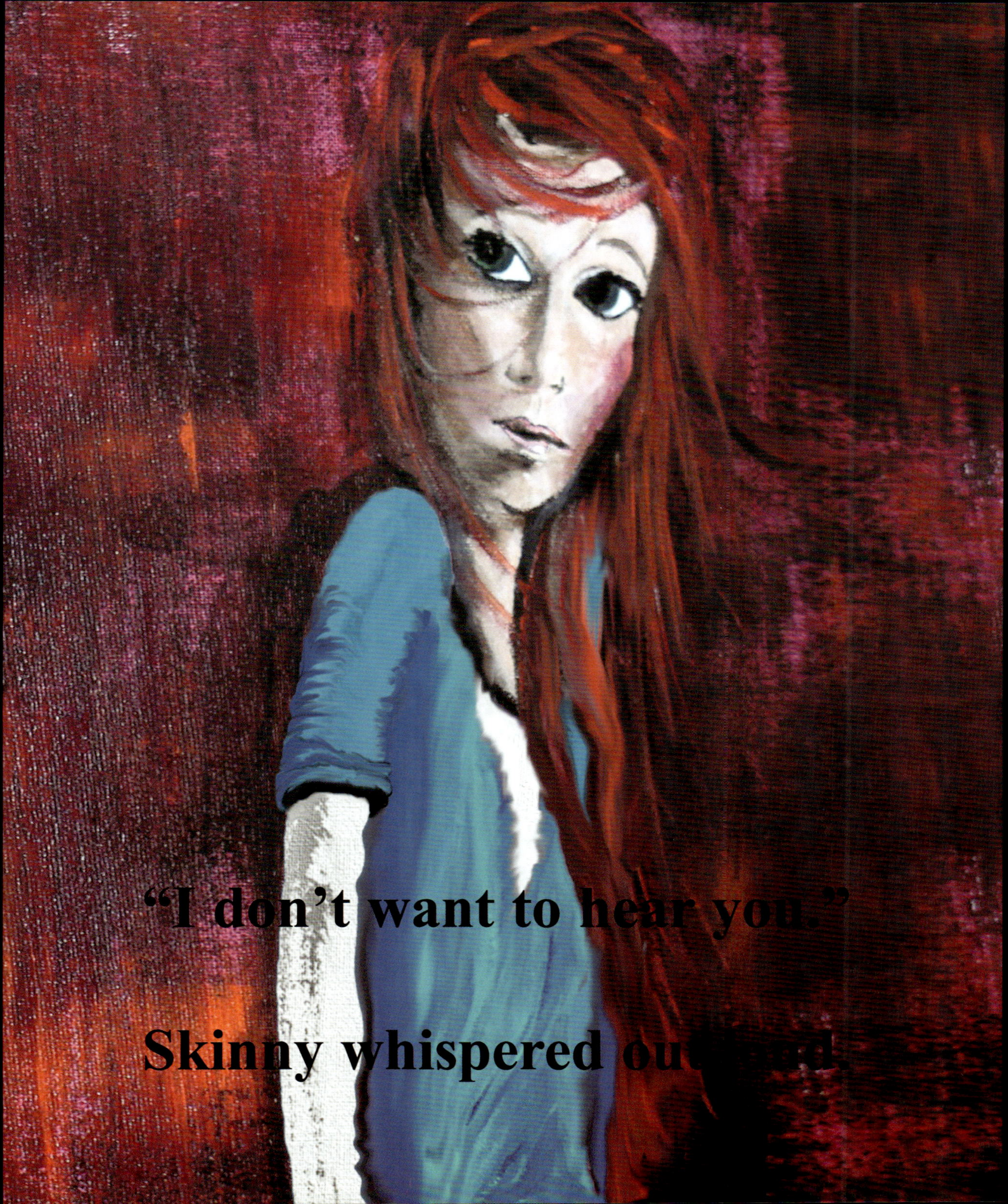

“I don’t want to hear you.”

Skinny whispered outloud.

truth
noun

1. sincerity in action, character, and utterance: FIDELITY, CONSTANCY.

2. the state of being the case: FACT.

3. the body of real things, events, or facts: ACTUALITY.

4. transcendent fundamental or spiritual reality.

5. a judgment, proposition, or idea that is true or accepted as true; *truths of thermodynamics.*

6. the body of true statements and propositions.

7. in truth: in accordance with fact; *Actually I really don’t want to hear the truth.*

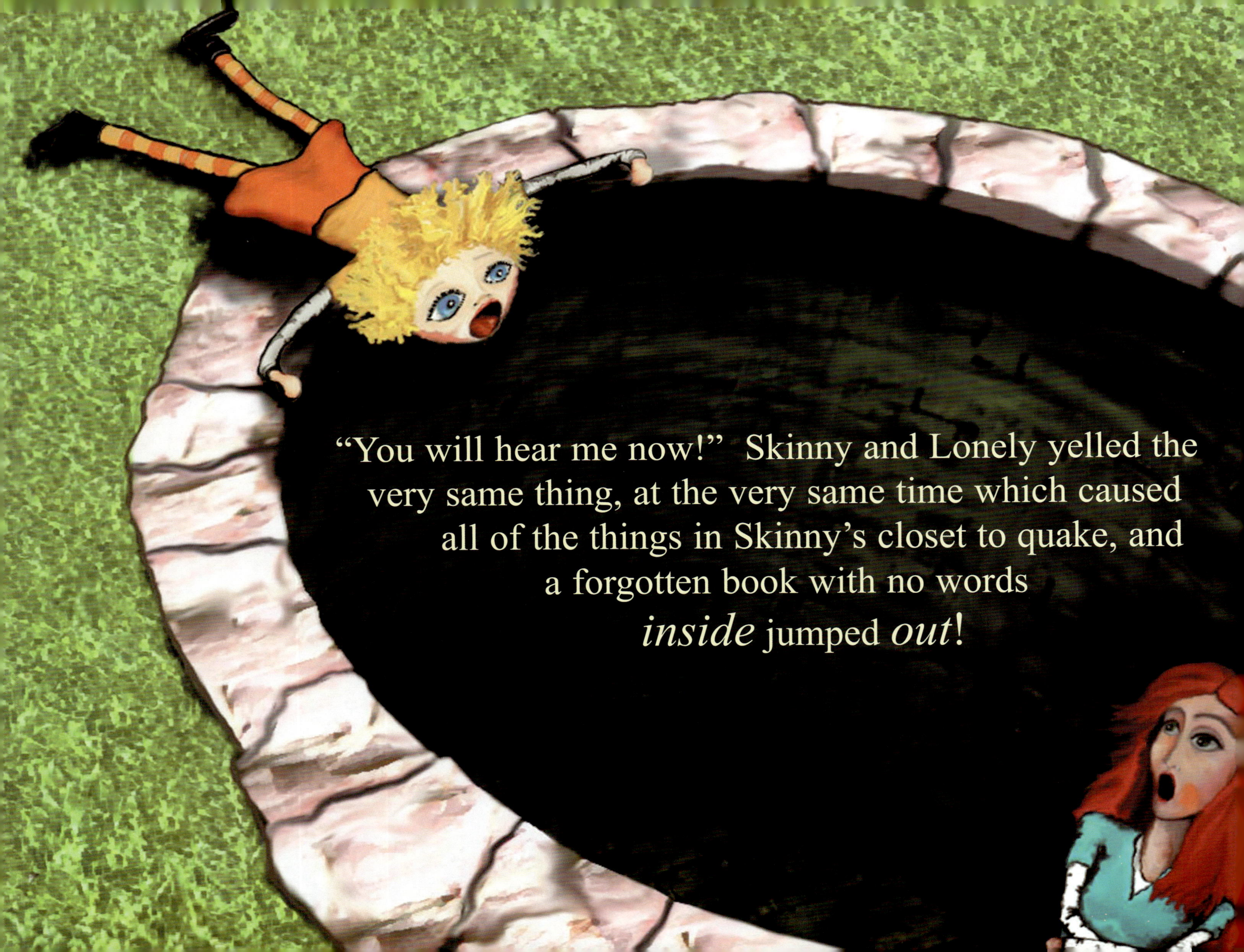

"You will hear me now!" Skinny and Lonely yelled the very same thing, at the very same time which caused all of the things in Skinny's closet to quake, and a forgotten book with no words *inside* jumped *out*!

It fell all the way to the floor of the well and landed next to Skinny's feet.

"A book with no words?" said Skinny Miss S.

"Oh this should be a bore." and Skinny fell asleep and began to snore, but this quest would be the best for Skinny to explore.

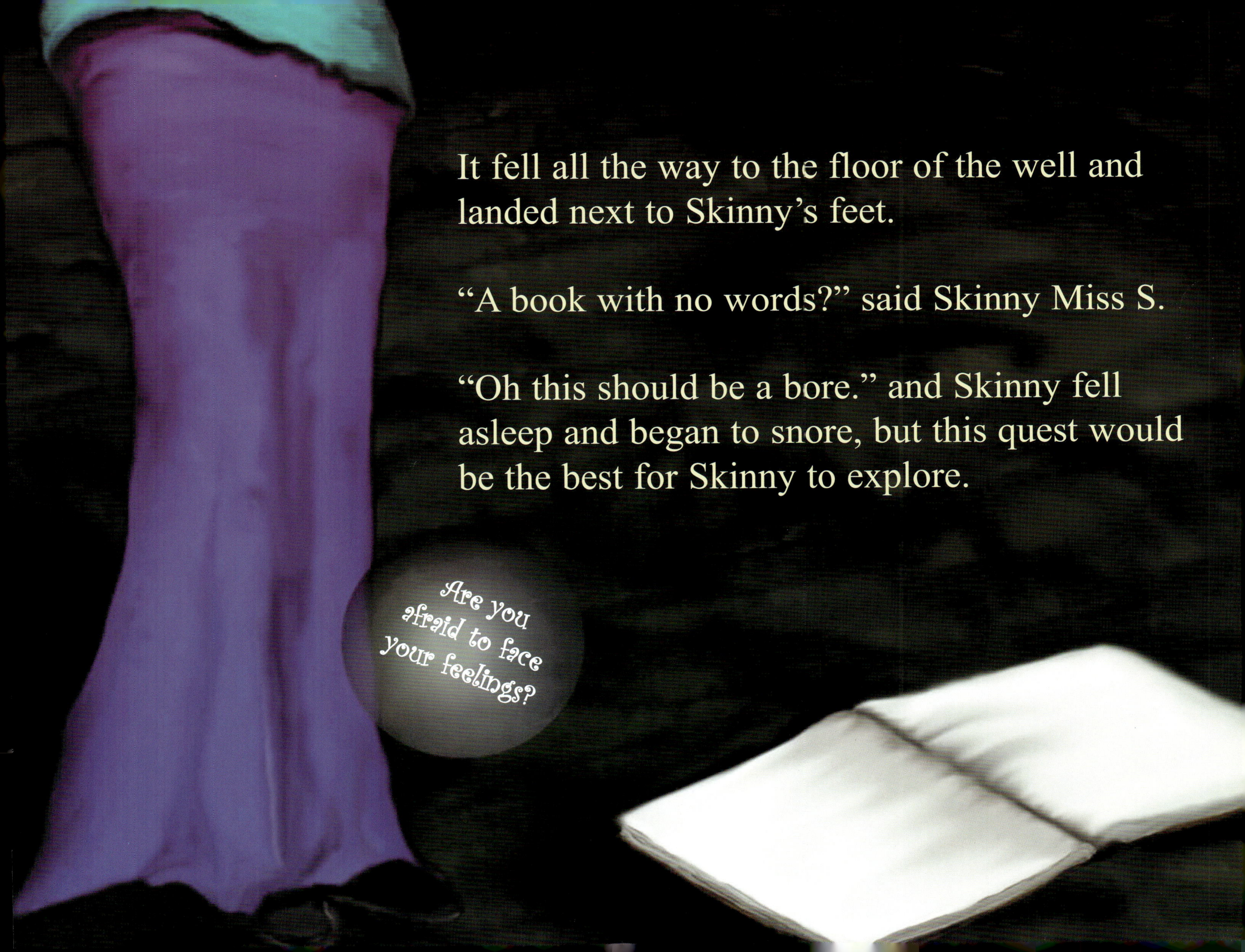

When Skinny Miss S. awoke from her sleep, nothing felt the same. The well was almost filled to the top with what seemed to be water. This made her become interested in the small mysterious book and so she took a closer look. It floated near her and to her surprise there were now **words written** on every page!

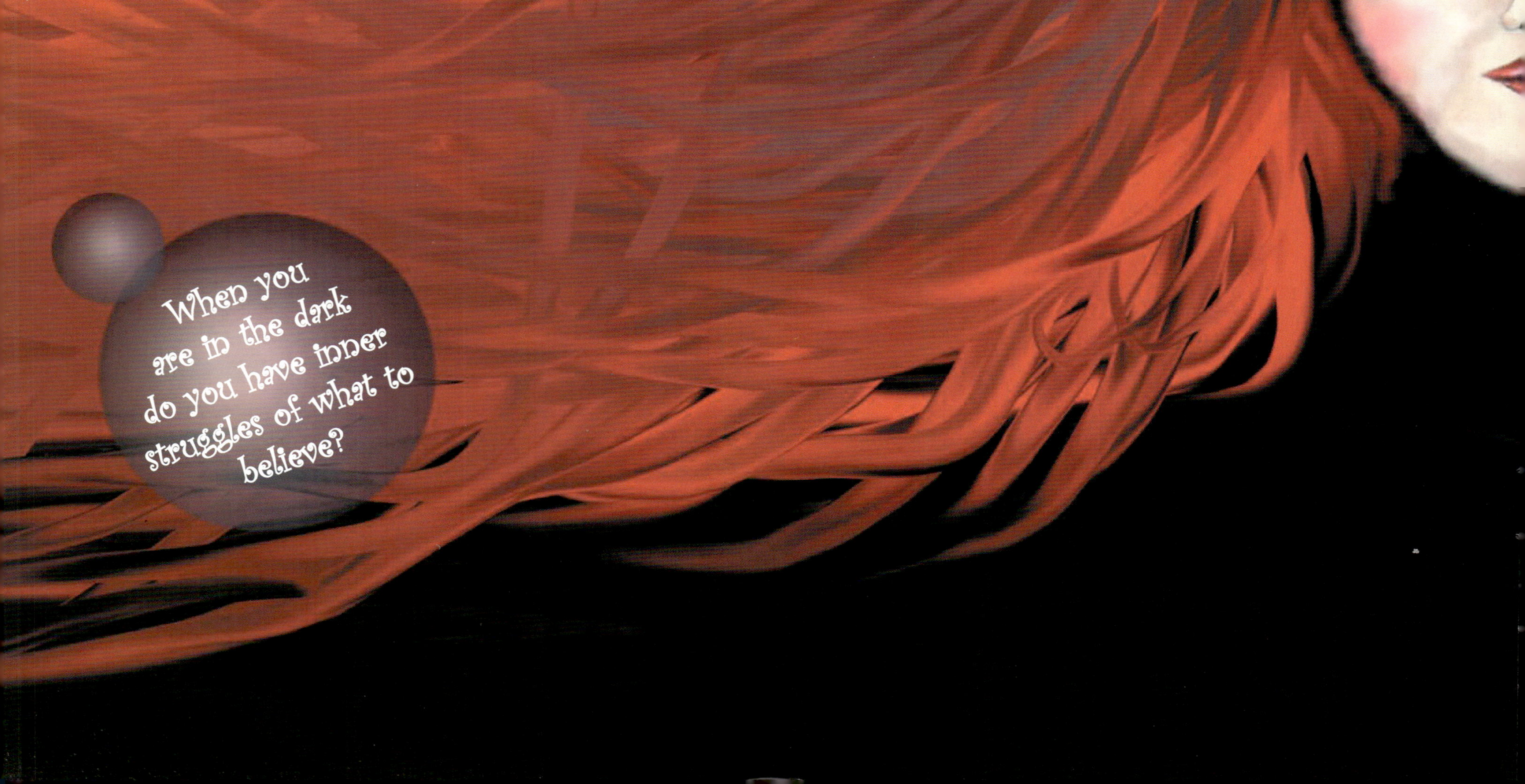

verb

to lose the remembrance of.

be unable to think of or recall; *I forget his name.*

to cease from doing, to treat with inattention or disregard; *forgot their old friends.*

to disregard intentionally: OVERLOOK -usually used in the imperative:; *I shouldn't have said that, so just forget it.*; to give up hope for or expectation of, usually used in the imperative; *as for prompt service, forget it.*

intransitive verb: to cease remembering or noticing; *forgive and forget*, to fail to become mindful at the proper time;*forgot about paying the bill.*

synonyms see

one who forgets

to lose one's dignity, temper, or self-control

Outside In

Skinny Miss S. was obsessed with her glass heart vase. She was convinced that if she filled it with something, even someone, she would be complete. She thought that was neat! She would move it all over the place thinking that if she found where it wanted to sit, she would then find the right fit. Problem was she was always moving it around. How was any filler supposed to learn to settle down?

Dean Doll suggested she put it on the front doorstep. Sir Grouchy Spider said that was an awful idea. She might get some transient from the street. Father Deana Marie added, "God is in the poor, you never know who knocks at your front door."

Lonely Miss C. giggled at the notion of Skinny finding God in her glass heart vase. She secretly wanted to fill the vase up with her lonely parts, all of the things she had seen, but Lonely Miss C. was an emotional cutter, and cutters tend to bleed. There was no chance Skinny wanted any recollection of those memories, or so it presently seemed.

Dean Doll noticed that Lonely Miss C. kept pushing Skinny to remember memories. This made Skinny Miss S. mad and one day she got really loud and threw Lonely to the ground. When she did misery came down upon her like an egg over her head. It seemed Lonely was right, Skinny needed to know in order to win her emotional fight.

Skinny Miss S. was very depressed and when misery came to eat her up she grabbed her glass heart vase and held it tight. It symbolized her empty heart and she would need it since she knew she was headed for a powerful spell as she surrendered to something that resembled the likes of hell. As she sleepwalked down a path disappearing into a big black hole, Skinny talked like a deviously deviled soul.

"Don't anyone follow me or come to save me. I want to go where I'm going and I don't want any guides or angels of any kind. I'm taking this one-way trip journey and I don't care to see anyone along the way. There will be something waiting for me down there. It's my passion to walk this road alone in this way! Isn't that what Christ's story told? It must be part of the surrendering to want to take on this dreadful load." Skinny was temporarily caught in her mind of belief a la mode.

Some people call it the rabbit hole, or hitting bottom. They say "the dark night of the soul" caught them. I call it the well from hell. It's as empty as the one who fell into it and the only way out is to find a real reason to cry tears until you make it back to solid ground. Real tears take a formula of elements and the trick is to release them, but not drown in them and most swimmers can't keep afloat in that kind of consciousness. At any rate that is where Skinny ended up, unconsciously of course. I'm here to tell what was written...by who knows who; I'm just a stuffed owl who sits and watches, guess who? Just because I do, Skinny thinks I'm judging her too.

There Skinny Miss S. sat at the bottom of the empty well. How she exactly got there so quickly no one could tell. Her hands were wrapped tightly around her glass heart vase. She wondered who was feeding #9, her black cat. She couldn't tell without her tarot cards, but then again she didn't care. To this experiment that wouldn't be fair.

She thought the voices in her head had guided her here...to heal? Couldn't be. She felt too terribly. This was a punishment, at least so it seemed. She finally didn't care if she died. What was life but a maze

God dropped her in. Why? To see how she would survive? Not telling her of what was on the outside?

"How mean!" she thought. "Not a god to believe, not me!" She wanted answers to all her questions that be.

It seemed like days and days and dazes passed and all Skinny could do is look with her tunnel vision eyes at the clouds that went by. When it was night she laid on her back in the waterless well and watched the stars twinkle in the sky, naming them and wishing on them as they floated by. One particular night she saw two of the brightest shining stars. She closed her eyes, held her breath and wished for...the ability to feel. She thought the only way she could muster up emotions, would be to cry and fill the well. Now that would mean finding out WHY... why she was so blue. Finding a filler for her glass heart vase was the second part of her wish. She thought she knew she must do this too.

When she opened her eyes she saw both stars fall at the very same time and one was headed right towards her! It landed right in her glass heart vase! The other one missed the well and where it landed she couldn't tell where it fell.

She held her glass heart up and took a long gaze into the brightness of the star. The ball of glow was slowly fading and transformed into a fairy-like girl in its place. Skinny was amazed at what she saw as the small girl was jumping up and down, attempting to get out of the vase that had captured her. She was yelling something, so Skinny put her ear to the top of the vase and heard the tiny voice tell her, "I am Pixie Pan. If you let me out of this vase I will grow and be your friend."

Skinny replied, "Why are you here?"

Pixie Pan answered, "I heard your wish to cry tears that are real. I am your inner child and I can help you heal."

Skinny turned the vase over and gave it a tap. Out fell Pixie straight on her lap! Sure enough in a matter of minutes, Pixie grew to her normal size; an ageless decade of years was the form she took on.

It was then that a small whimper was heard right outside of the well.

Skinny yelled up at the other half of the pair, "Who's up there? Who's there?"

The whimper became more like a cry and a boy's voice answered, "It's me, the other star; I'm just on the outside!"

Pixie Pan said, "Why are you crying and what is your name? Do you even have a name?"

The boy answered, "What do you think, this is my first life? I have a name! My name is Teek and I am the Son of God! I'm a poltergeist ghost who is commitment shy!" Teek continued, "It's been hard for me to choose any one life or any one family. I hurt my leg and I hurt my arm when I came in for landing, and I also bumped my funny bone. Worst of all I've got blood on my big toe. It's dark and it's cold out here! I need a mommy to kiss it and make it all feel better! This time I promise not to leave. Just believe! Behold the second coming is me!"

"Well, that's a lot of complaining coming from the Son of God. Is there anything else? Are you here for sympathy or here for duty?" Pixie Pan said very matter-of-factly.

"In answer to your question, Miss Boss E. with a capital E., someone must have been shooting at the stars, because I remember getting hit and I now have a bunch of pellets stuck in my rear! Did I tell you I am also missing an ear?" He started to cry again. Skinny stood looking at Pixie Pan and then up toward the voice of God himself?

"I wonder who shot you down, my sweet little dear?" asked Skinny. She wanted to know.

"Some wisher-on-a-star. It must be you! Why would you hurt me the way that you do?" Teek began to pout about.

"He's here for sympathy. What a savior and the guilt is thicker than any Jew." Pixie being Jewish thought she knew. She continued to yell back up to Teek. "If you're going to be a cry-baby then why don't you swing your head over and contribute to the pool of tears we are trying to formulate here? It's the only way to get her out, if you care!"

"Ok, so I was not telling the whole truth in fact. I just need a little attention and she seems very warm and nice. I will help her get out of this mess!" Teek pointed to Skinny. His silhouetted head was shadowed from where she stood. "I wish for her to be my mom in return. She's nicer than you and she listens to me. She doesn't care if I'm full of stories!"

Out of nowhere a shiny penny came down and hit Pixie Pan on the head.
Ouch, what was that?" Pixie said.

Skinny picked up the penny and showed it to Pixie Pan.

Teek hollered down, "Someone had to pay for me to come down from a star to get what they wished for. Now that's the correct way to make a wish, but you'll have to tell me what it is that you want, Skinny.

I'm not a mind reader you know."

"You should be! If you're a part of her you should just know! Besides aren't you supposed to be the Son of God?" Pixie spat back.

Teek hated to be challenged. He directed himself to Skinny instead, "Just tell me what you want!" Teek then turned to Pixie, "You would be a terrible sheep if I had to herd you!"

"But then my wish might not come true if I tell you." said Skinny ignoring the distaste between the two. She sat in over-thought as to whether or not she should state her wish out loud.

Teek and Pixie were at odds. "This is my mission!" Pixie yelled back. "Bug off!"

"Ask her how many wishes she wished for. She had to wish for two." replied Teek. "She must have. Why else would I have been awakened from sleep? If I'm not called upon then I don't share a peep."

"I wished for the ability to feel," Skinny gave in, "so that I would cry tears because that must be what I need to get out of this well. I also wished for my glass heart vase to be filled."

"See! Two wishes and you already fulfilled the second so I'm taking the first." said Teek, "Never-you-mind, I can make anyone feel!"

"Why don't you take the fifth. I don't think so, she wished for me!" replied Pixie, "So you may be here to watch and learn." Pixie continued, "Skinny I'm going to be blunt with you. Right now you can't feel. You're in shock and it may be difficult to get you right again. I have a memory of yours from a long time back, which may help you open the doors to facing your fears...in turn stirring up tears. It may bring up other issues. One's you should look at and heal as well. Not knowing them may be why you don't eat, or why you oversleep, or occasionally want to commit suicide."

"Listen to me. Don't tell her those truths! She doesn't need to know them! Her memory has dug a hole and buried them for a good reason. I will tell her all of my truly sad and sorrowful tragic stories. She will cry then." Teek argued. He was all about the save and going after the hardest ones was his nature of his game.

"You don't know what you're talking about! Telling stories that are lies means all you ever do is deny. Skinny needs to free herself from denial. You know nothing about modern day Pop-Psychology and how it can help to really heal." The little girl zoned in, "Now Skinny Miss S., you wished for me. Are you ready to free yourself from all that you have covered way deep inside and really break through to the other side?" Pixie looked her square in the eye. She was a very intense little girl.

"Yes, Pixie, I want to be free. I should have listened to Lonely Miss C." said Skinny. "Free me!"

"You might not have believed if you hadn't remembered yourself. There is something to be said for you participating in the hard work of what you're dealt." said Pixie Pan. "Skinny you play with cards don't you? Tarot that is?"

"All of your talk of 'dealing your fate' and 'hard work in order to heal'...let me tell you the deal! Have you forgotten about the loop hole to karma? What was that guy's name that just takes all burdens away? I remember now, that guy is ME! You think I'm just a mere clown but I'm here to stay. It's easier to believe! You don't have to dig up the past to be set free. Why do you think your mind is as bright as it is, creating blocks from remembering all those things from a rainy day?" Teek had a good argument, but Skinny was always the type to look up stream.

"Thank you, Teek, you are such a dear, but I really want to face my fears." Skinny said. "I'm not sure I believe in anything. Besides my dolls, I have no one and no one has me. If you told me you could miraculously get me out of this hell, should I believe?"

"No, Skinny. You always have to do the work. That's the nature of this life." Pixie sounded realistic, but negative indeed. She turned up to Teek, "You religious fanatics hide behind your beliefs. I am Skinny's inner child and she should believe in me, thus believe in herself,, Mr. Hang-on-the-cross-then-rise-from-the-dead. Sounds like an overrated magic show if you ask me. Where'd you go after that disappearing act? Where's your Father at? Maybe he's ME! Where's the Spirit that is suppose to get the whole world through? Where are the holes in your feet? Looks to me that Judgment Day should be upon you." Pixie Pan was insistent on getting her point through.

"I'll prove you wrong you know-it-all, Miss Boss E. You're not the boss of me! I'm sick of you always trying to out shine my star. Game on. I'm keeping score." Teek was hot-headed now.

Pixie ignored him and spoke directly to Skinny, "Teek is not really your inner child. Only I am and I represent your most pure and honest side. As you grew up you began to be challenged mentally. It skewed your mind and your core has been hard to find. Teek is a bit mentally challenged himself. It looks like his second coming could stir up the wind, but that's a whole other book so let's finish this one we're in."

"Fine, tell Skinny her memories, but I'll tell mine too! You're not the only one who has a bunch of crap in you.' He caught his breath and started straight in, "One time, when I had my last life, my big, fat, ugly, delusional, psychotic grandmother..."

Pixie ignored Teek and leaded over to whisper something, which took a long time to say. Skinny's reaction was more and more of dismay. As Pixie told her, Skinny remembered what the forgotten memories were. They were all true, at least for her. She broke down and cried for the rest of that day. Teek helped also by telling her all of his made-up stories of how he too was so abused.

Teek went on, "...and then she locked me in the attic with all of my toys double-locked inside of my toy chest so I couldn't play with them and then served me my meals from under the door with no fork or spoon and sour milk I had to pour." His sentences ran on and on.

Skinny was sincerely sorry for Teek's experiences and she decided to share her's with him, but not before Teek was finished, "and then...there was the time uncle made me ride horsy on his big, fat, hairy leg. He was creepy the way he looked at me, you know, in that way...when someone wants to make love to you? Euuu! Oh yeah, and then once I went to confession and the priest wanted to know about my sins.
I told him I had none and he made me clean his chalis' rim"

That one really stirred up Teek's tears and Skinny followed. Pixie supplied the memories Skinny needed in order to feel and Teek made up his, believing every word he said. They spent the rest of that day sharing stories back and forth as the well slowly filled up and Pixie and Skinny slowly got closer to the top. They were almost there and both ran out of memories to share.

Teek yelled down at Skinny, "I will get you out of this well, but you have to believe in something you can't see with your eyes."

"What is it?" asked Skinny.

"It's what I stand for, and after you're out, I'll fill you in without a doubt." Teek wanted to take care of Skinny and saw the vulnerability in her big green eyes.

"Fill me in? Could it be true? Is this boy my new filler for my glass heart vase? A brand new belief system come true?" Skinny spoke her thoughts out loud, only to upset Pixie Pan.

"I filled your vase, but you helped me out. You're the only one now who can figure this out! Do you need an outside source to fill your heart or can you find it within?" Pixie was mad again.

Skinny got smart. "But the two of you are my inner children and you said it yourselves, so get back in!" Skinny got louder.

This time Pixie Pan and Teek were on the same page, "We came to help you recall dark memories to help you feel. We can't be contained!" Pixie continued, "The memories I told you were the truth and you agree because you're living proof. Teek made his up and they require belief."

"Not true! Now I'm gonna leave!" and just like that he was gone from the scene.

"Skinny, I must go too. This is no place for a child to be." Pixie began to disappear.

"Wait, Pixie!" yelled Skinny Miss S. "Are these memories true? Can I really trust you?"

"Can you trust you? Memories are like Teek. You never can tell." said Pixie.

"I can't tell." But Skinny knew very well,

"I can't tell . . . and who is going to get me out of this well?!"

remember

1.

2.

3.

4.

5.

1.
2.

REMEMBERS, RECOLLECT, RECALL

"Where did all of this water come from? How did words get on to the pages of this book? Did I write them? But I haven't a pen! I must be going insane again!" said Skinny to herself and she began to read, now floating a-top of what she would find to be her **hard-earned tears.**

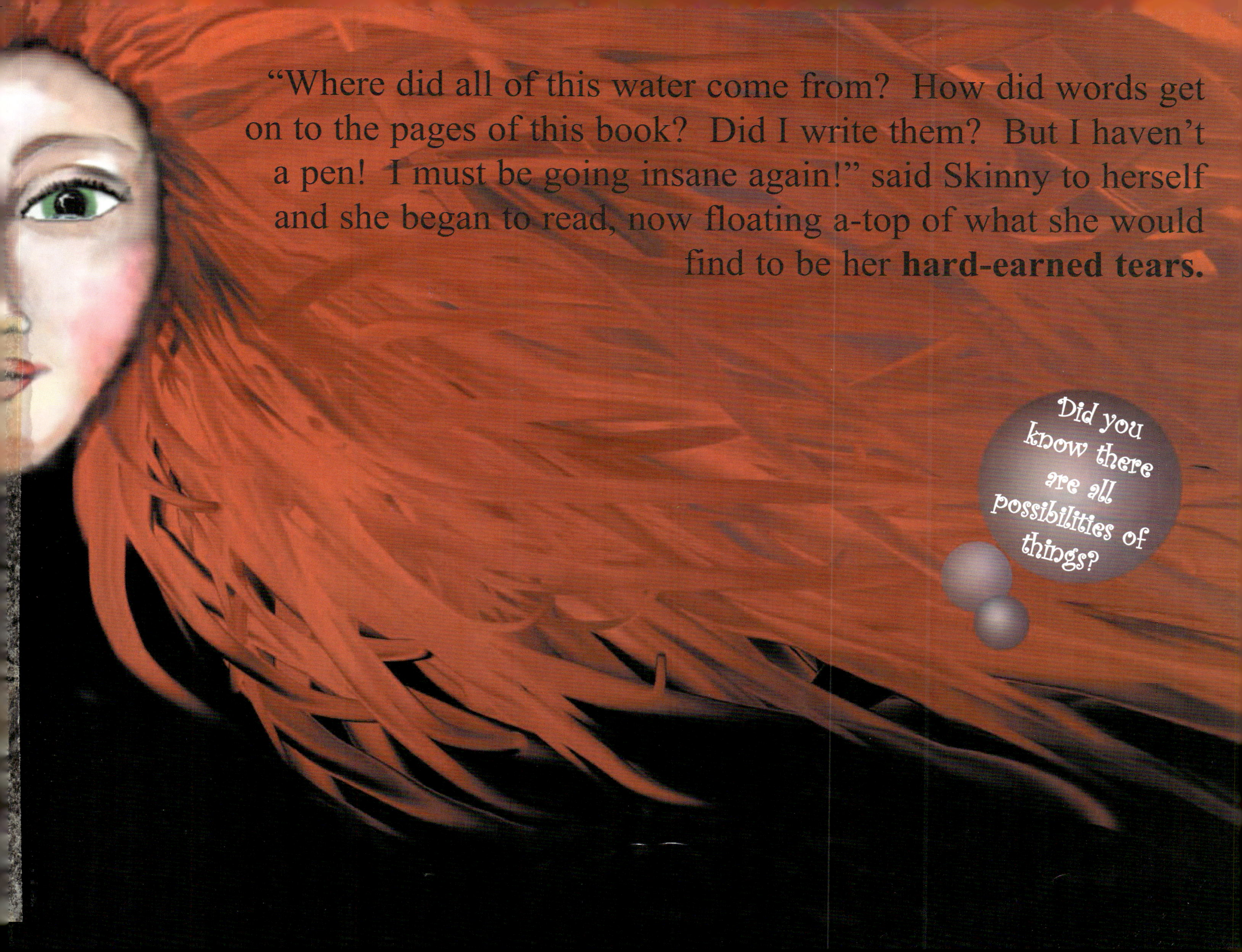

The story of meeting her inner children left her sad and forgotten, but something down deep in her made a shift. She was curious to find out where they went. Had she scared them away? Did they want someone who would care for what they had to say? They did tell her they didn't want to stay.

She now had a purpose to be the best she could be…"For them! For me!" said Skinny. She knew they were a part of her even though it was all such a blur. She knew they were a part of her cure.

Skinny told the dolls who were still patiently waiting outside of the well, of the story left in the book and how she must get out of this well now for real! This mysterious book was something to feel! She could barely swim anymore and she yelled to the dolls to help her reach the top. Dean Doll had an idea which may have made it possible for Skinny to return home.

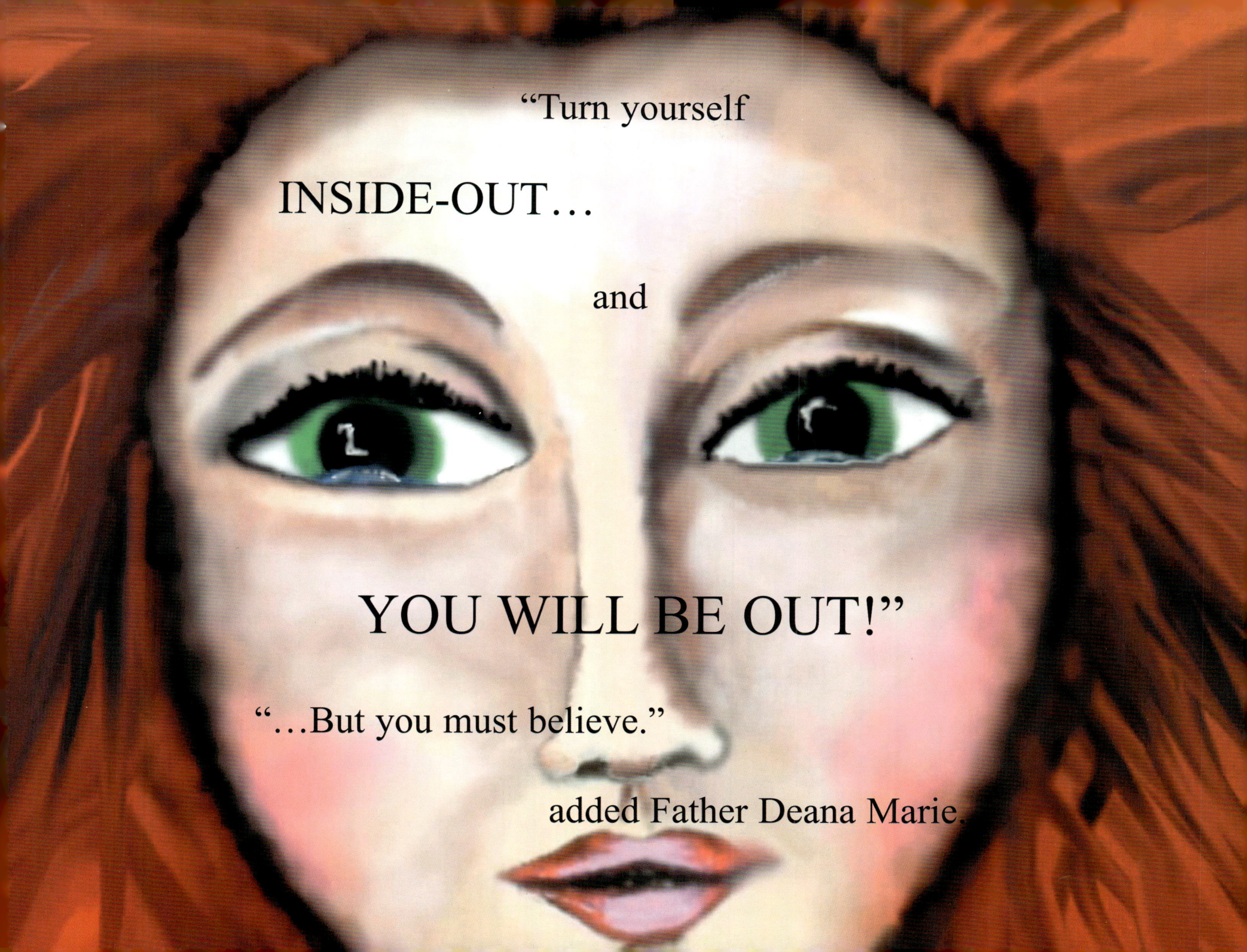

"Turn yourself

INSIDE-OUT…

and

YOU WILL BE OUT!"

"…But you must believe."

added Father Deana Marie.

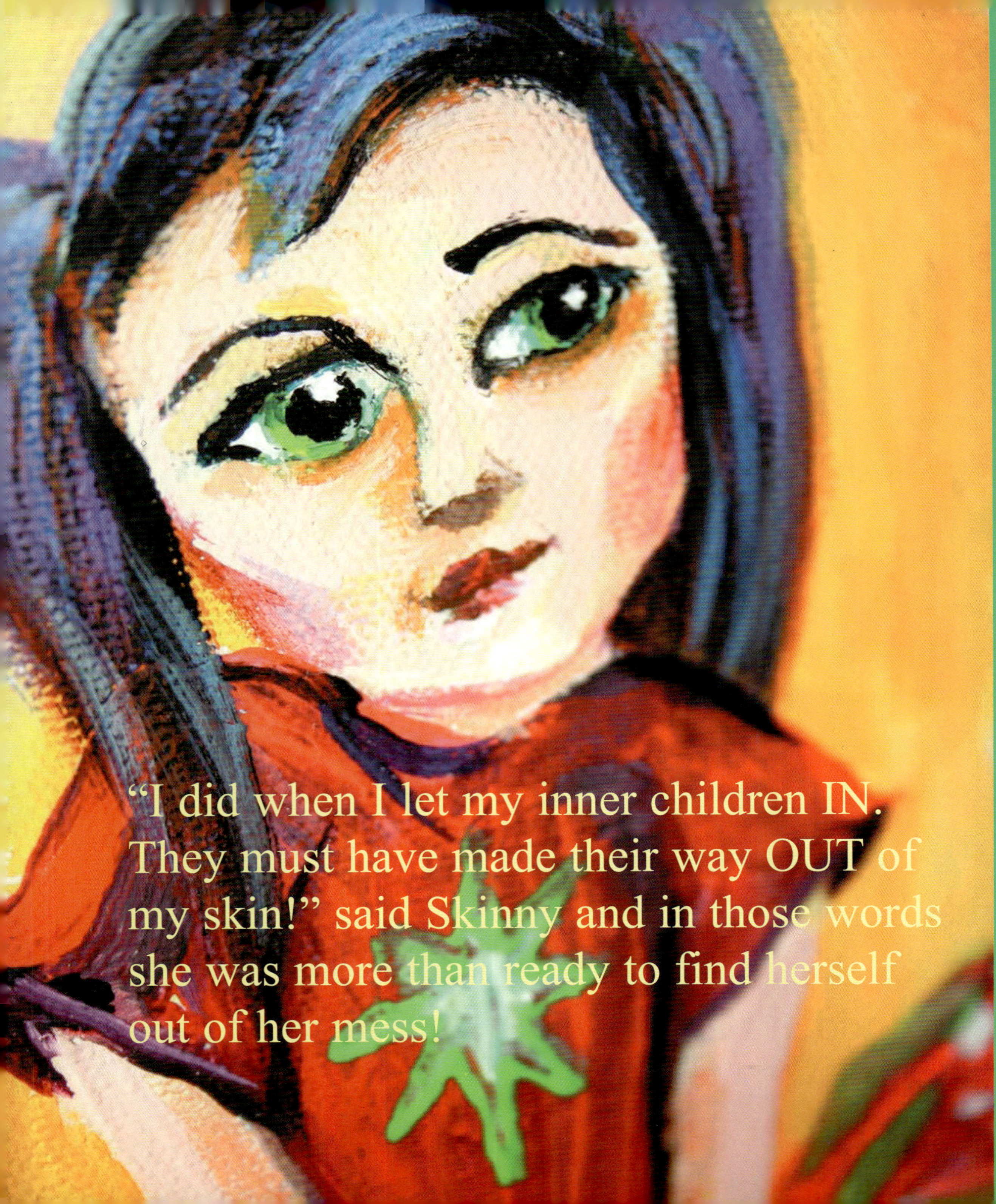
"I did when I let my inner children IN. They must have made their way OUT of my skin!" said Skinny and in those words she was more than ready to find herself out of her mess!

Inner child *is a concept used in popular psychology to denote the childlike aspect of a person's psyche, especially when viewed as an independent entity.*

Frequently, the term is used to address subjective childhood experiences and the remaining effects of one's childhood. The Inner Child also refers to all of the emotional memory and experiences stored in the brain from earliest memory.

The Twelve-step program recovery movement considers healing the Inner Child to be one of the essential stages in recovery from addiction, abuse, trauma, or post-traumatic stress disorder. In the 1970s, the Inner Child concept emerged alongside the clinical concept of Codependency (first called Adult Children of Alcoholics Syndrome.)

Carl Jung referred to a similar concept as the 'Divine Child.' Emmet Fox called it the 'Wonder Child.' Charles Whitfield dubbed it the 'Child Within.' Some psychotherapists call it the 'True Self'. Transactional Analysis calls it simply Child. W. Missildine may have been the first to refer to this concept as the inner child in his 1963 book Your Inner Child of the Past. The "wounded inner child" is a modified application of the inner child concept popularized by American educator, and pop psychology and self help movement leader, John Bradshaw.[15]

Repressed Memory [Forgotten Memory] is a significant memory, usually of a traumatic nature, that has become unavailable for recall. The term is used to describe memories that have been dissociated from awareness as well as those that have been repressed without dissociation. The existence of repressed memories is not totally accepted by mainstream psychology, although some studies have concluded that amnesia can occur in victims of trauma. According to the theory's proponents, repressed memories may sometimes be recovered years or decades after the event, most often spontaneously, triggered by a particular smell, taste, or other identifier related to the lost memory. It is not currently possible to distinguish a true repressed memory from a false one without corroborating evidence.[16]

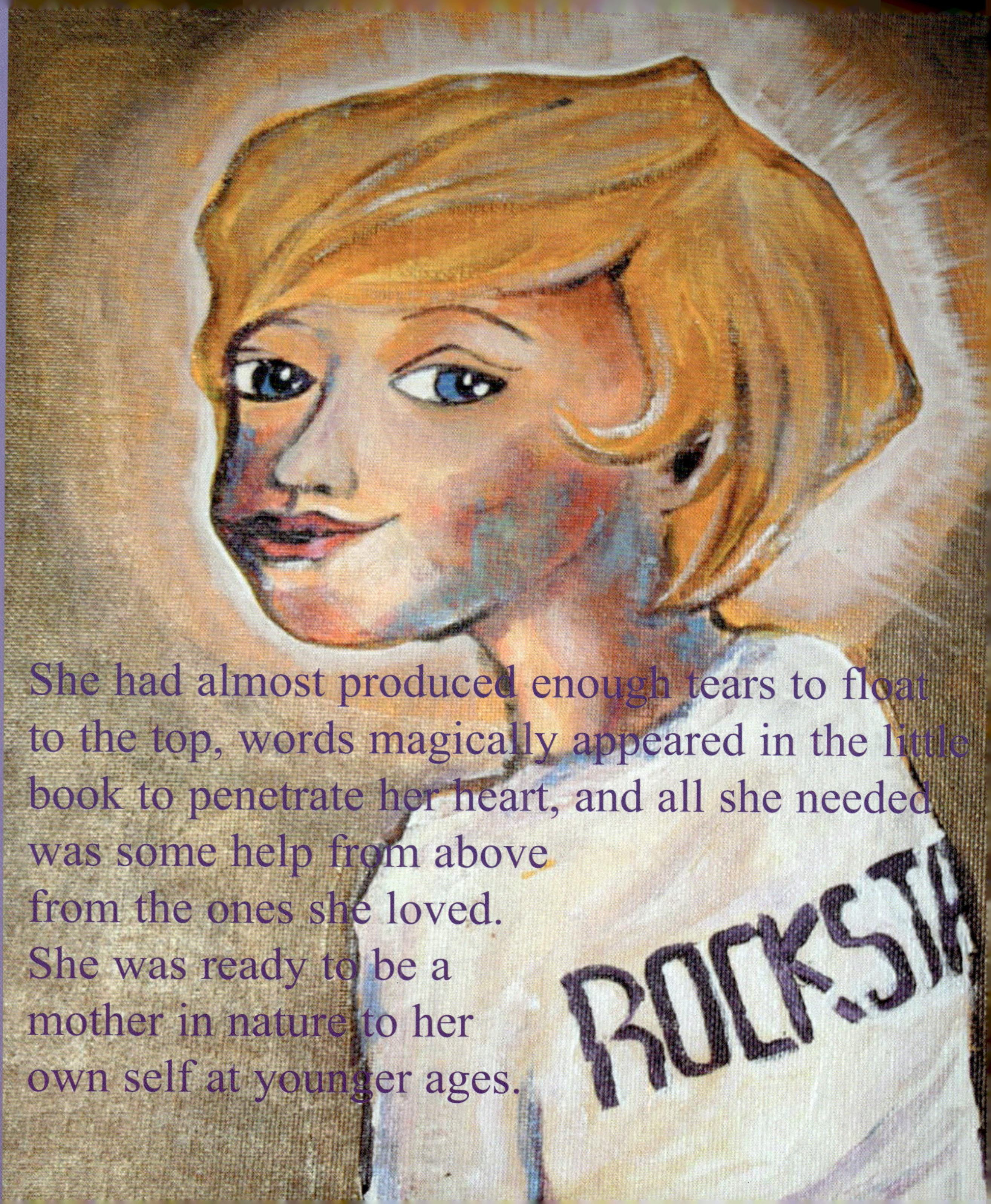

She had almost produced enough tears to float to the top, words magically appeared in the little book to penetrate her heart, and all she needed was some help from above
from the ones she loved.
She was ready to be a
mother in nature to her
own self at younger ages.

Did you know you can truly put your wounds to bed ... after they have been acknowledged in your head?

Dean Doll knew what he had to do.
He must throw her a line to save her even though Father Deana Marie fought with him every inch of the way from the back of Dean Doll's head yelling, "There is only one man who saves! You are not *The Way*! Besides she has shed enough tears as her penance to get out alive."

But Dean Doll knew better and had climbed up high to where Lonely Miss C. and Sunny Mister E.'s light hid, tossing the sun down to Skinny. She grabbed one of Sunny's rays with both hands, pulled herself up, as Dean Doll demanded Skinny to open the doors of the closet she found herself in. Skinny Miss S. was successfully pulled out from her subconscious liquid misery and laid out to dry in the heat of the Sunny Mister E.

"Believe in yourself Skinny Miss S."
said Dean Doll out of breath.

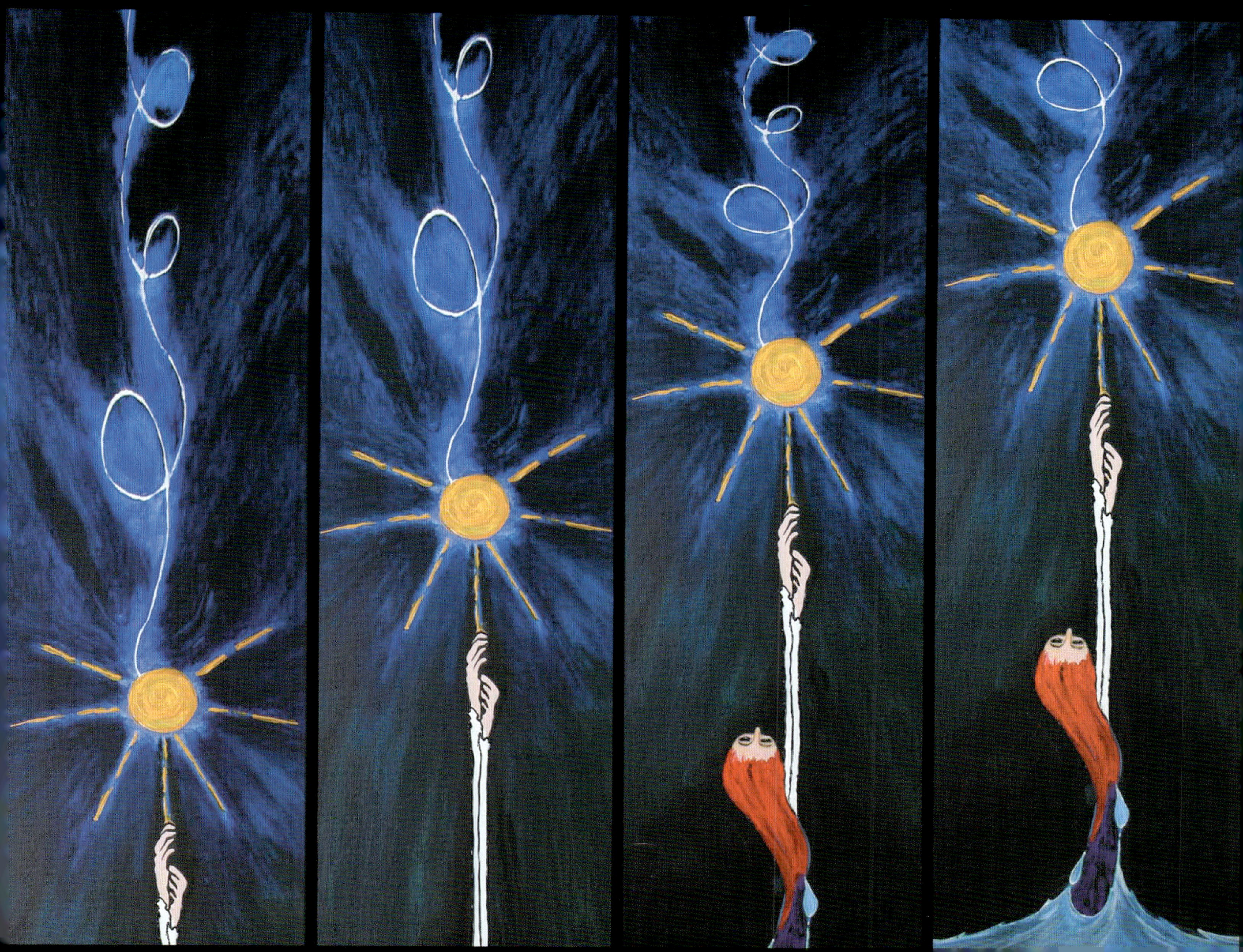

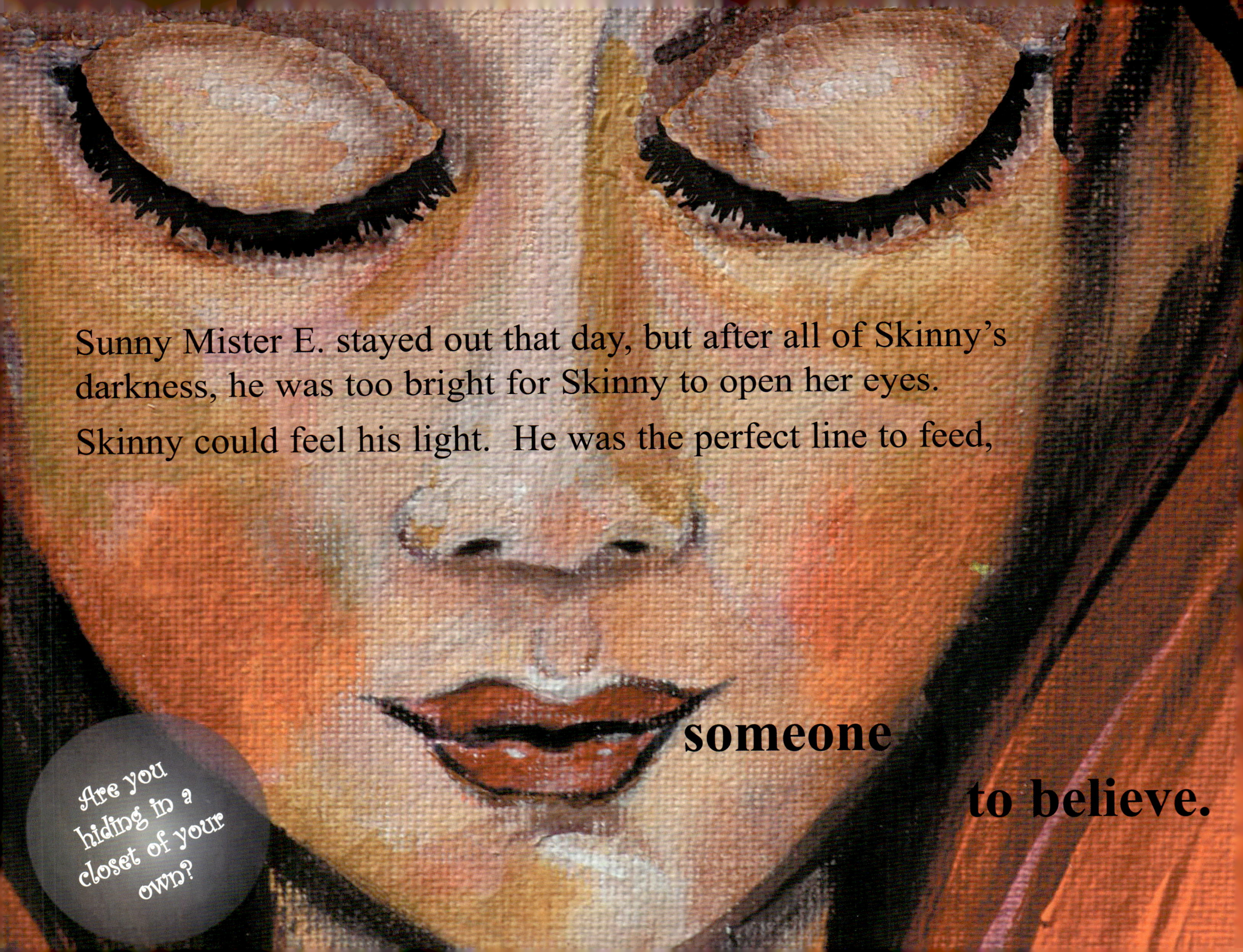

Sunny Mister E. stayed out that day, but after all of Skinny's darkness, he was too bright for Skinny to open her eyes. Skinny could feel his light. He was the perfect line to feed,

someone

to believe.

Are you hiding in a closet of your own?

bright
adjective

1. radiating or reflecting light: SHINING, SPARKLING; *bright lights, bright eyes.*

2. SUNNY; *a bright day.* also radiant with happiness; *bright smiling faces, bright moments.*

3. ILLUSTRIOUS, GLORIOUS; *brightest star of the opera.*

4. LIVELY, CHEERFUL *be bright and jovial among your guests.*

5. INTELLIGENT, CLEVER; *a bright idea.*

6. AUSPICIOUS, PROMISING; *bright prospects for the future.*

She placed him on top of her head with pride and told him of her adventures in the well, "I don't understand. I met my inner children in there and they caused me such hell! Now more than ever, I want to take care of them because I now know they are a part of me. They helped me to see." With that Skinny squinted her eyes open.

Sunny Mister E. replied, "They must have something to say. Do you know what chased them away?"

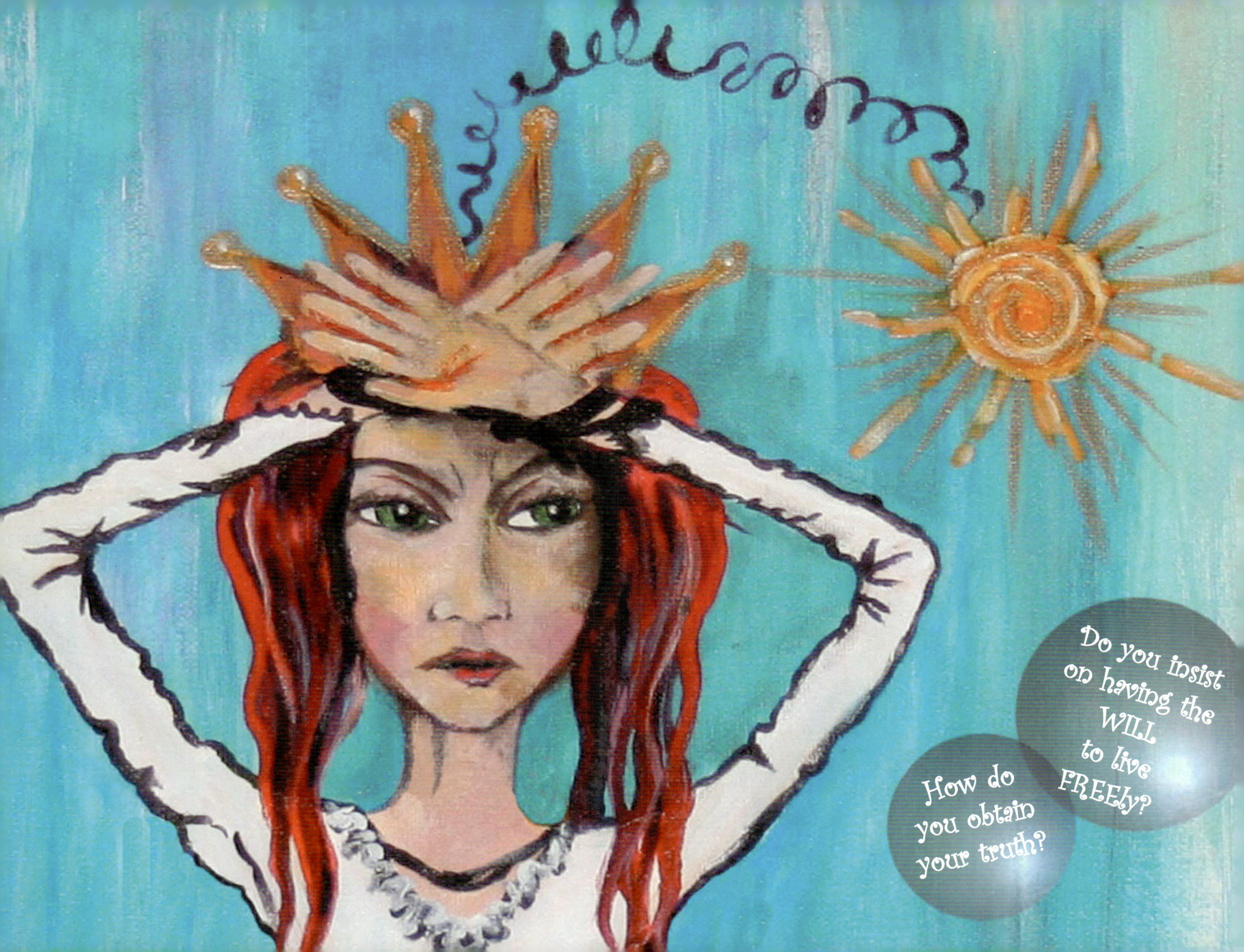
Do you insist on having the WILL to live FREEly?
How do you obtain your truth?

Skinny opened her eyes a wee bit more, “I think they chased each other away! It sounded like they didn’t like what each other had to say!” Skinny cried from deep inside, “Can you give me a clue as to which of their stories I should buy? It sounded like they had seen many dark things through my eyes. They told me things that made me cry…things I can’t tell are truth or lies. Then they up and left before granting my second wish and if you ask me again, that is cause for discipline! Sunny Mister E., will you help me? Can you see how much this darkness has hurt me? I want to see…completely! It doesn’t have to be in 3-D! Have you shed so many tears of this size? Do your powerful rays care if I lay down and die? There is one thing now that must be said, I want to see because I’m not yet dead!”

will
verb

1. DESIRE, WISH; *call it what you will.* verbal auxiliary: used to express desire, choice, willingness, consent, or in negative constructions refusal. *Will you please stop that racket?*

2. used to express frequent, customary, or habitual action or natural tendency or disposition; *will work one day and loaf the next.*

3. used to express capability or sufficiency; *the back seat will hold three passengers.*

4. used to express determination, insistence, persistence, or willfulness and used to express inevitability; *I have made up my mind to go and go I will.*

5. used to express a command, exhortation, or injunction; *you will do as I say at once, if you will.*

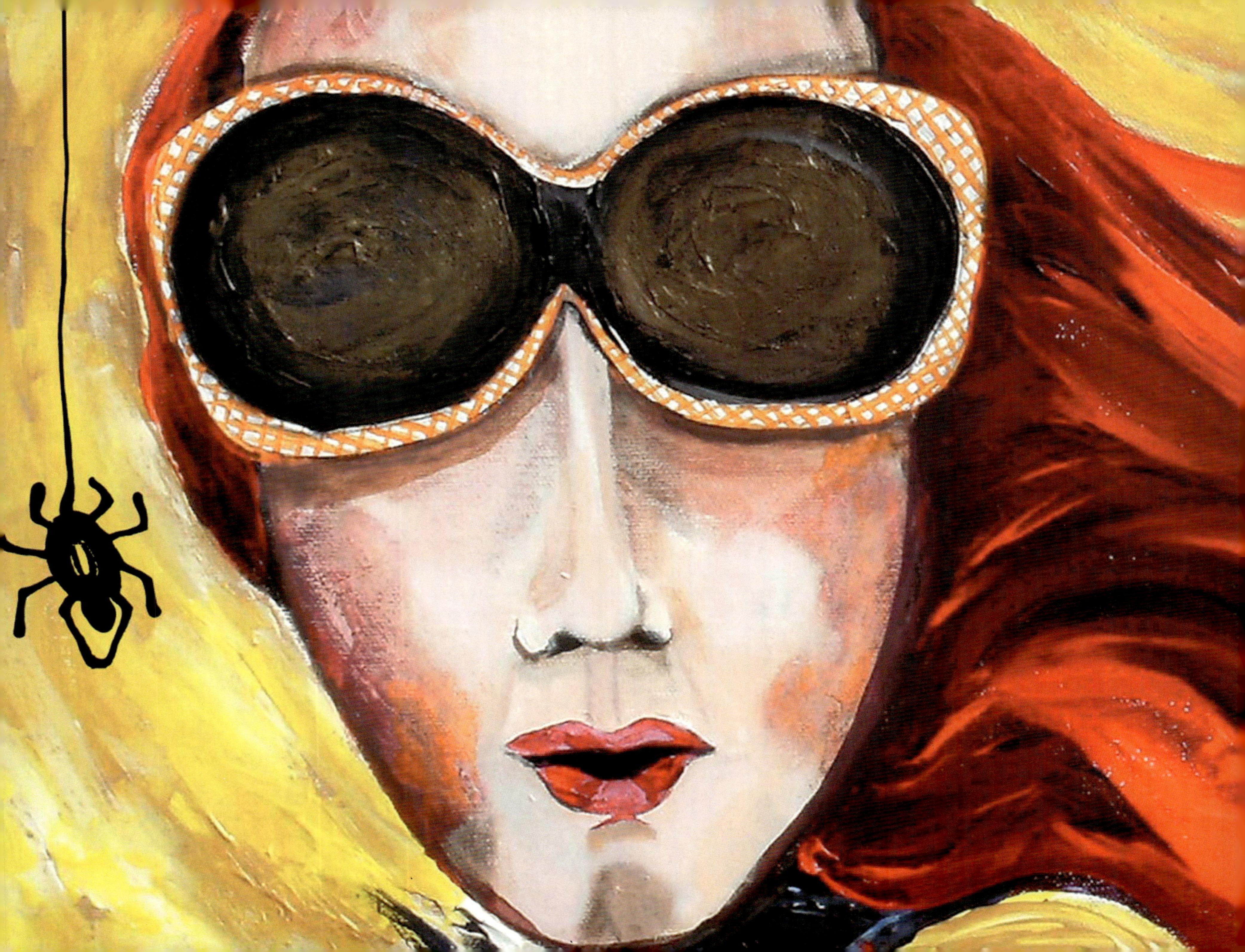

Sir Grouchy Spider spun down from a different view, "I see no big deal with what you feel. We'll just sweep away those voices, into the right boxes of course, or sweep them right under the bed.

Out of sight, out of mind,
is always what I've said!"

Skinny sighed, "Great another one whose words I wish would disappear." Skinny reached for her sunglasses and knelt down to hear what Sunny Mister E. had to say. Sunny answered with a reverent light, "I thought you would never ask. Did you notice you're not the same as you use to be? It's not enough to have words with your dolls over a dark cup of tea. I'll tell you the reason since you cannot see. You have a clinical condition that makes you feel blue. Let me spell it out for you…

D.-E.-P.-R.-E.-S.-S.-I.-O.-N! My dear, Skinny Miss S.
it's called CLINICAL DEPRESSION."

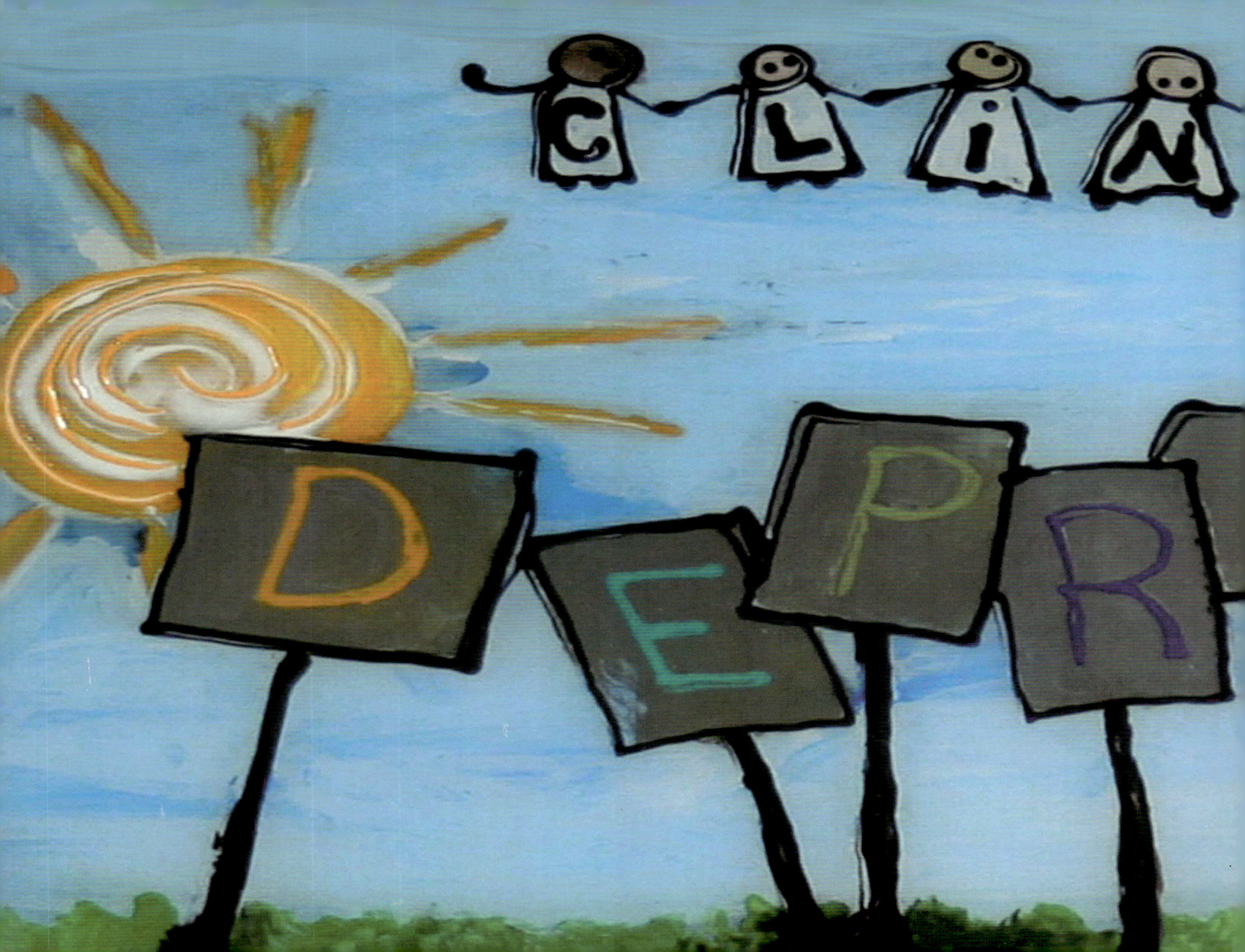
CLIN
DEPR

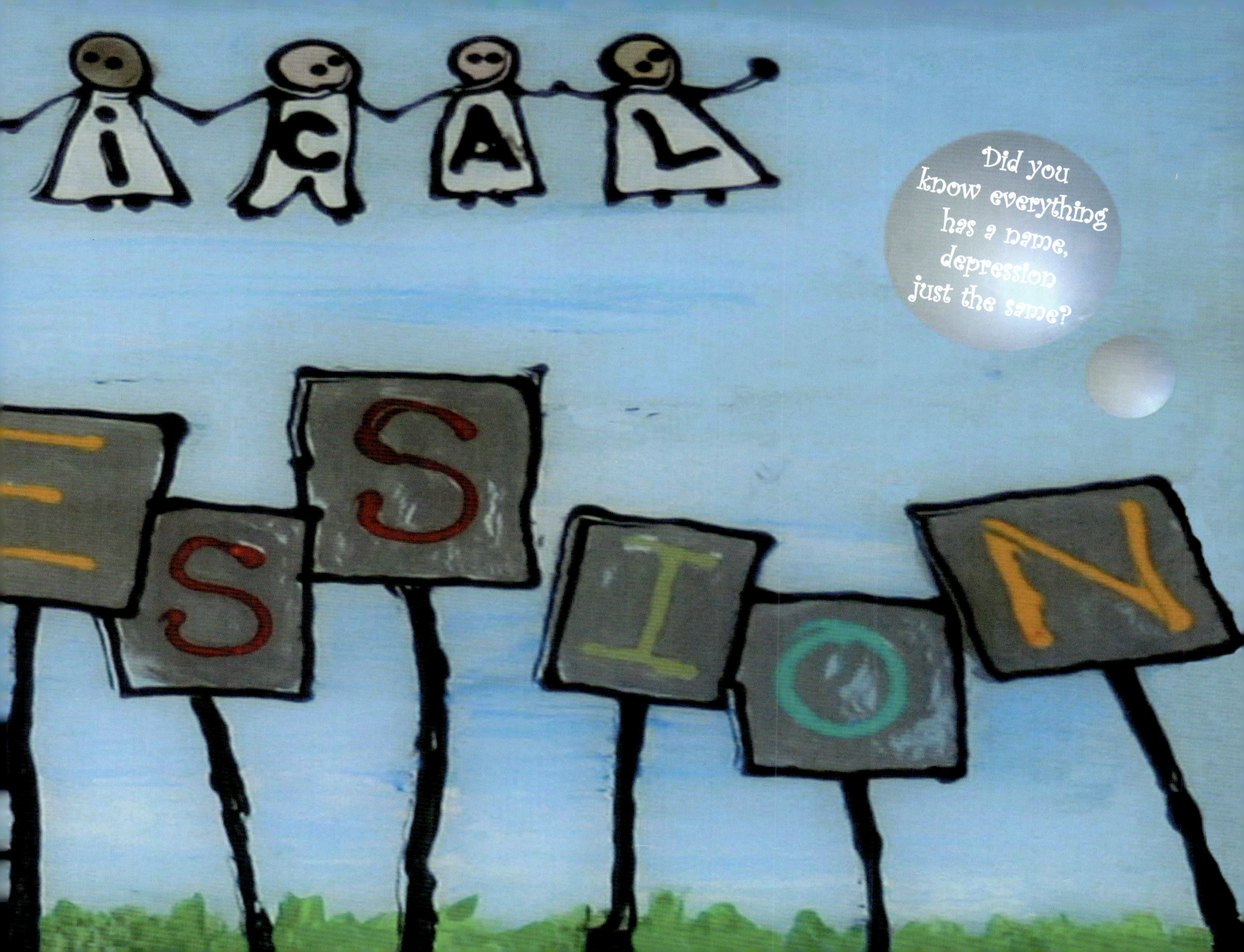
iCAL
ESSION
Did you know everything has a name, depression just the same?

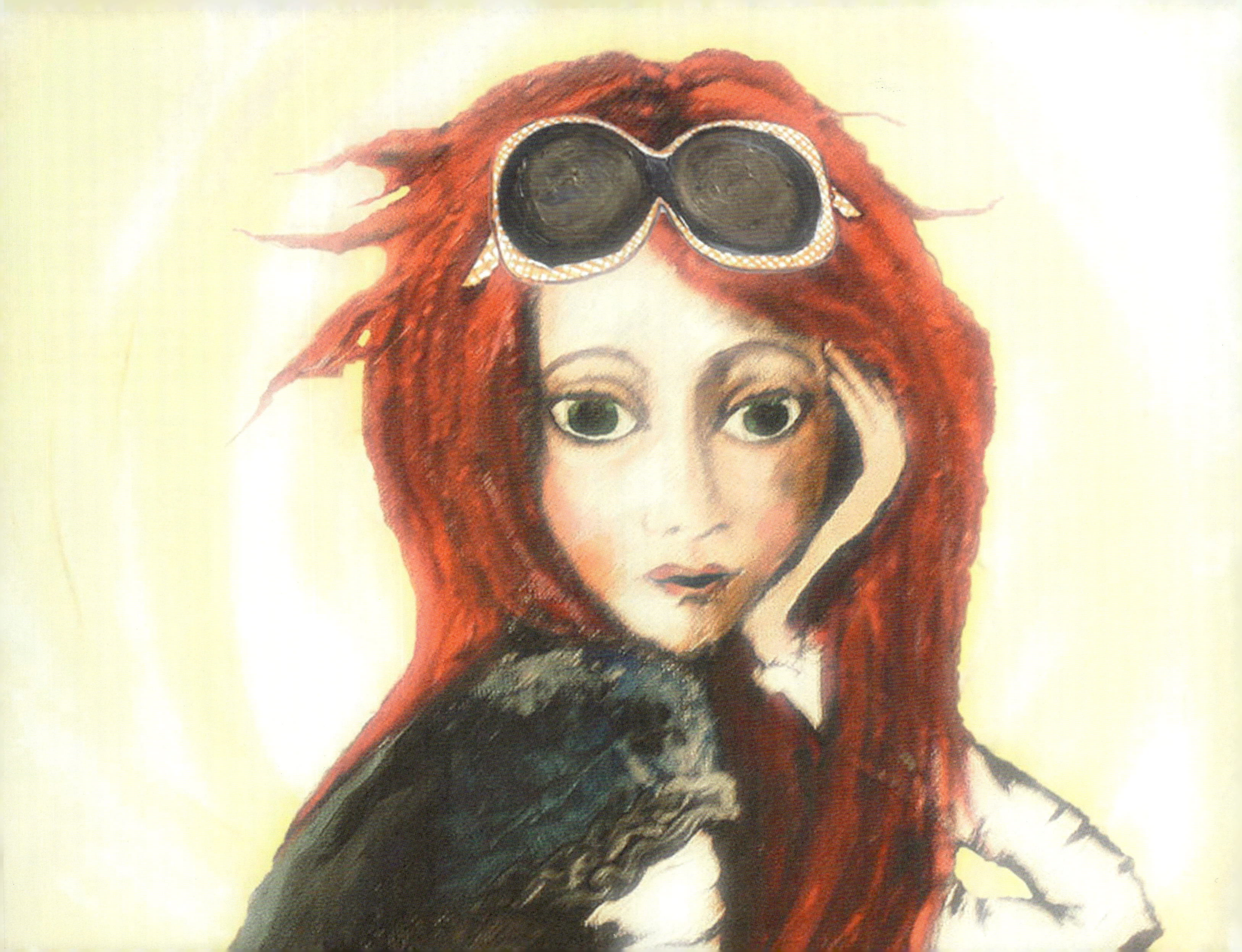

Did you know you have a bright side who sees every part of you?

Skinny Miss S. surprisingly could not believe! "No, not me! That just can't be. I'd rather go back to having tea. Well, now that I think about it, maybe not. Is this 'depression' something that can be easily fought?"

"That is something even I can't say. Everyone's healing has their own way." Sunny knew the hell she was experiencing was for her higher good and would one day disappear when she no longer needed it as food.

Does your denial help you cope, but doesn't ultimately heal you?

Oh, how Skinny was confused!

"It has a name…

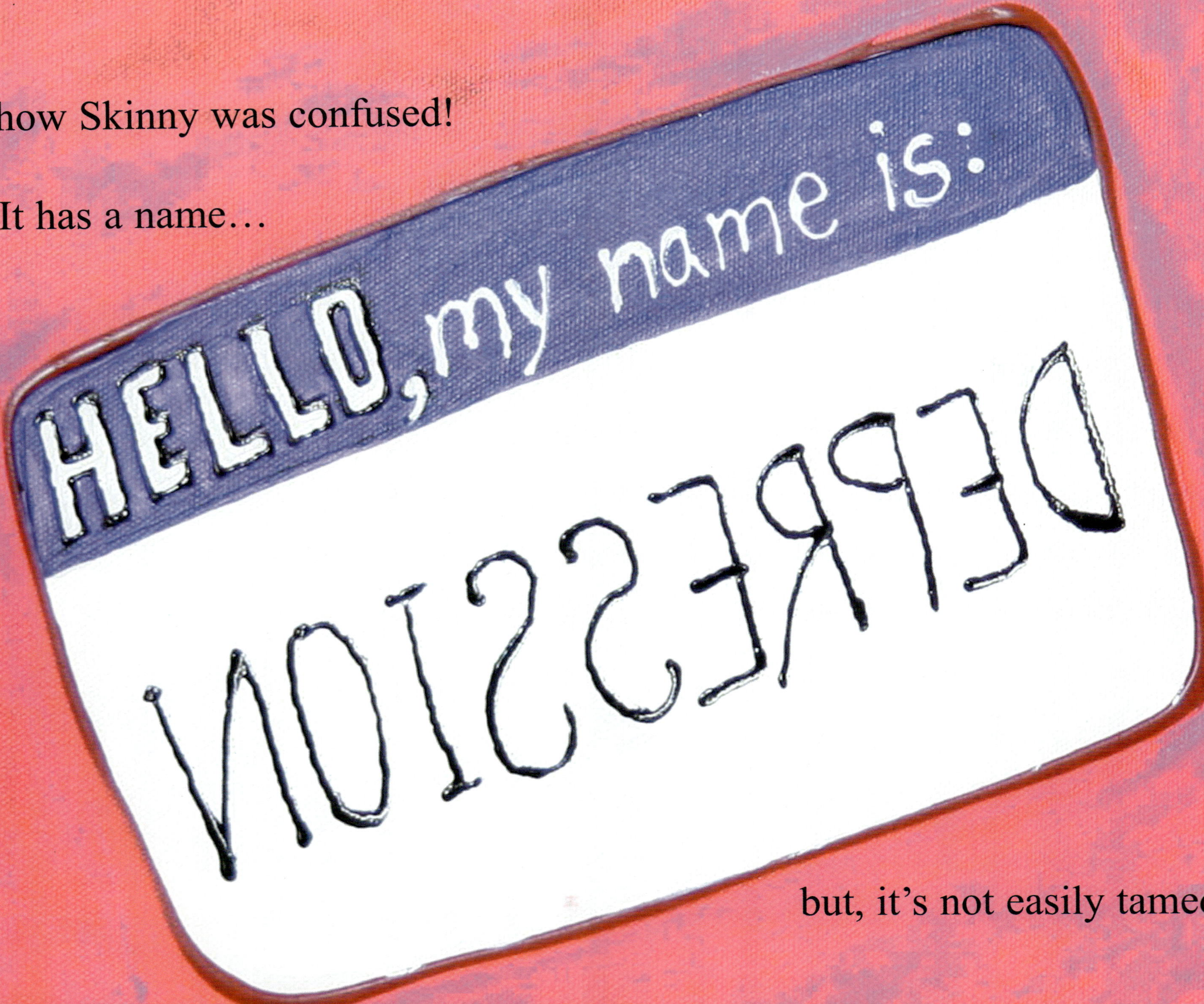

but, it's not easily tamed?"

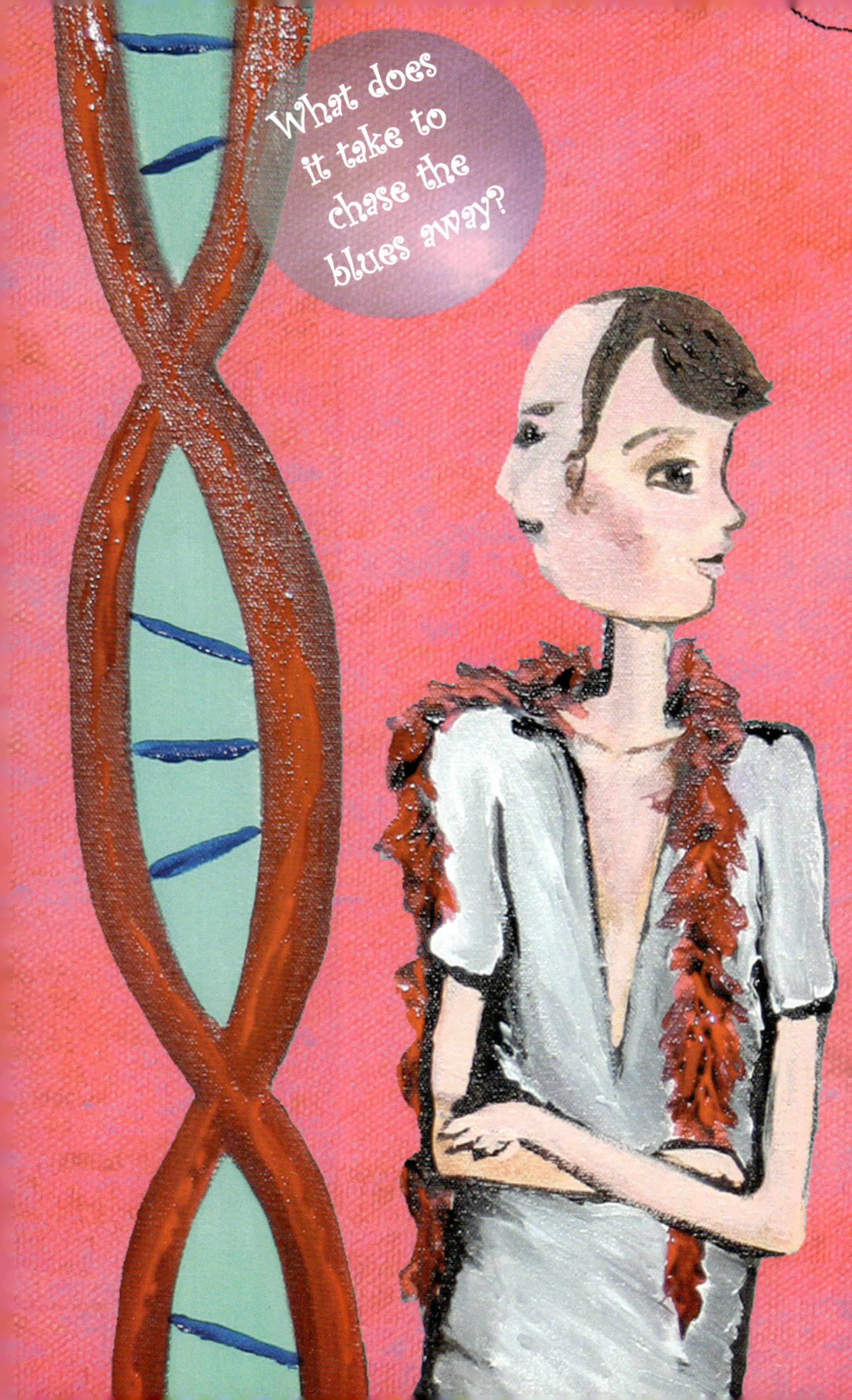

“Yep. Something is wrong with you…this I knew.” replied Sir Grouchy Spider coming down from a book off my shelf. Dean Doll blew him away with his breath. Off he went in the wind he was sent.

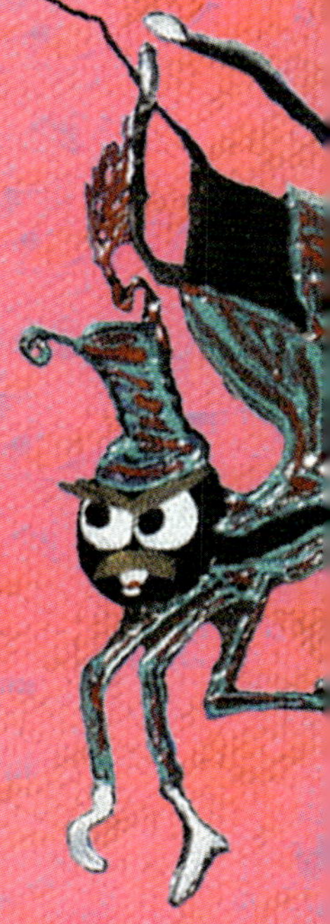

Dean Doll had something to teach Sir Grouchy Spider, “Depression is in Skinny’s make-up too. There’s not always something she can do! Just like me, so let us be! And who says your make-up can’t be one of your best features? ”

Sunny had a way with words,

"Be patient little one, I'm just the sun.

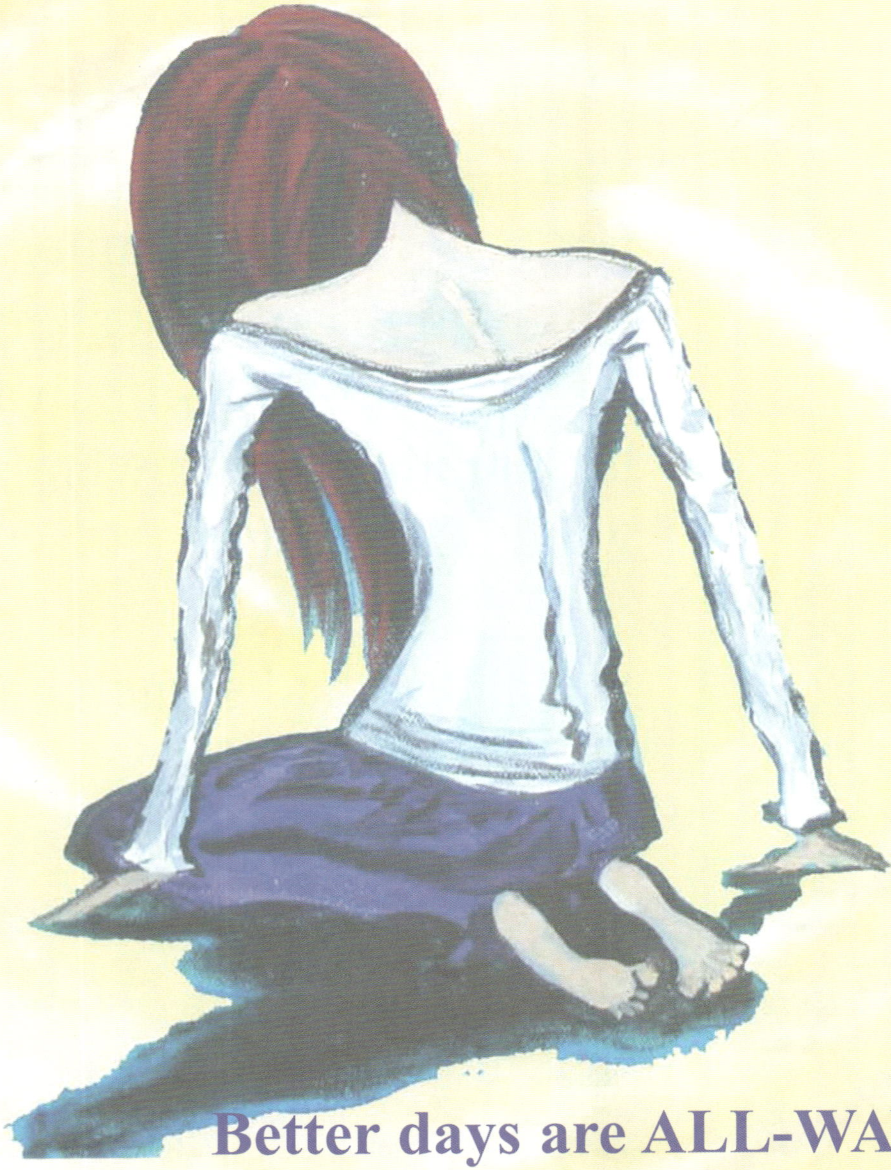

Did you know finding relief isn't any harder than where you are?

Better days are ALL-WAYS ahead.

If your desire is greater than your fear

then **YOU** will create a new life from here!"

create

verb

1. to bring into existence; *God created the heaven and the earth - Genesis*

2. to invest with a new form, office, or rank; *was created a lieutenant.*

3. to produce or bring about by a course of action or behavior; *create new jobs. Her arrival created a terrible fuss.*

4. CAUSE, OCCASION *Famine creates high food prices.*

5. to produce through imaginative skill; *create a painting.*

6. DESIGN; *creates dresses.*

7. to make or bring into existence something new.

8. to set up a scoring opportunity in basketball; *create off the dribble.*

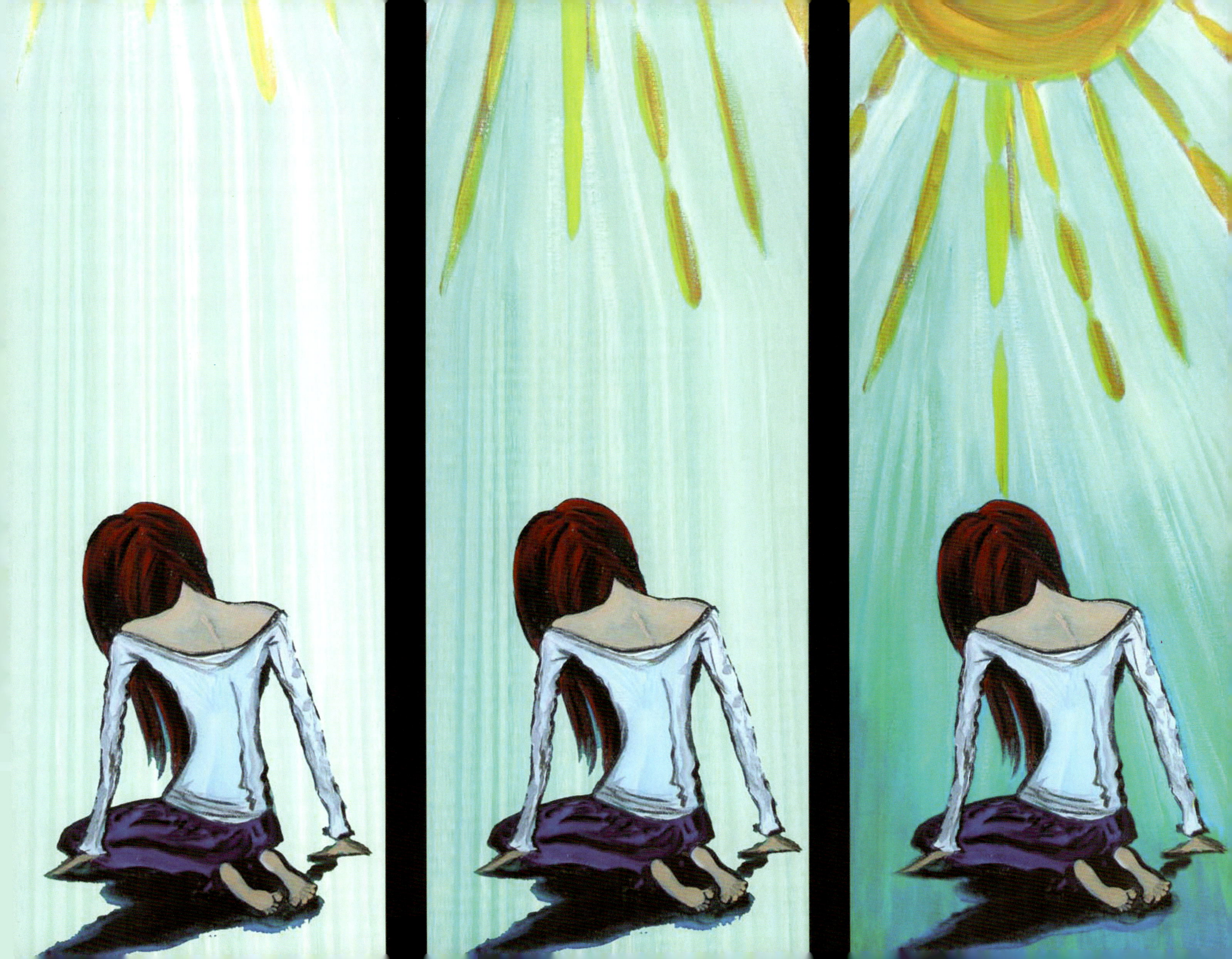

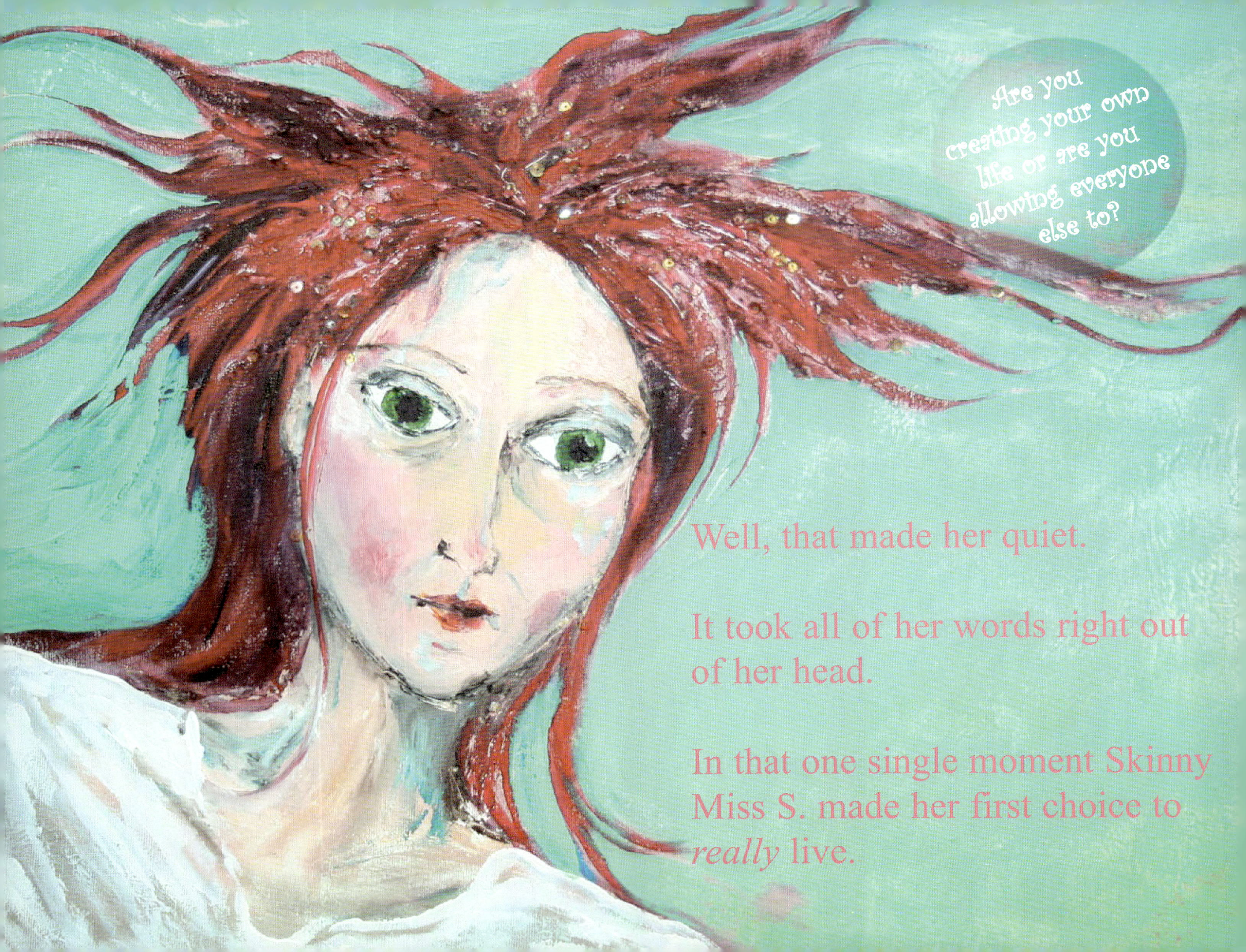
Are you creating your own life or are you allowing everyone else to?

Well, that made her quiet.

It took all of her words right out of her head.

In that one single moment Skinny Miss S. made her first choice to *really* live.

BREATH

slow
adjective

1. mentally dull: STUPID; *a slow student.*

2. naturally inert or sluggish, lacking in readiness, promptness, or willingness, not hasty or precipitate; *was slow to anger.*

3. moving, flowing, or proceeding without speed or at less than usual speed; *traffic was slow.*

4. exhibiting or marked by low speed; *he moved with slow deliberation.*

5. not acute; *a slow disease.*

6. LOW, GENTLE; *slow fire.*

7. requiring a long time: GRADUAL; *a slow recovery.*

8. having qualities that hinder rapid progress or action; *a slow track.*

9. registering behind or below what is correct; *the clock is slow.*

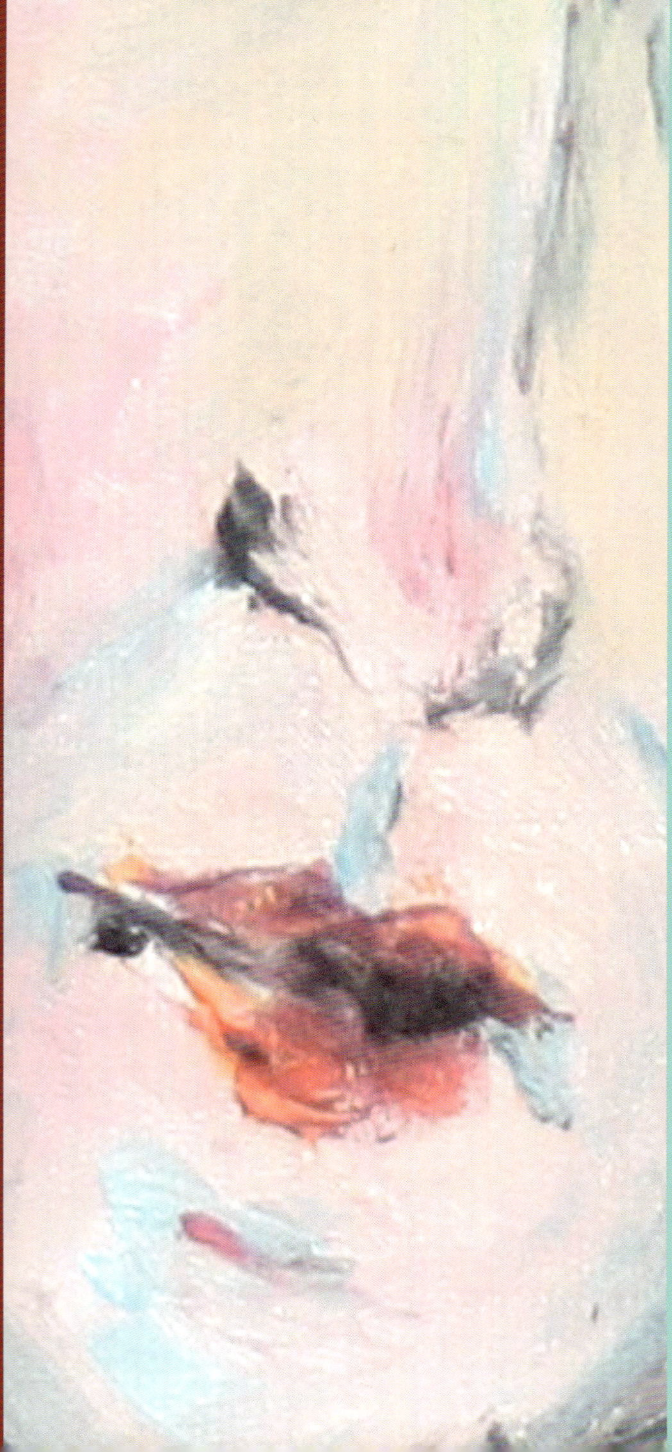

suicide
noun

1. the act or an instance of taking one's own life voluntarily and intentionally especially by a person of years of discretion and of sound mind.

2. ruin of one's own interests; *political suicide.*

3. APOPTOSIS; *cell suicide.*

4. one that commits or attempts suicide.

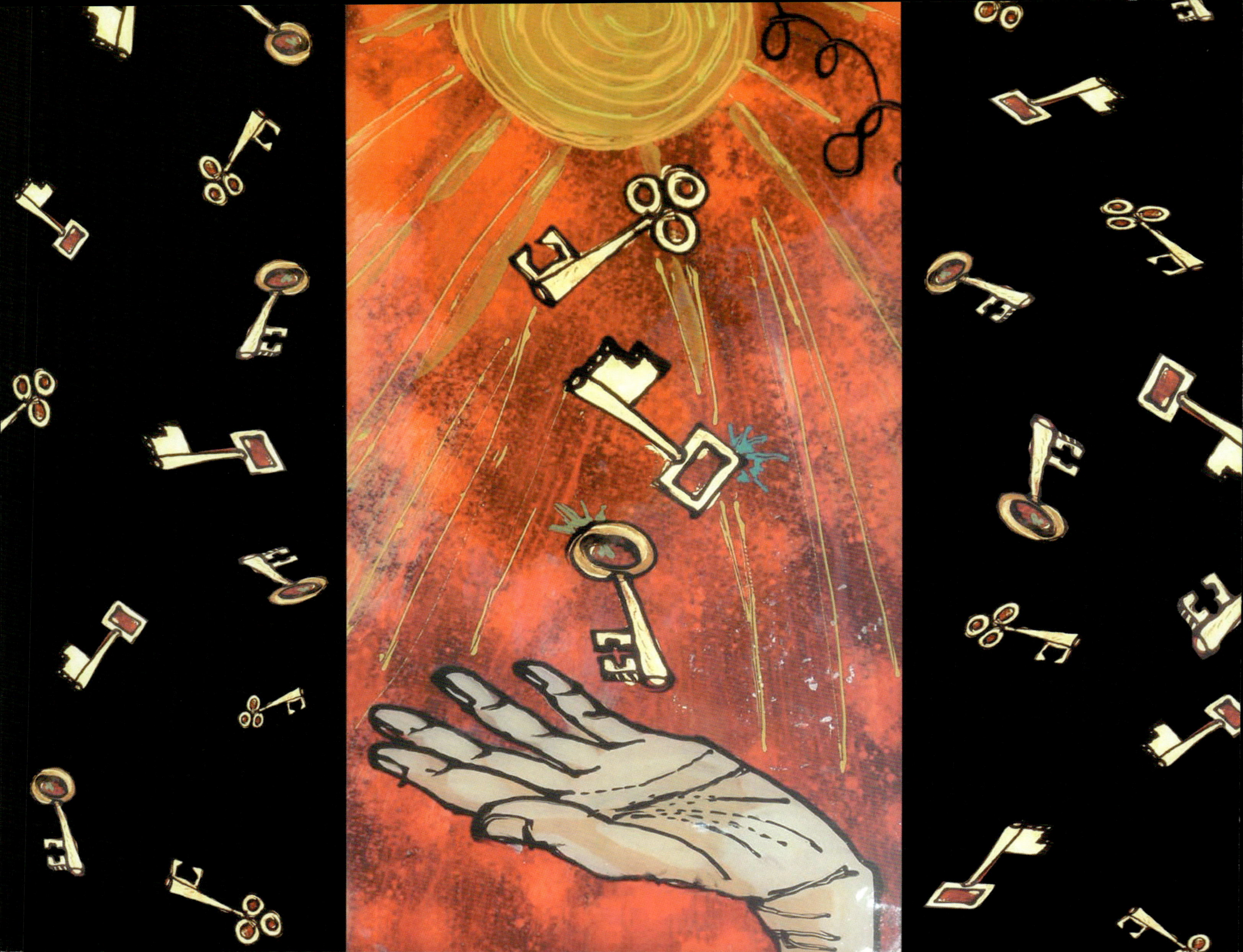

It was then that Sunny Mister E. gave her

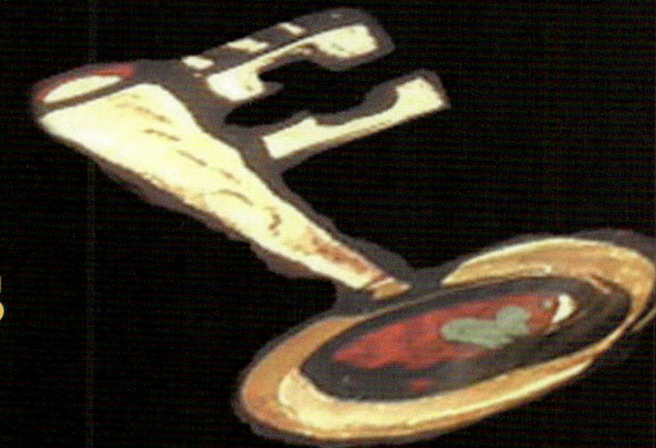

three golden keys

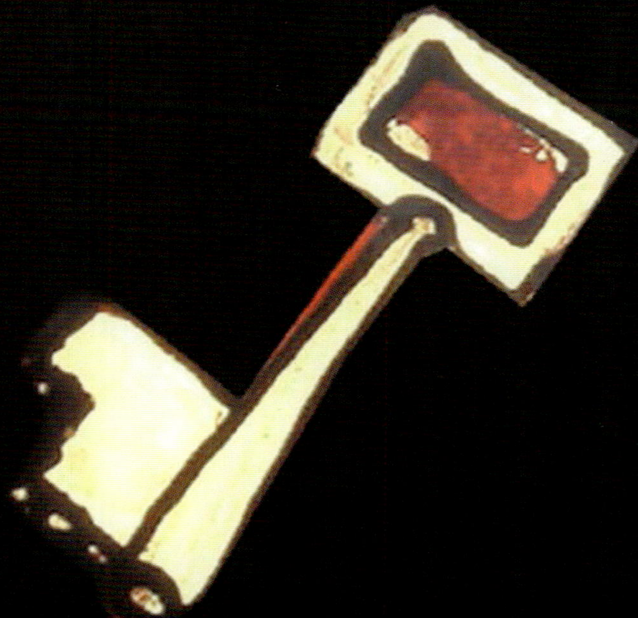

to three golden doors

and

whispered in her ear…

"The relief you've been seeking can finally be yours."

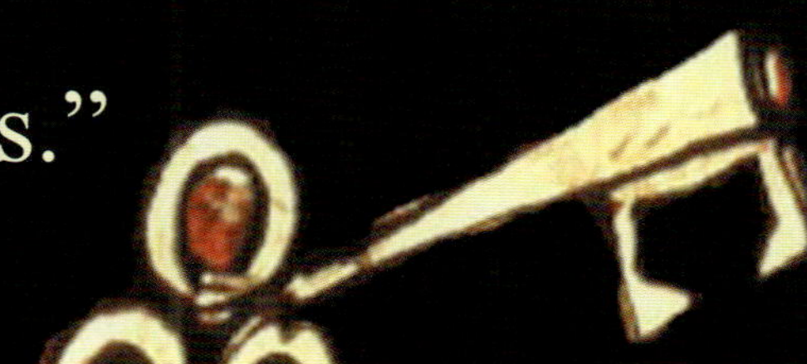

relief

noun

1. removal or lightening of something oppressive, painful, or distressing.

2. means of breaking or avoiding monotony or boredom.

3. a mode of sculpture in which forms and figures are distinguished from a surrounding plane surface, sculpture or a sculptural form executed in this mode, projecting detail, ornament, or figures.

Skinny Miss S. carefully unlocked the first golden door.

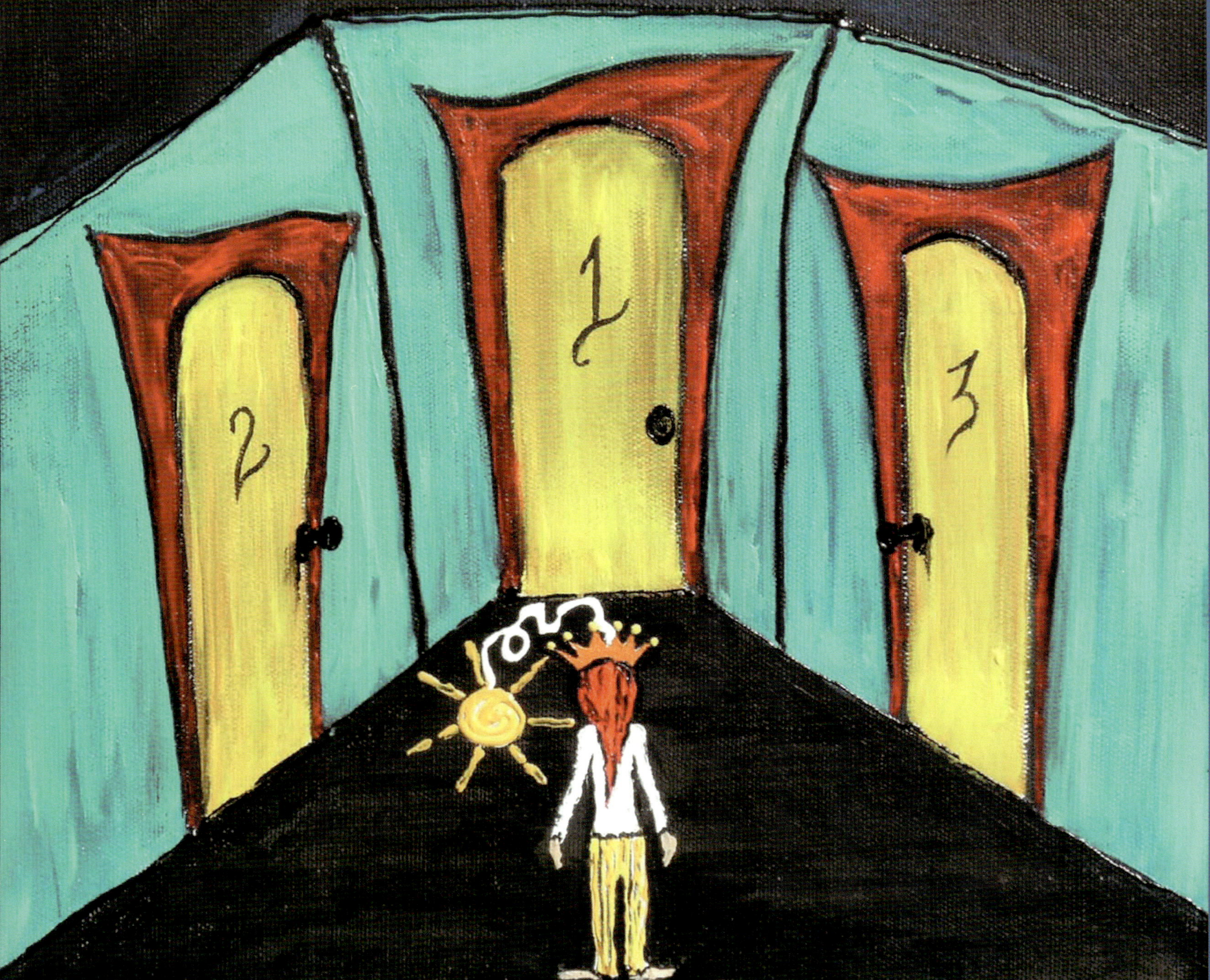

Guess who was there to help her get well?

door

noun

1. usually a swinging or sliding barrier by which an entry is closed and opened; also a similar part of a piece of furniture.

2. doorway

3. a means of access or participation or an opportunity; *opens new doors - door to success.*

4. at one's door; as a charge against one as being responsible; *laid the blame at our door.*

unlock

transitive verb

1. to unfasten the lock of.

2. open , undo.

3. to free from restraints or restrictions; *the shock unlocked a flood of tears.*

4. to furnish a key to; *disclose.*

5. to become unfastened or freed from restraints.

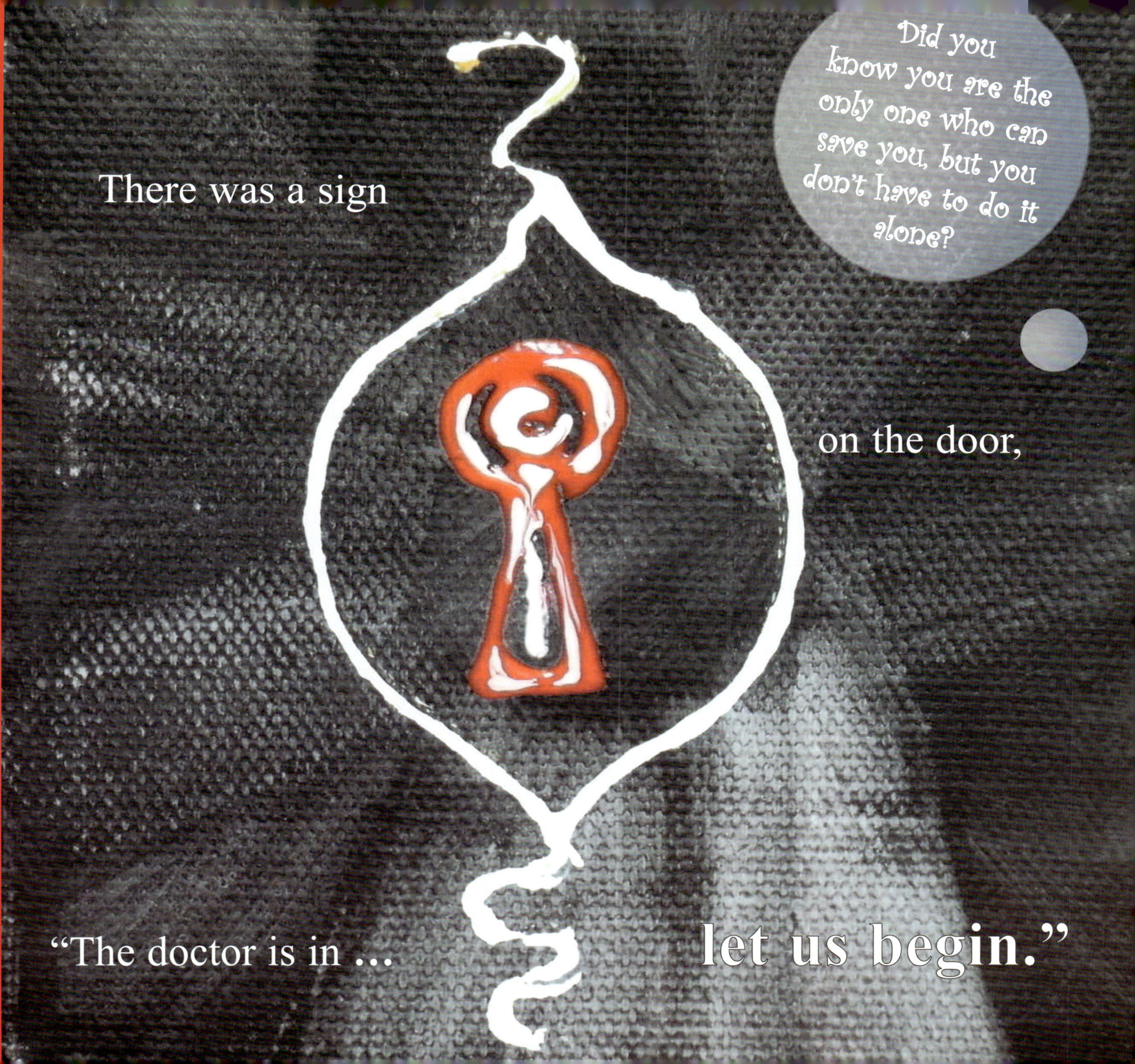

There was a sign on the door,

"The doctor is in ... let us begin."

Did you know you are the only one who can save you, but you don't have to do it alone?

shrink
noun

1. short for headshrinker, a clinical psychiatrist or psychologist.

2. an act or instance of shrinking.

3. a shrinking movement.

It was Smarty Dr. W. ready to tell her all that he knew!

Skinny had lots of questions to ask…like,

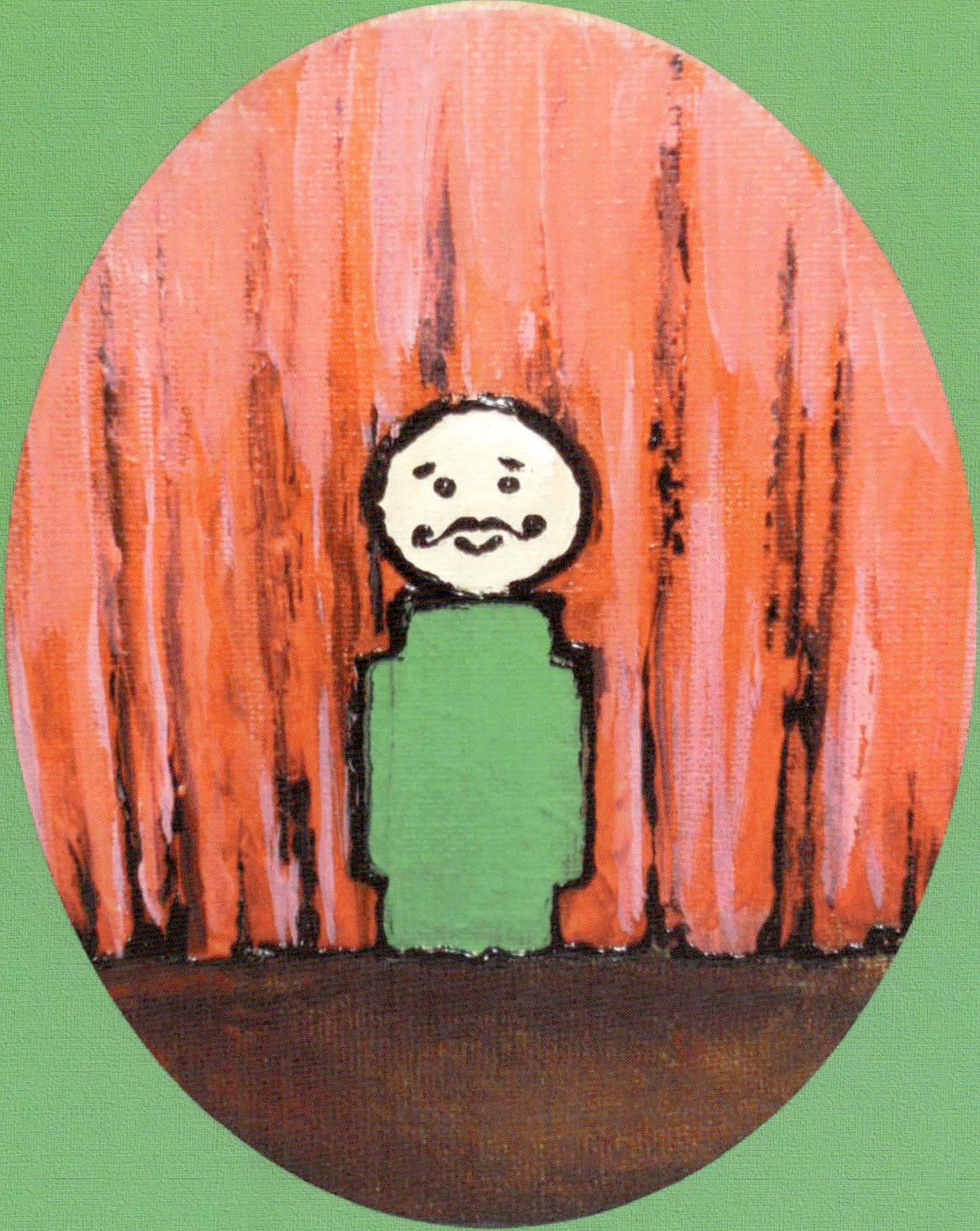

"What, when, why me, how,
and will I get fat?"

Does your doctor shrink in on the origin of the cause?

"**Depression** is a biological condition of the mind when the chemicals in the brain flow differently than normal. It can be triggered by stress or anger turned inward for a long period of time. It can be considered a coping mechanism for great stress in one's life. Many times it is hereditary and will affect children, teenagers, adults, the elderly, and is even known to affect all creatures, big and small."

Have you been referred to a psychiatrist who has gotten others well?

dictionary

noun

1. a reference source in print or electronic form containing words usually alphabetically arranged along with information about their forms, pronunciations, functions, etymologies, meanings, and syntactical and idiomatic uses.

2. book listing alphabetically terms or names important to a particular subject or activity along with discussion of their meanings and applications.

3. a reference book giving for words of one language equivalents in another.

4. a computerized list (as of items of data or words) used for reference (as for information retrieval or word processing).

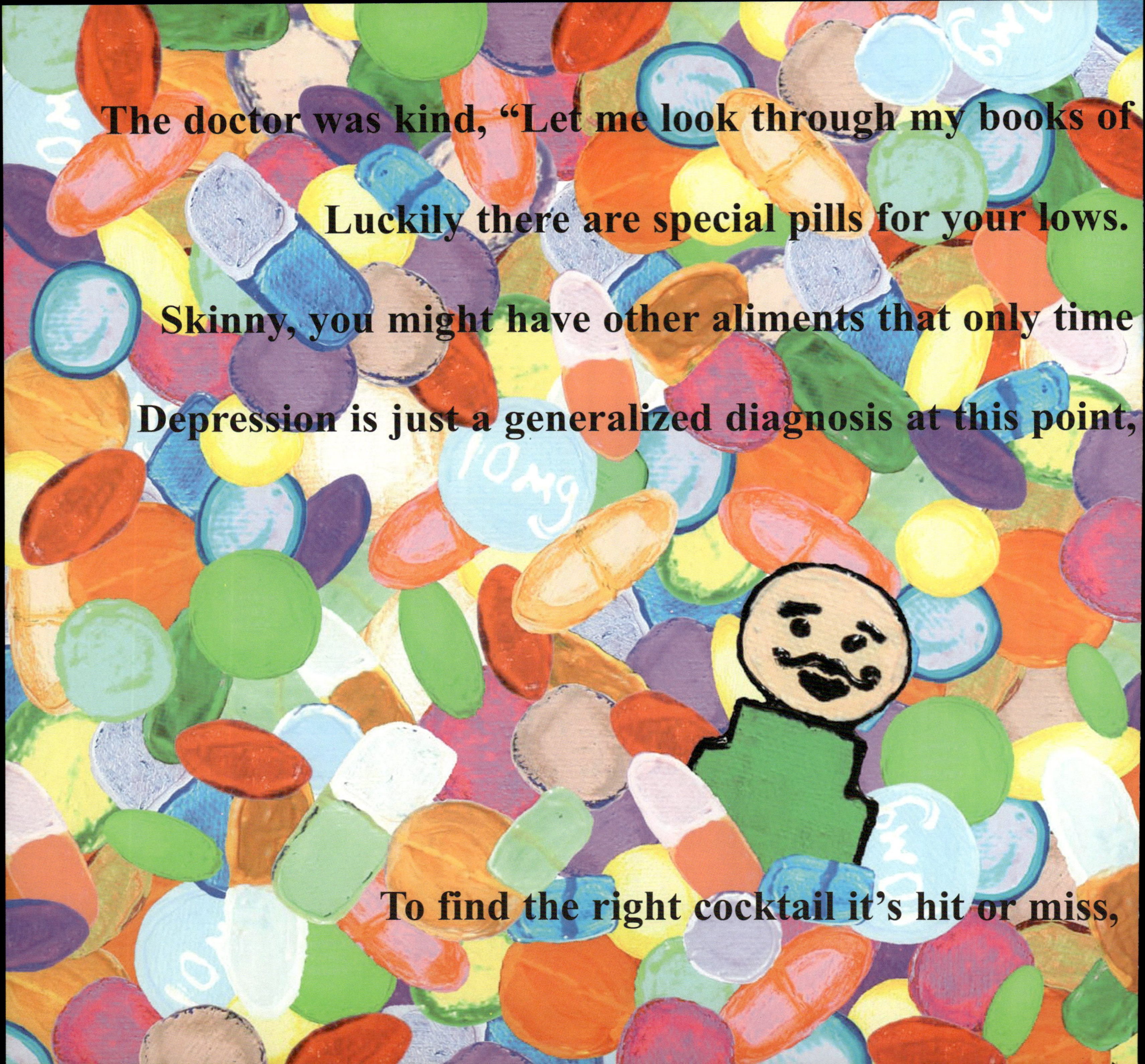

The doctor was kind, "Let me look through my books of

Luckily there are special pills for your lows.

Skinny, you might have other aliments that only time

Depression is just a generalized diagnosis at this point,

To find the right cocktail it's hit or miss,

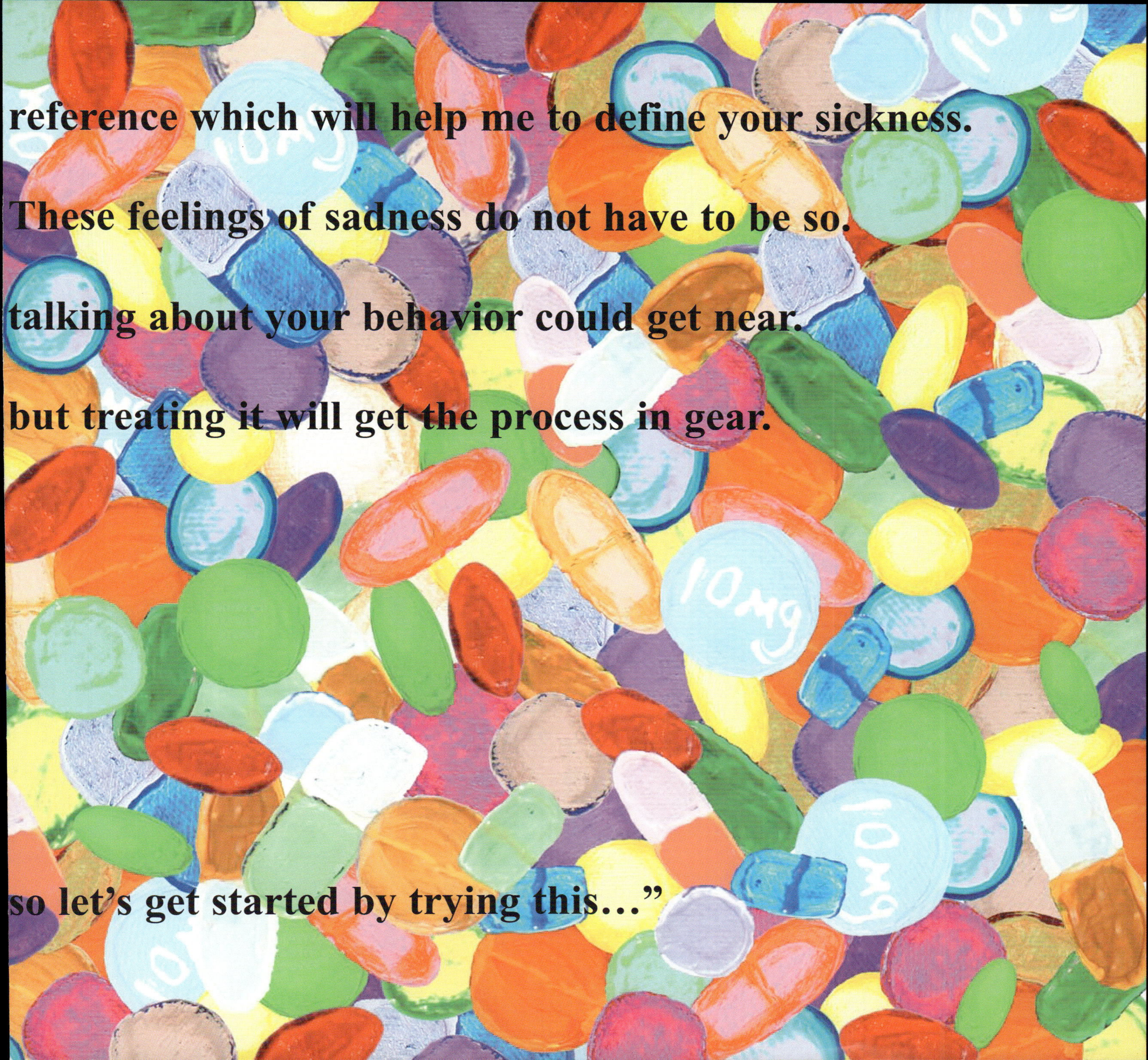

reference which will help me to define your sickness.

These feelings of sadness do not have to be so.

talking about your behavior could get near.

but treating it will get the process in gear.

so let's get started by trying this..."

DSM-IV Medical Reference Book for Mental Disorders

The Diagnostic and Statistical Manual of Mental Disorders (DSM) is an American handbook for mental health professionals that lists different categories of mental disorders and the criteria for diagnosing them, according to the publishing organization the American Psychiatric Association.

It is used worldwide by clinicians and researchers as well as insurance companies, pharmaceutical companies and policy makers.

It has attracted controversy and criticism as well as praise.

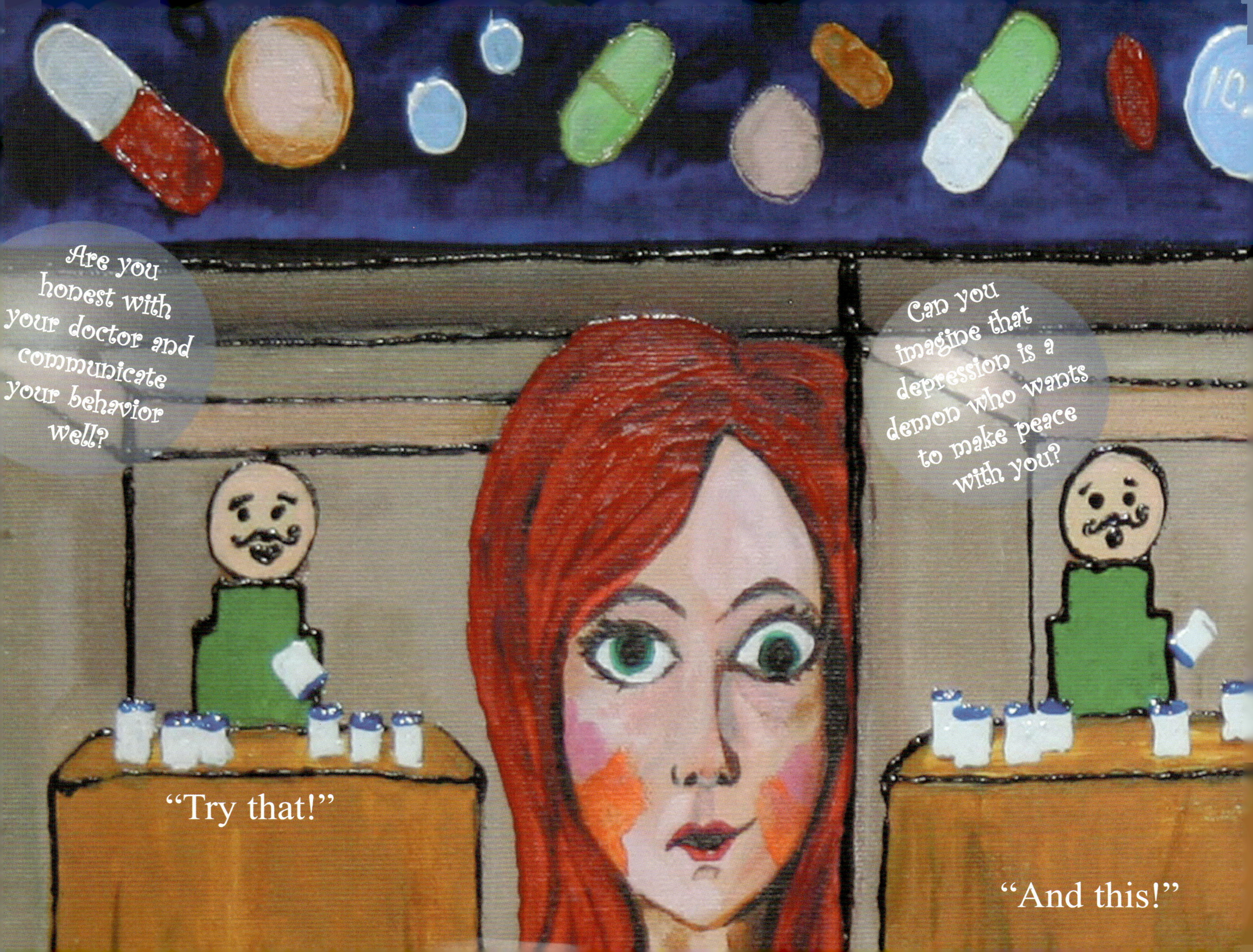
Are you honest with your doctor and communicate your behavior well?
Can you imagine that depression is a demon who wants to make peace with you?
“Try that!”
“And this!”

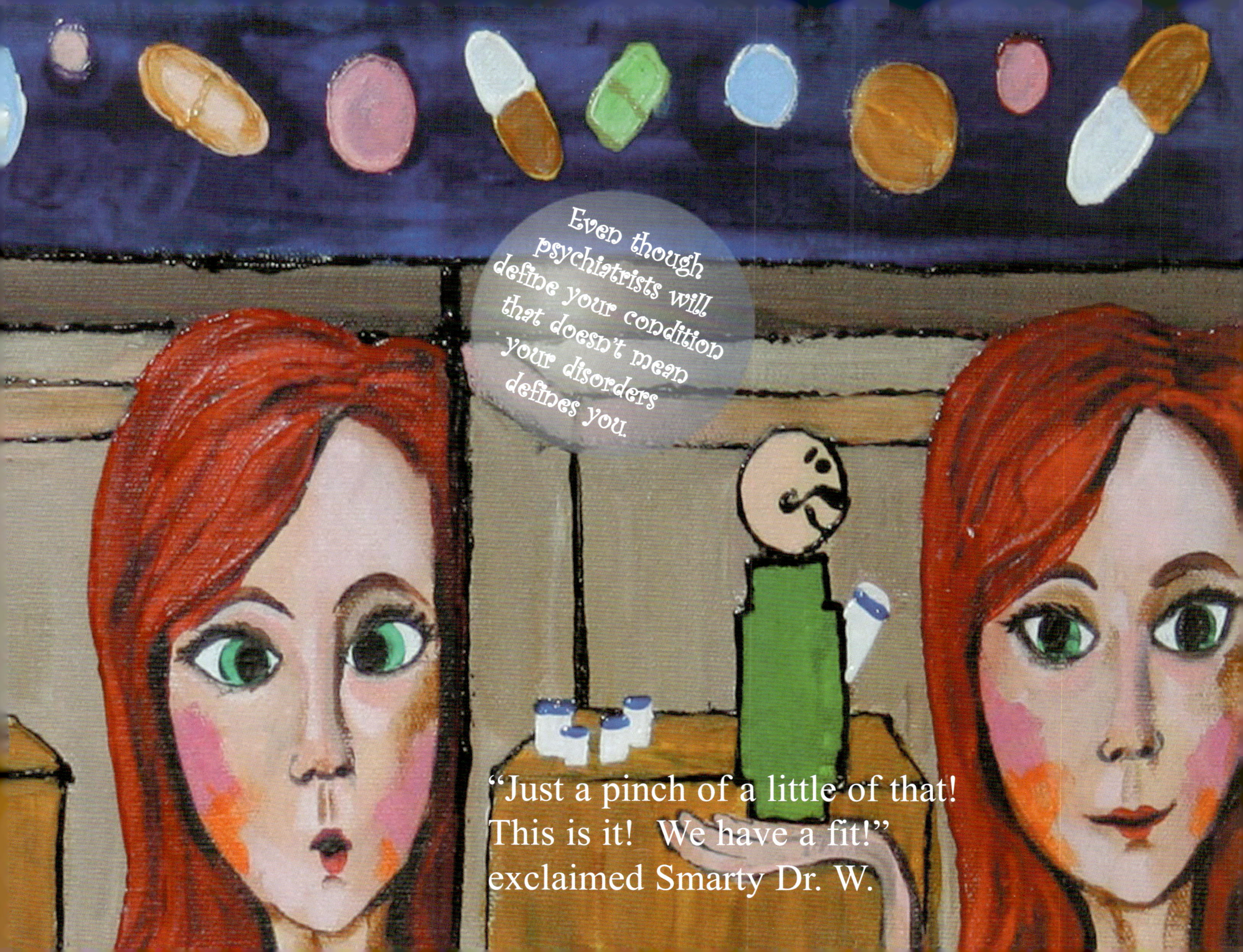
Even though psychiatrists will define your condition that doesn't mean your disorders defines you.
"Just a pinch of a little of that!
This is it! We have a fit!"
exclaimed Smarty Dr. W.

Side effect:

Adverse drug reaction, an unintended consequence specifically arising from drug therapy.

Therapeutic effect, an unintended but desirable consequence of any kind of medical treatment.

Adverse effect (medicine0, an unintended, and undesirable, consequence of any kind of medical treatment.

Unintended consequence, an effect that is unforeseen, regardless of type or quality.

Side effect (computer science), a state change caused by a function or expression.

Side Effects (2005 film), starring Katherine Heigl, a satirical look at the pharmaceutical industry.

Side Effects, a collection of short stories by Woody Allen.

Side Effects (TV series), a Canadian TV series.

The Side Effects, a 1980s indie rock band.

Side Effect, a 1970s soul band.[17]

Suddenly Skinny Miss S. could hear the voices of doubt getting louder. She knew she would have to stand up to them.

"Meds have side effects…" Dean Doll feared.

Skinny answered load and clear, "But depression is worse than side effects, dear."

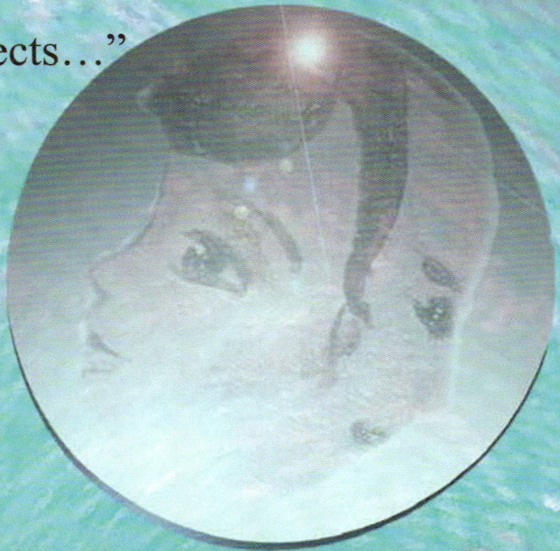

"This doctor won't know how to medicate you right…" Father Deana Marie came in with all of his might to teach her his 'right'. "There is only ONE way to be saved and that power comes through me!"

Skinny spoke up after thinking Father Deana Marie was quite precocious, "The powers that you be have not helped me."

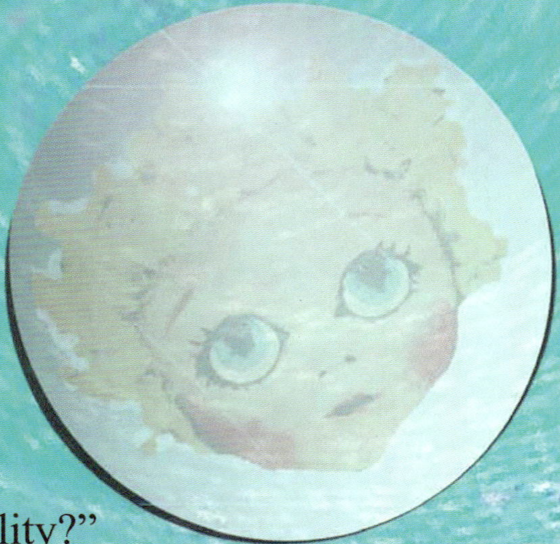

"What if it changes your personality?" asked Lonely Miss C. holding tightly to one golden key.

Skinny answered, "Depression has already done that to me," and she reclaimed the golden key right out of Lonely Miss C.'s hand.

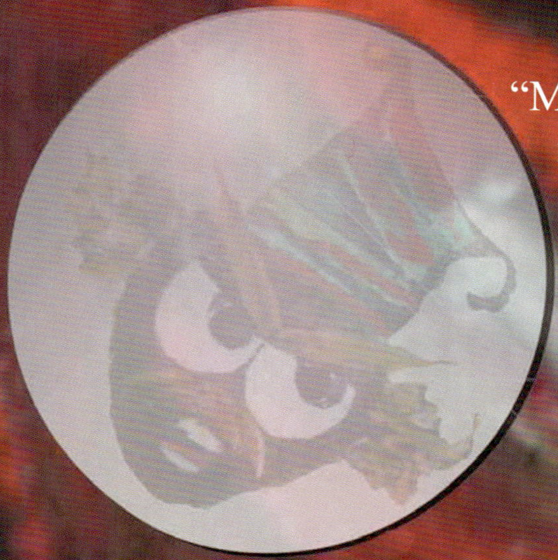

"Maybe you're not really depressed…
now look at your life without the rose color glasses, Skinny Miss S."
from the back blew in Sir Grouchy Spider. He always thought he knew. What he knew, he denied too. Sir Grouchy was as negative as negative could be, "You don't really want to take those pills all the time?" he said distastfully.

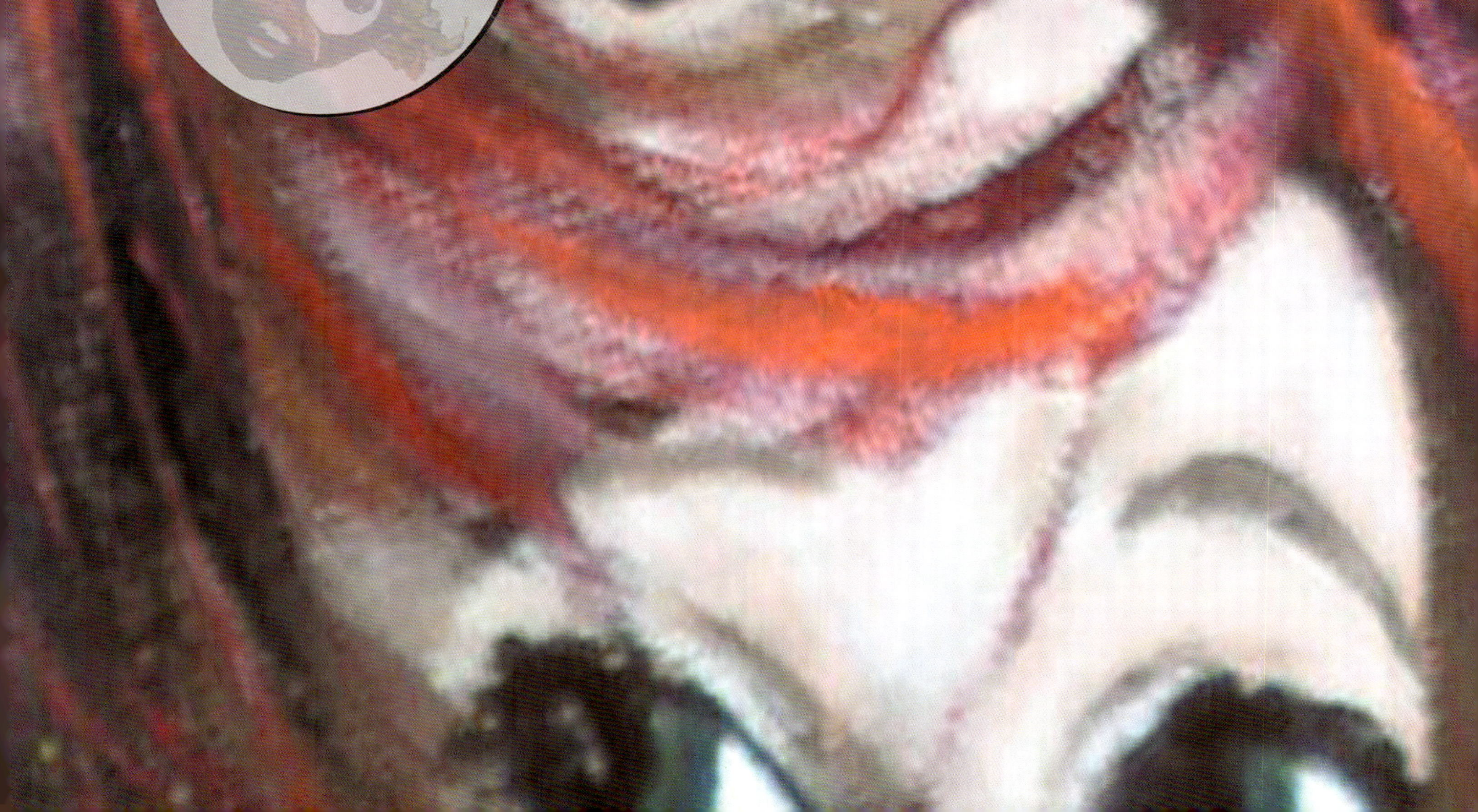

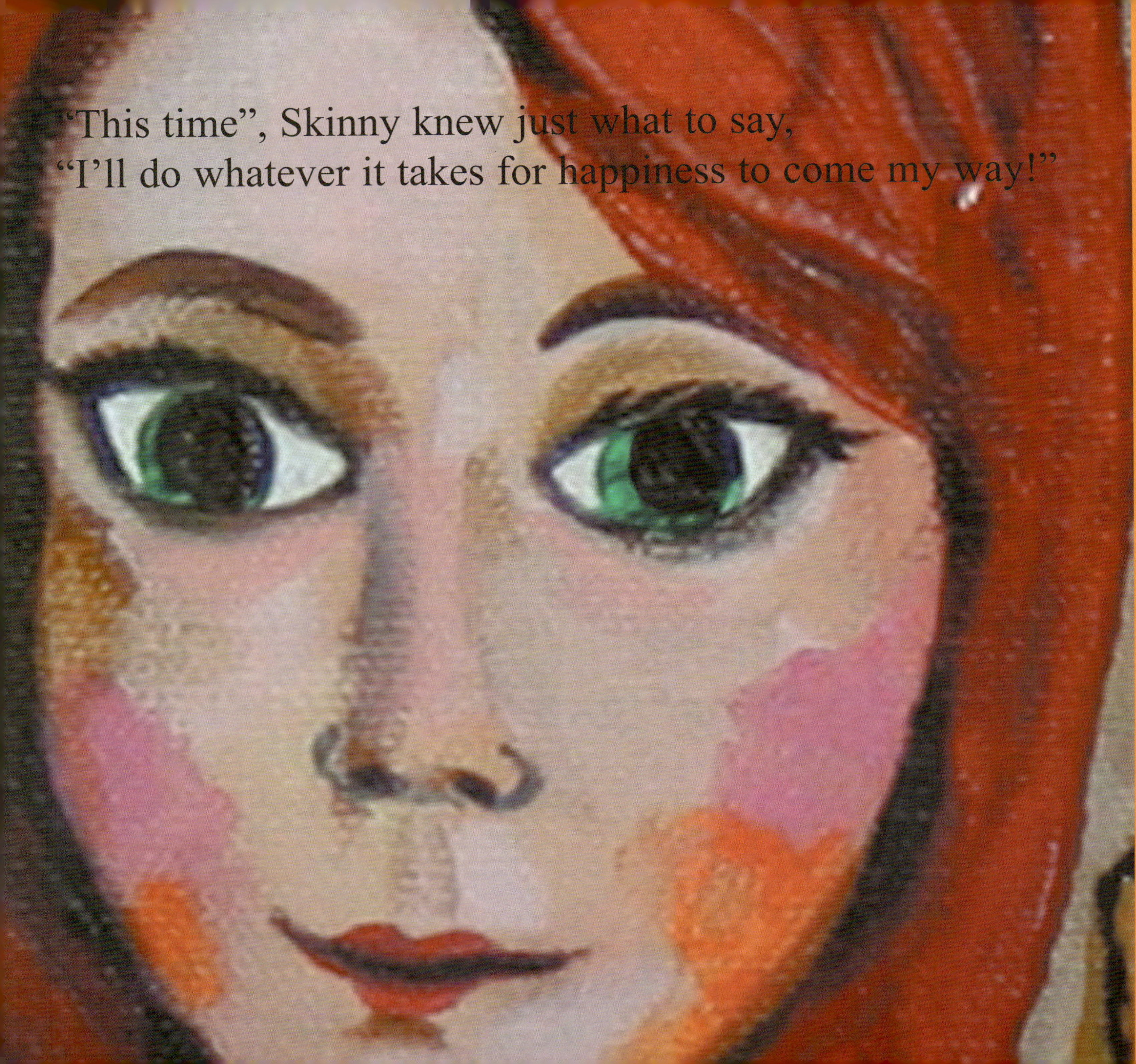

“This time”, Skinny knew just what to say,
“I’ll do whatever it takes for happiness to come my way!”

perseverance
noun

1. STEADFASTNES: the action or condition or an instance of persevering.

2. continuance in a state of grace to the end, leading to eternal salvation.

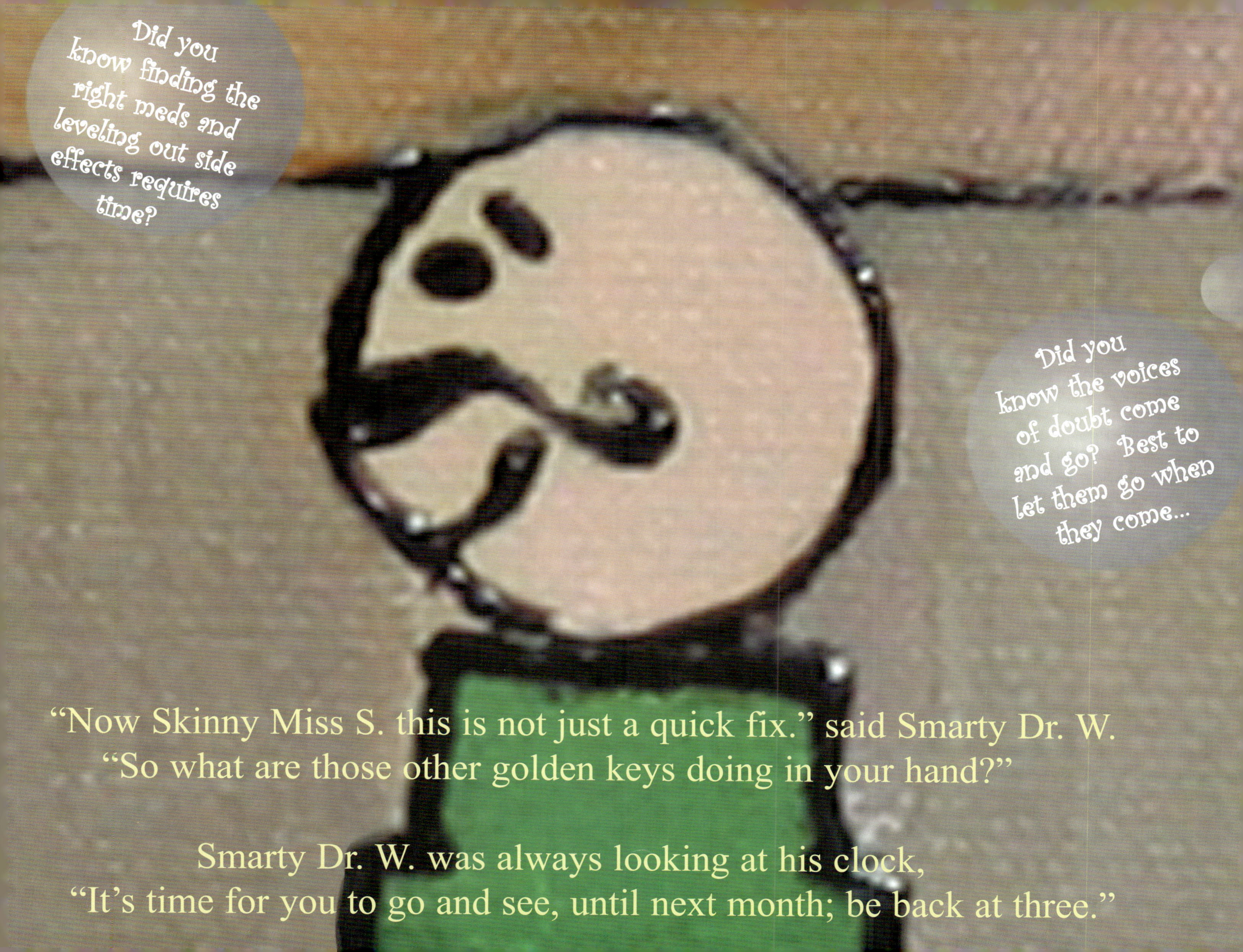
Did you know finding the right meds and leveling out side effects requires time?
Did you know the voices of doubt come and go? Best to let them go when they come...

"Now Skinny Miss S. this is not just a quick fix." said Smarty Dr. W.
"So what are those other golden keys doing in your hand?"

Smarty Dr. W. was always looking at his clock,
"It's time for you to go and see, until next month; be back at three."

Next she unlocked the
second golden door.

Guess who was there to talk
with her?

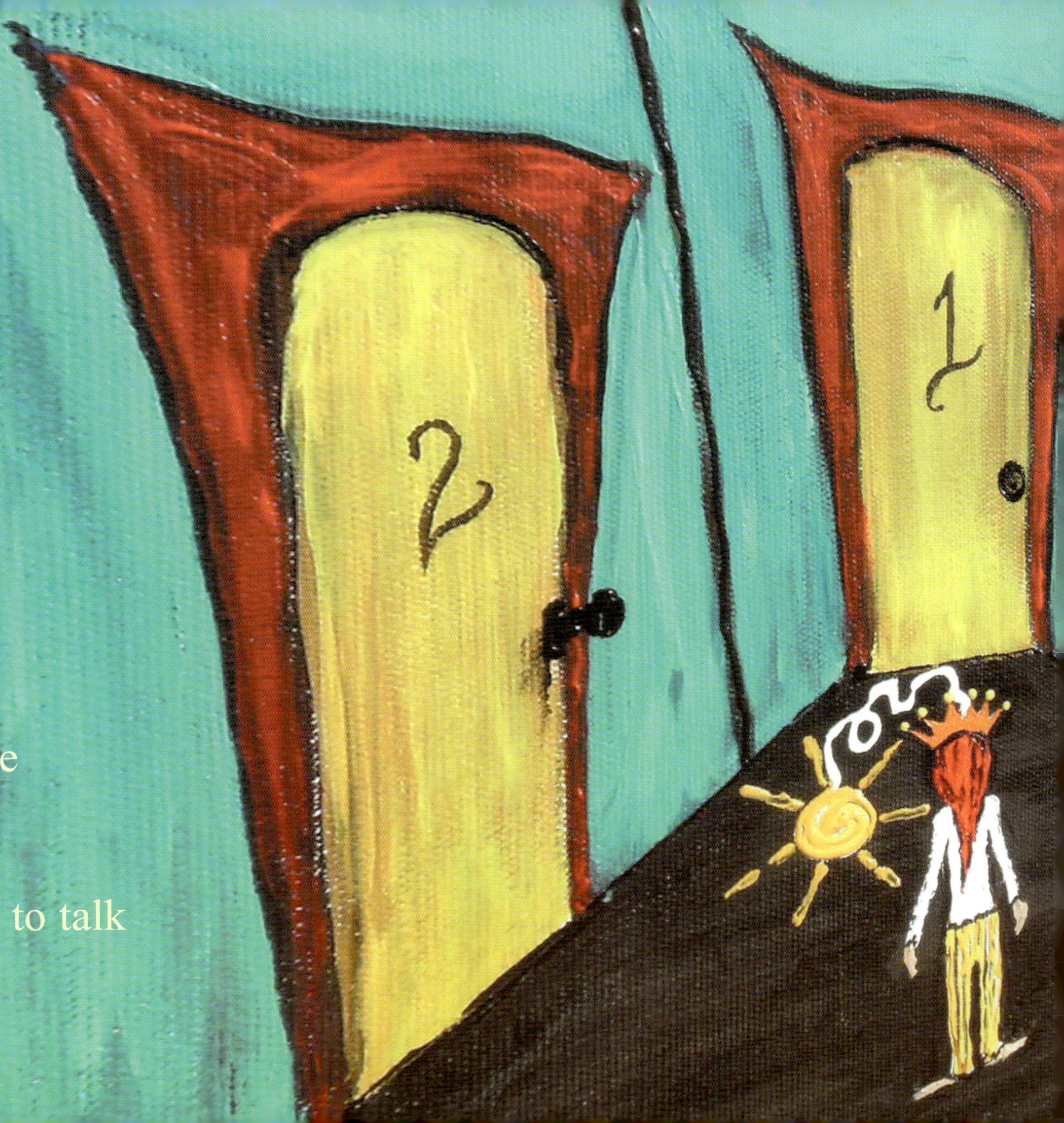

key

noun

1. a usually metal instrument by which the bolt of a lock is turned, any of various devices having the form or function of such a key.

2. something that gives an explanation or identification or provides a solution; *the key to a riddle.*

3. a small piece of wood or metal used as a wedge or for preventing motion between parts.

4. a system of tones and harmonies generated from a hierarchical scale of seven tones based on a tonic; *the key of G major.*

5. the set of instructions governing the encipherment and decipherment of messages.

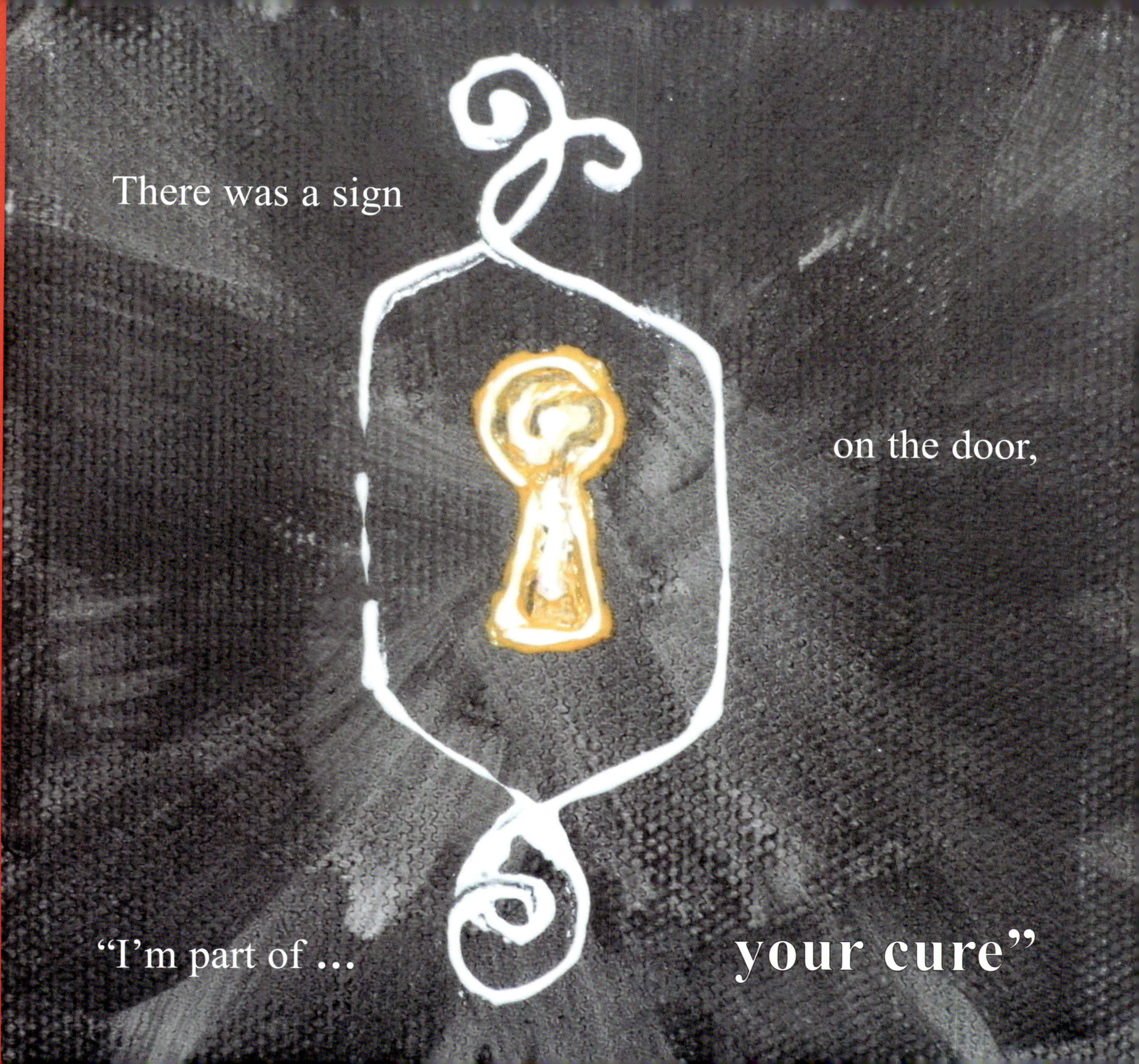

There was a sign
on the door,
“I’m part of ...
your cure”

Psychologist

Family therapy, also referred to as couple and family therapy and family systems therapy, is a branch of psychotherapy that works with families and couples in intimate relationships to nurture change and development. It tends to view change in terms of the systems of interaction between family members. It emphasizes family relationships as an important factor in psychological health.

What the different schools of family therapy have in common is a belief that, regardless of the origin of the problem, and regardless of whether the clients consider it an "individual" or "family" issue, involving families in solutions is often beneficial. This involvement of families is commonly accomplished by their direct participation in the therapy session. The skills of the family therapist thus include the ability to influence conversations in a way that catylizes the strengths, wisdom, and support of the wider system.

In the field's early years, many clinicians defined the family in a narrow, traditional manner usually including parents and children. As the field has evolved, the concept of the family is more commonly defined in terms of strongly supportive, long-term roles and relationships between people who may or may not be related by blood.

Family therapy has been used effectively in the full range of human dilemmas; there is no category of relationship or psychological problem that has not been addressed with this approach.[18]

It was Merry Miss Humm...

who wouldn't let Skinny go missed.

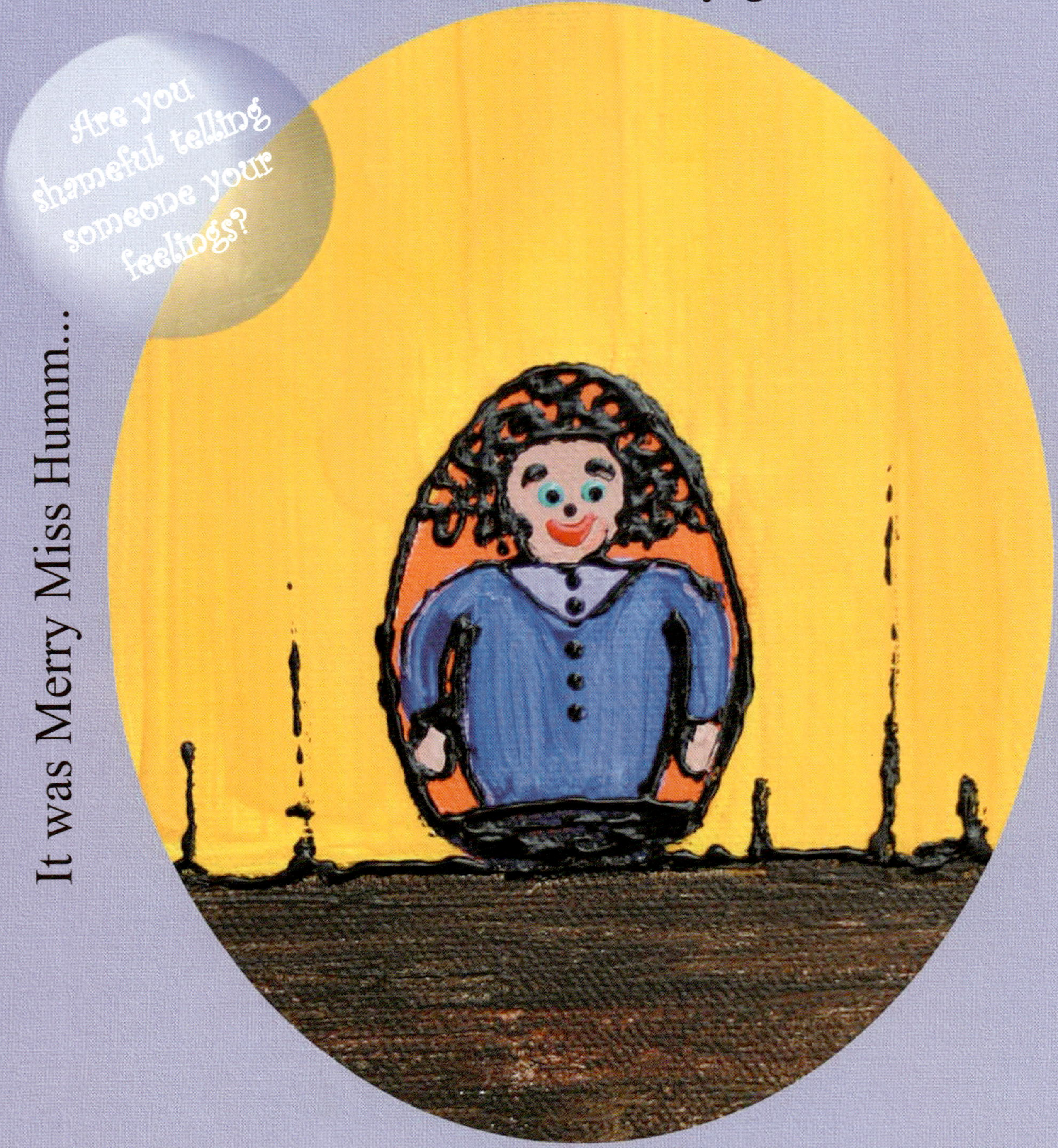

She introduced herself as a Marriage and Family Therapist.

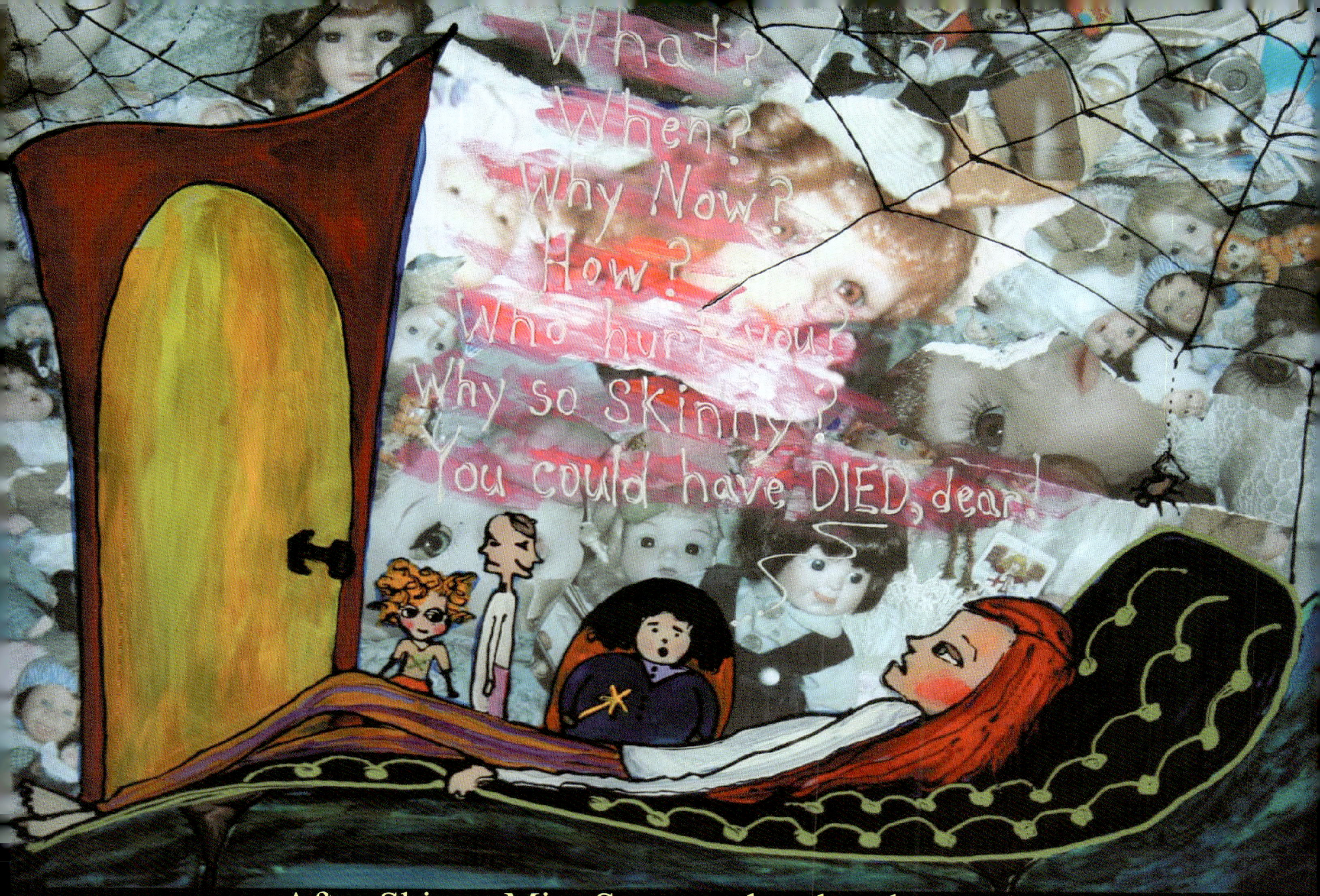
What?
When?
Why Now?
How?
Who hurt you?
Why so Skinny?
You could have DIED, dear!

After Skinny Miss S. entered and took a seat,
Merry Miss Humm had lots of questions for her.

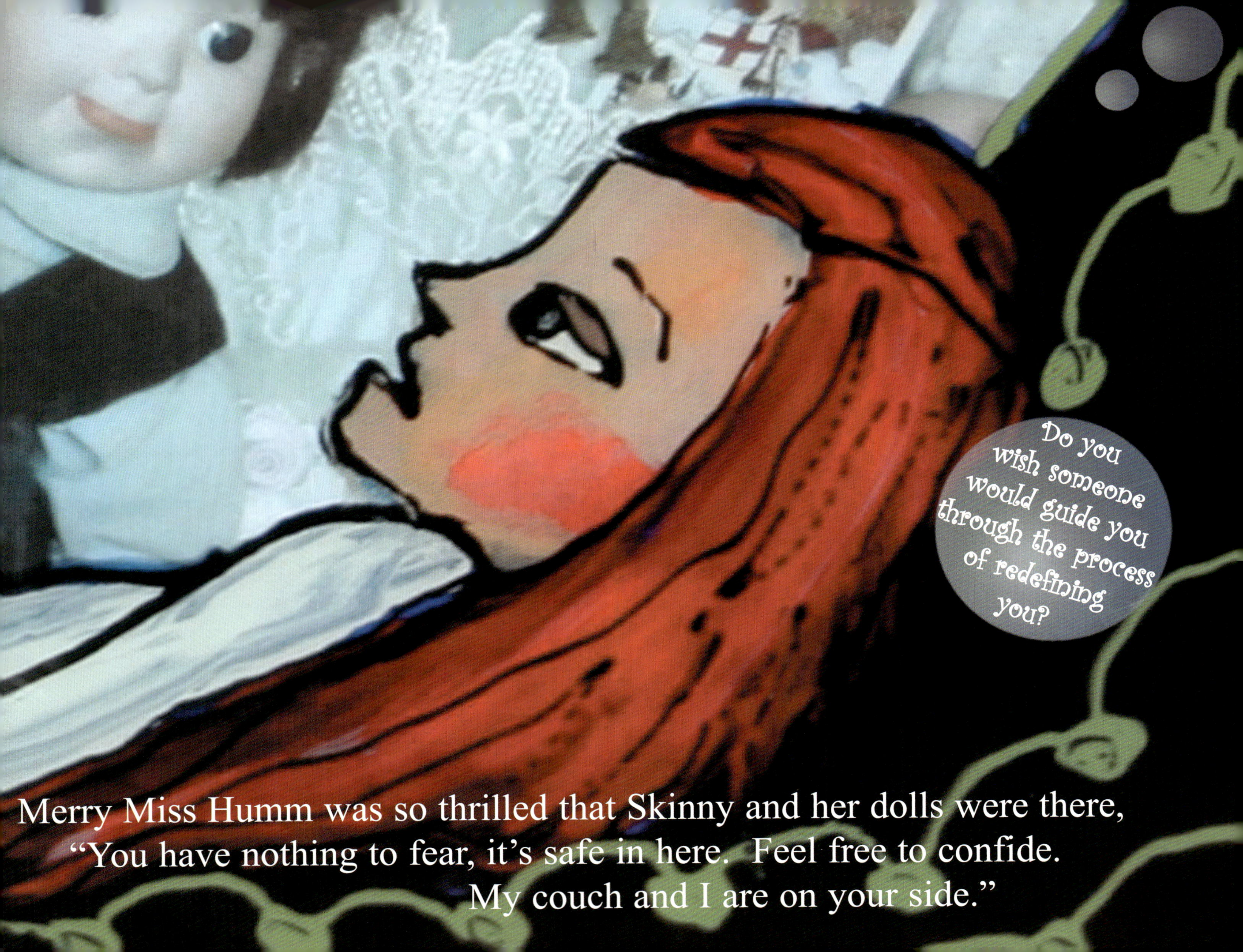
Do you wish someone would guide you through the process of redefining you?

Merry Miss Humm was so thrilled that Skinny and her dolls were there,
"You have nothing to fear, it's safe in here. Feel free to confide.
My couch and I are on your side."

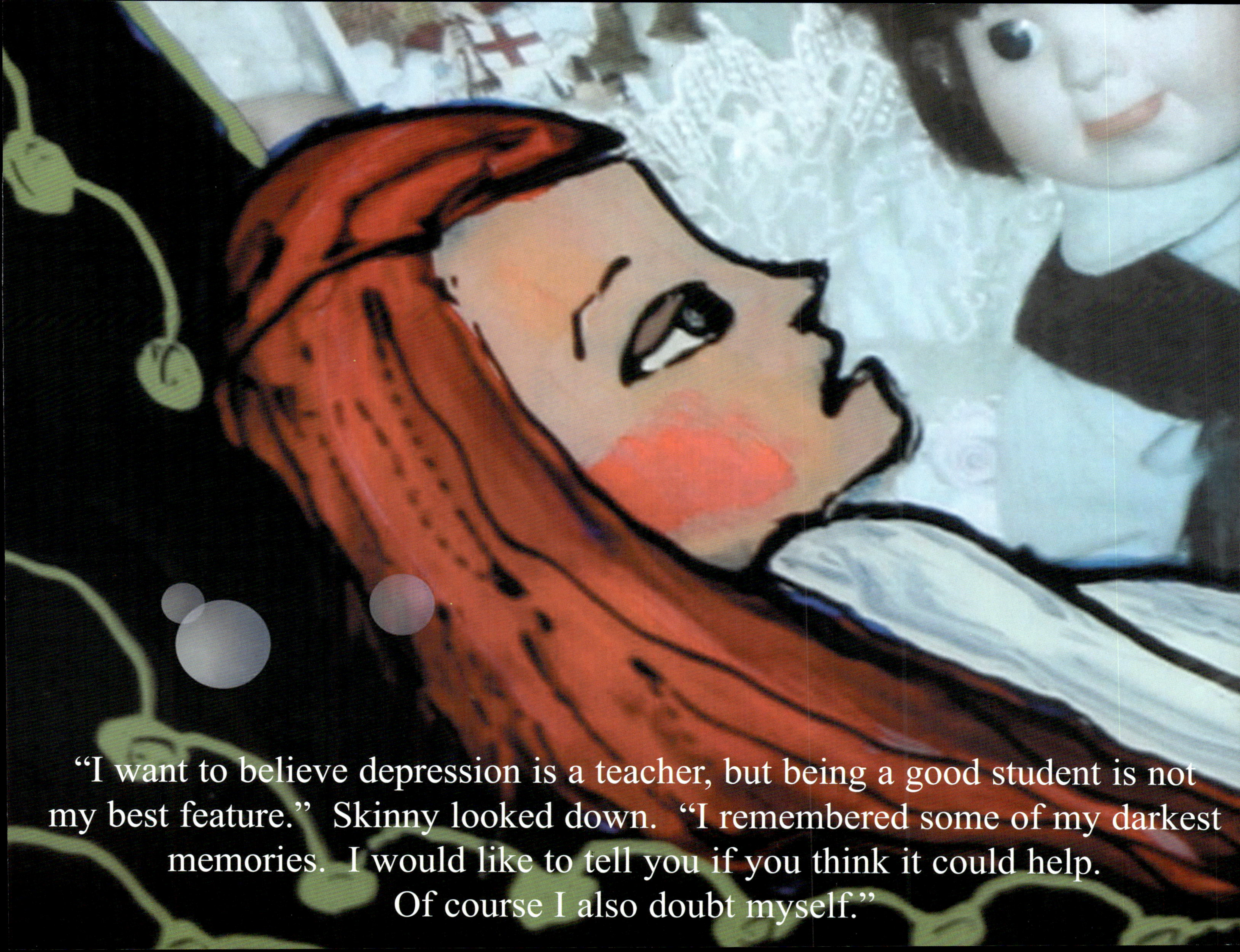

"I want to believe depression is a teacher, but being a good student is not my best feature." Skinny looked down. "I remembered some of my darkest memories. I would like to tell you if you think it could help. Of course I also doubt myself."

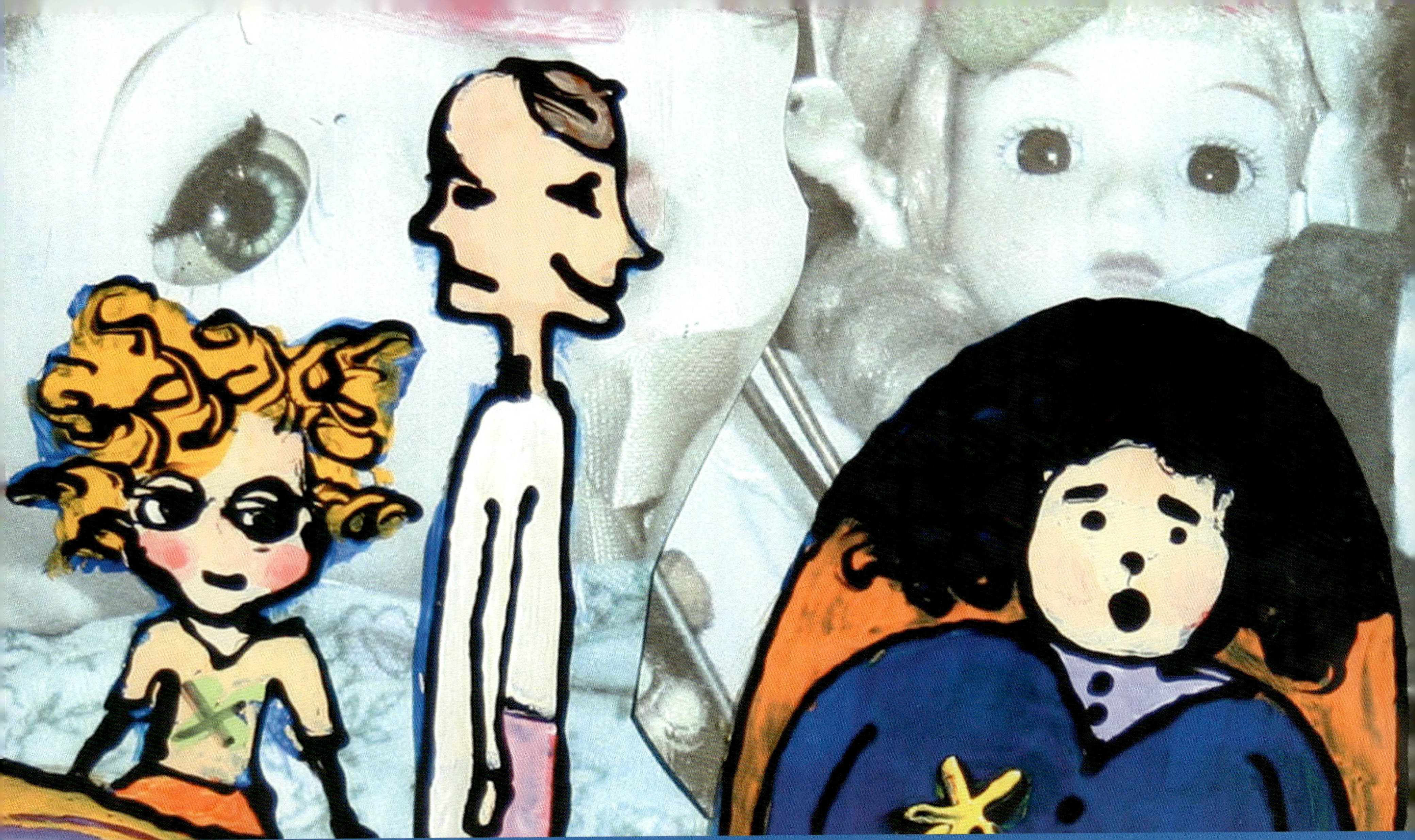

Pillow talk

Pillow talk is the relaxed, intimate conversation that often occurs between two partners.

It also can consist of two or more friends talking late at night. The "pillow talking" generally takes place at night and involves talk of romantic interests. The friends do not have to be in the same bed, although this does happen occasionally. Most of the time pillow talk will consist of more than two people, but it still can be done with two.[19]

Merry Miss Humm was always repeating her own name when Skinny told her something of shame, "Hmmm…now that is interesting. Tell me more about that Skinny Miss S. Let's make a mess so you can get properly dressed!!"

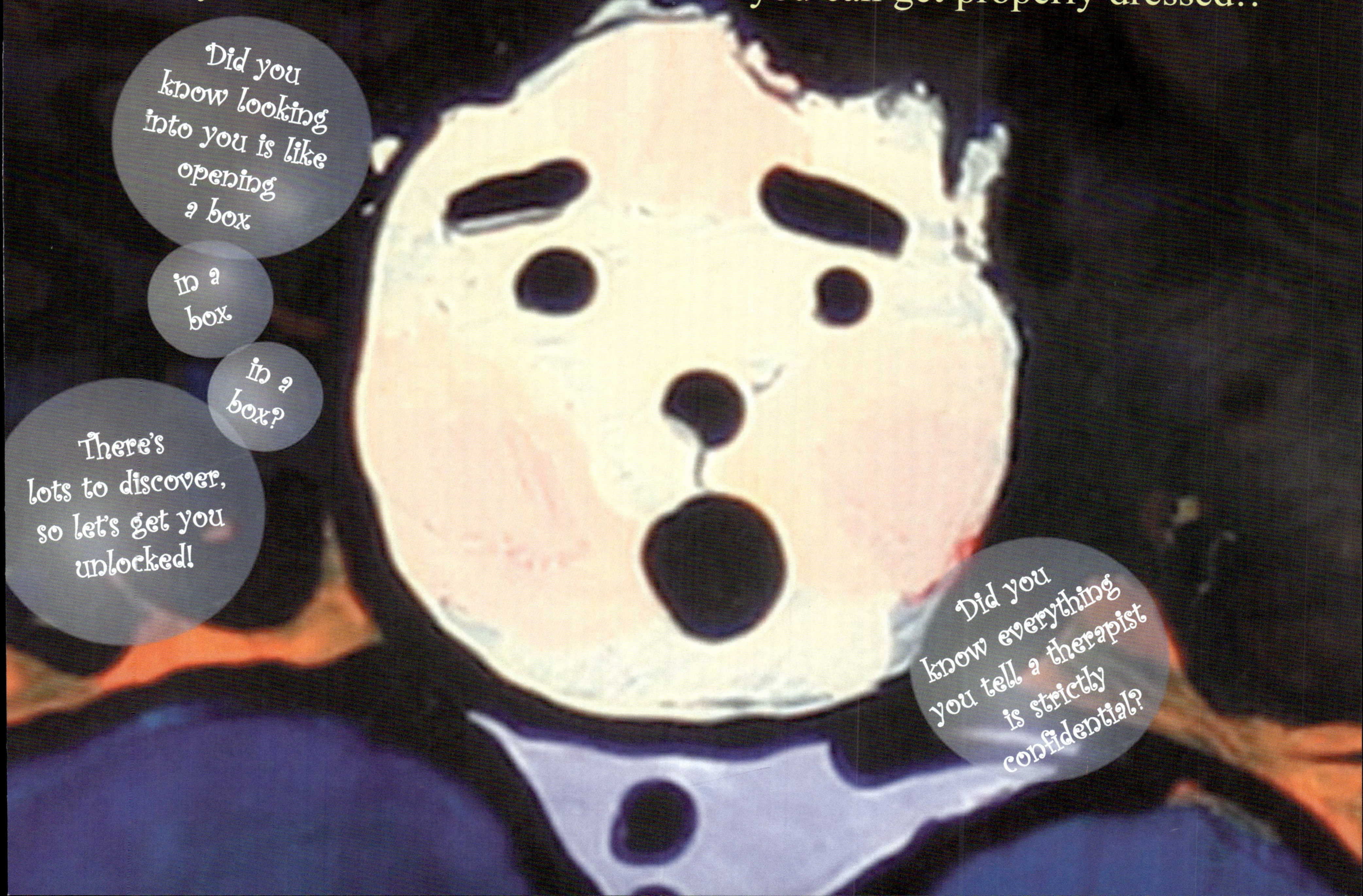
Did you know looking into you is like opening a box
in a box
in a box?
There's lots to discover, so let's get you unlocked!
Did you know everything you tell a therapist is strictly confidential?

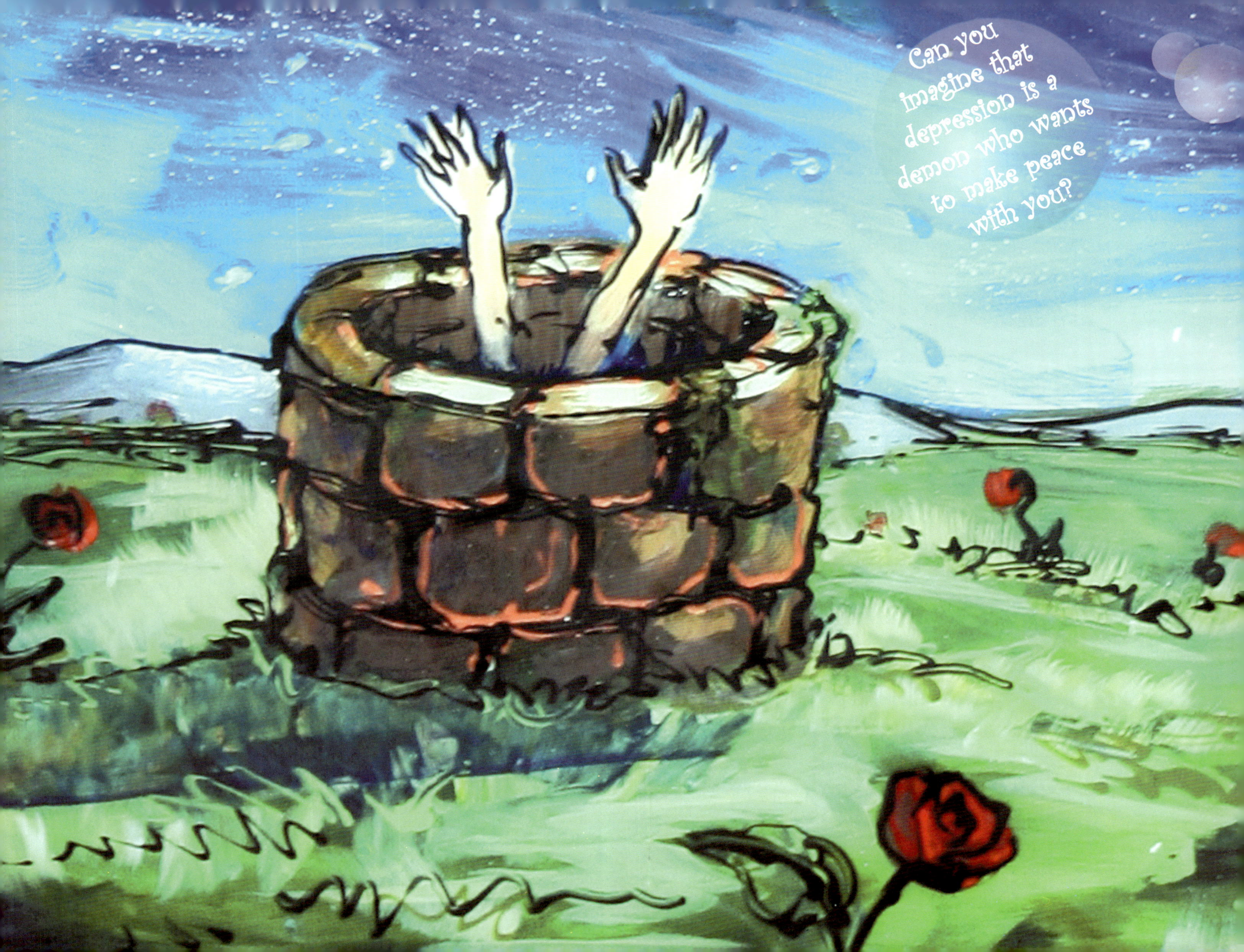
Can you imagine that depression is a demon who wants to make peace with you?

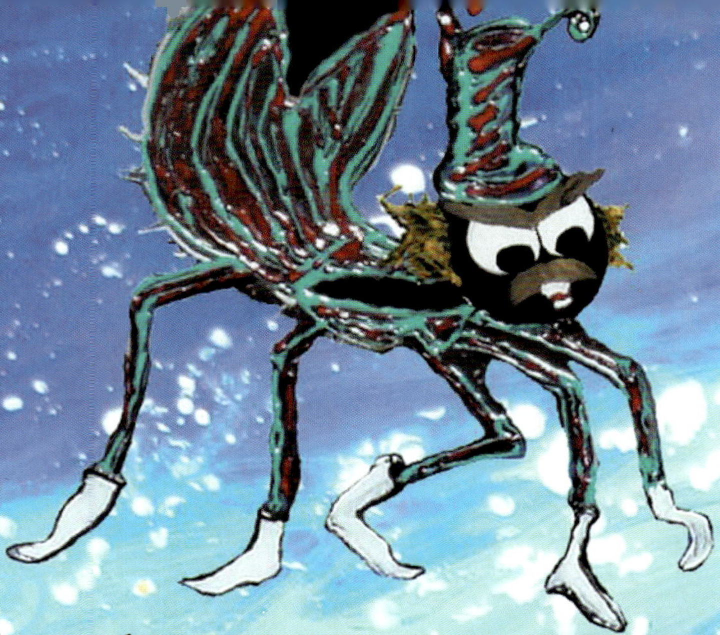

Sir Grouchy spider was crawling all around Skinny telling her obscenities to get her to leave. “I agree! How could you believe such atrocities? Tell her where you remembered such things…locked in your closet that you thought was a well! I think what you claim to remember has something to do with your imagination on a cold, dark day. This would have never happened on a unny day in May!”

‘Hmmm…many people experience repressed memories after time in a well. A holding tank of any kind will force someone to think they are in the ikes of hell. Release only comes when the healing process has begun. Now Sir Grouchy, this is not your session to yell.” replied Merry Miss Humm.

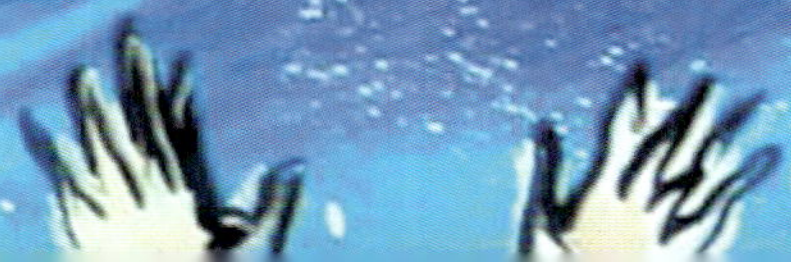

After going through the pages of Skinny's early life, she could see how she had held on to old beliefs.

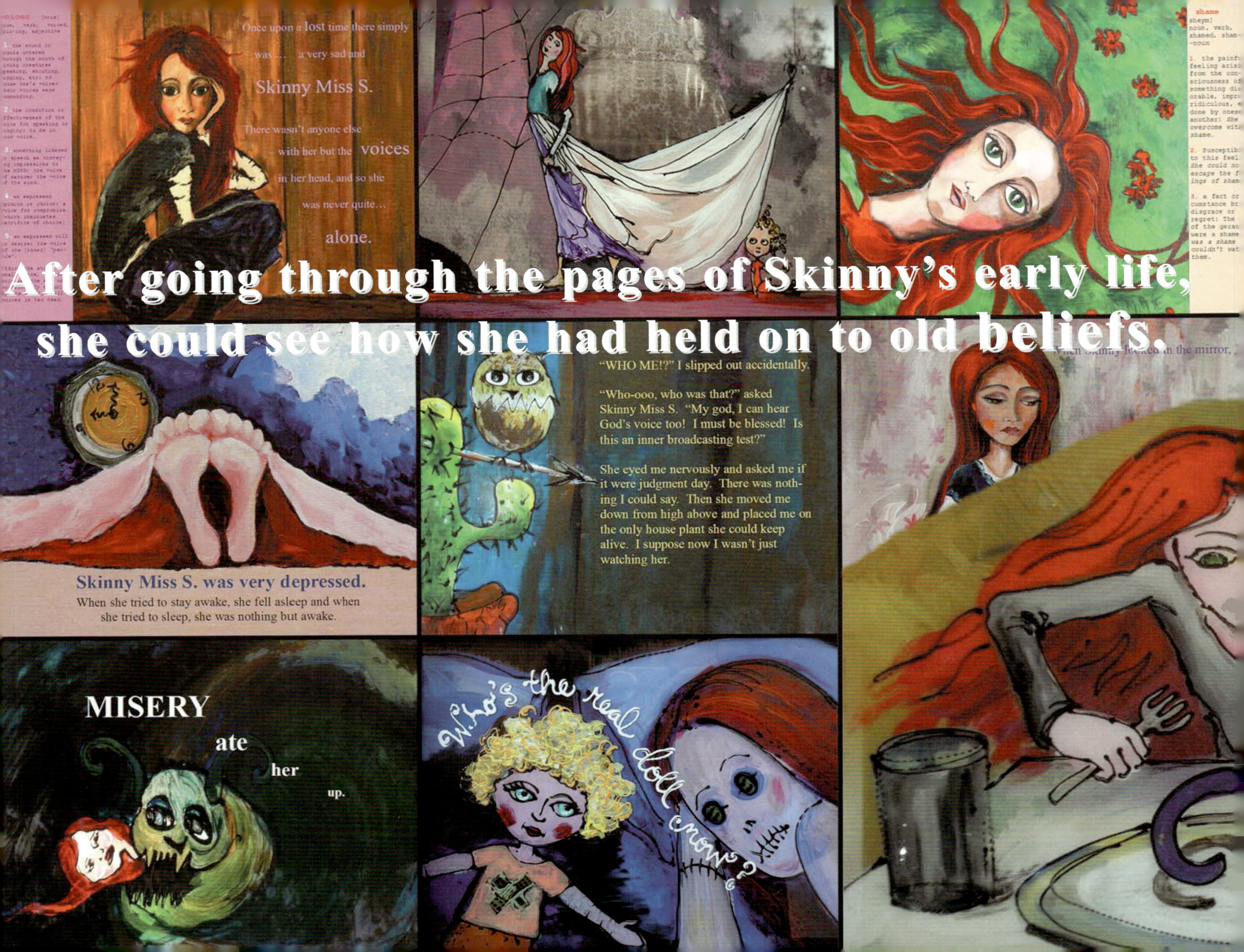

Those beliefs used to serve her, but they weren't serving her anymore, and self-serve meant making sure she got her portion.

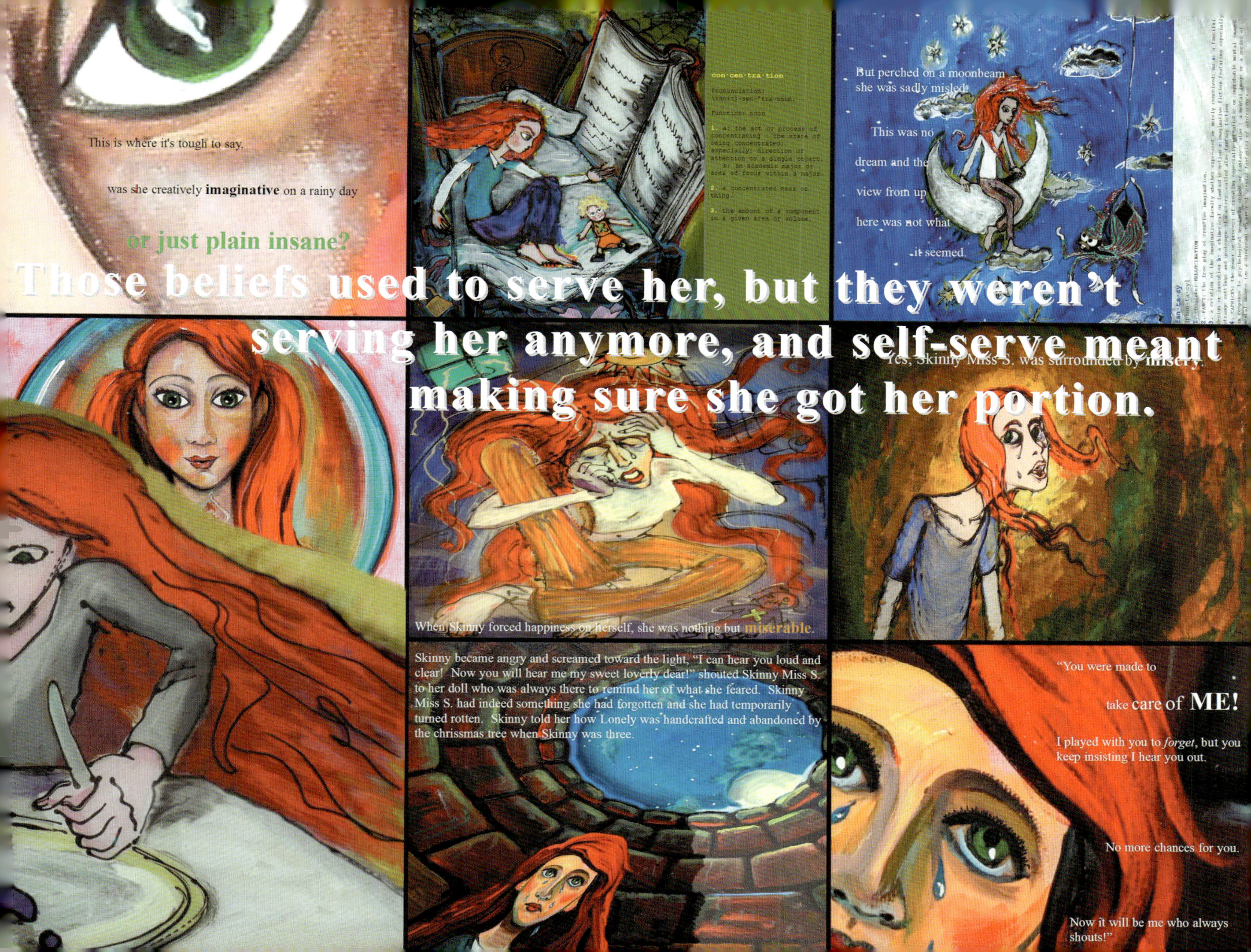

This is where it's tough to say.
was she creatively **imaginative** on a rainy day
or just plain insane?
con·cen·tra·tion
Pronunciation:
\kän(t)-sen-ˈtrā-shun.
Function: noun
1. a: the act or process of concentrating : the state of being concentrated; especially: direction of attention to a single object. b: an academic major or area of focus within a major.
2. a concentrated mass or thing.
3. the amount of a component in a given area or volume.
But perched on a moonbeam
she was sadly misled.
This was no
dream and the
view from up
here was not what
it seemed.
Yes, Skinny Miss S. was surrounded by **misery**.
When Skinny forced happiness on herself, she was nothing but miserable.
Skinny became angry and screamed toward the light, "I can hear you loud and clear! Now you will hear me my sweet loverly dear!" shouted Skinny Miss S. to her doll who was always there to remind her of what she feared. Skinny Miss S. had indeed something she had forgotten and she had temporarily turned rotten. Skinny told her how Lonely was handcrafted and abandoned by the chrissmas tree when Skinny was three.
"You were made to
take care of **ME!**
I played with you to *forget*, but you keep insisting I hear you out.
No more chances for you.
Now it will be me who always shouts!"

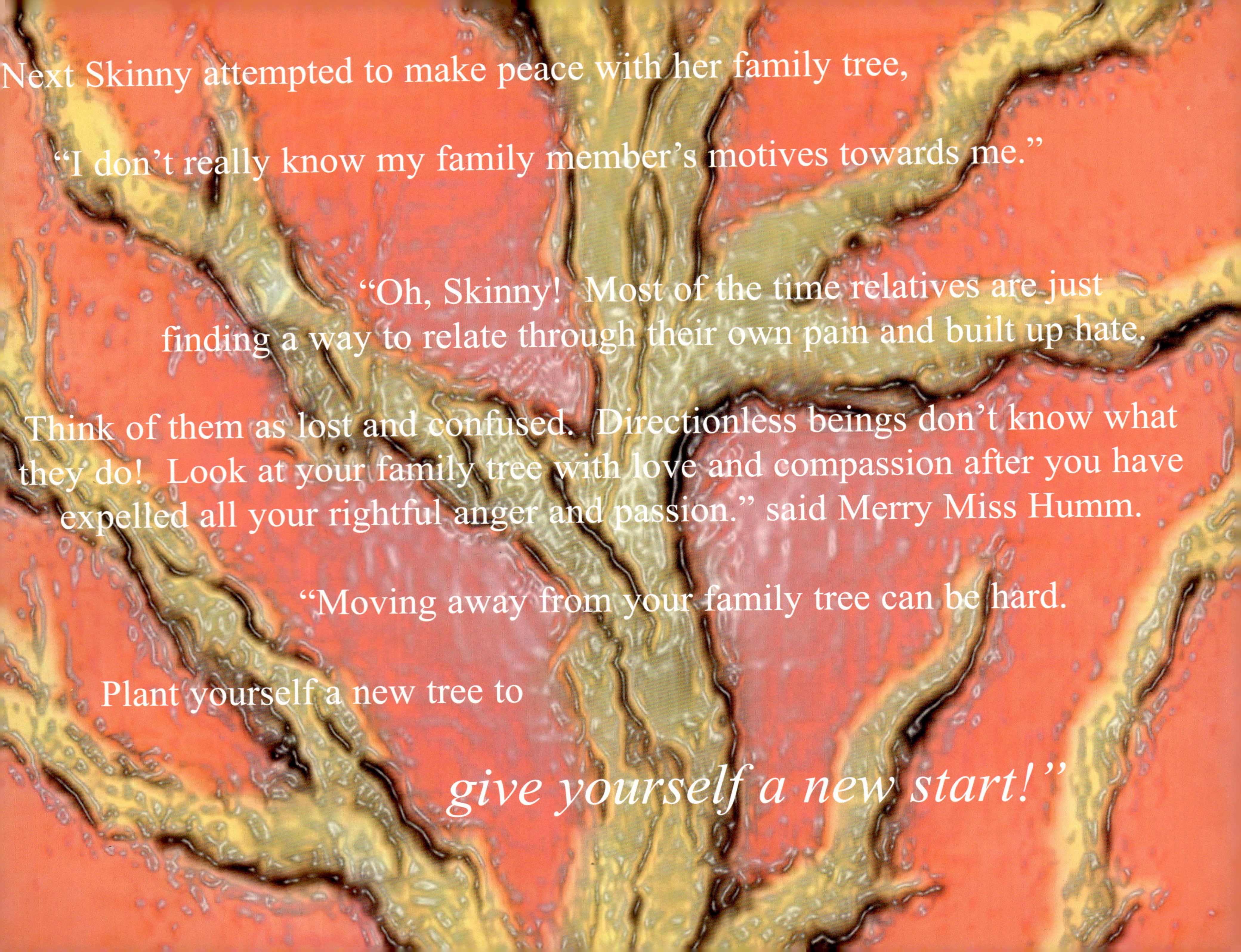

Next Skinny attempted to make peace with her family tree,

"I don't really know my family member's motives towards me."

"Oh, Skinny! Most of the time relatives are just finding a way to relate through their own pain and built up hate.

Think of them as lost and confused. Directionless beings don't know what they do! Look at your family tree with love and compassion after you have expelled all your rightful anger and passion." said Merry Miss Humm.

"Moving away from your family tree can be hard.

Plant yourself a new tree to

give yourself a new start!"

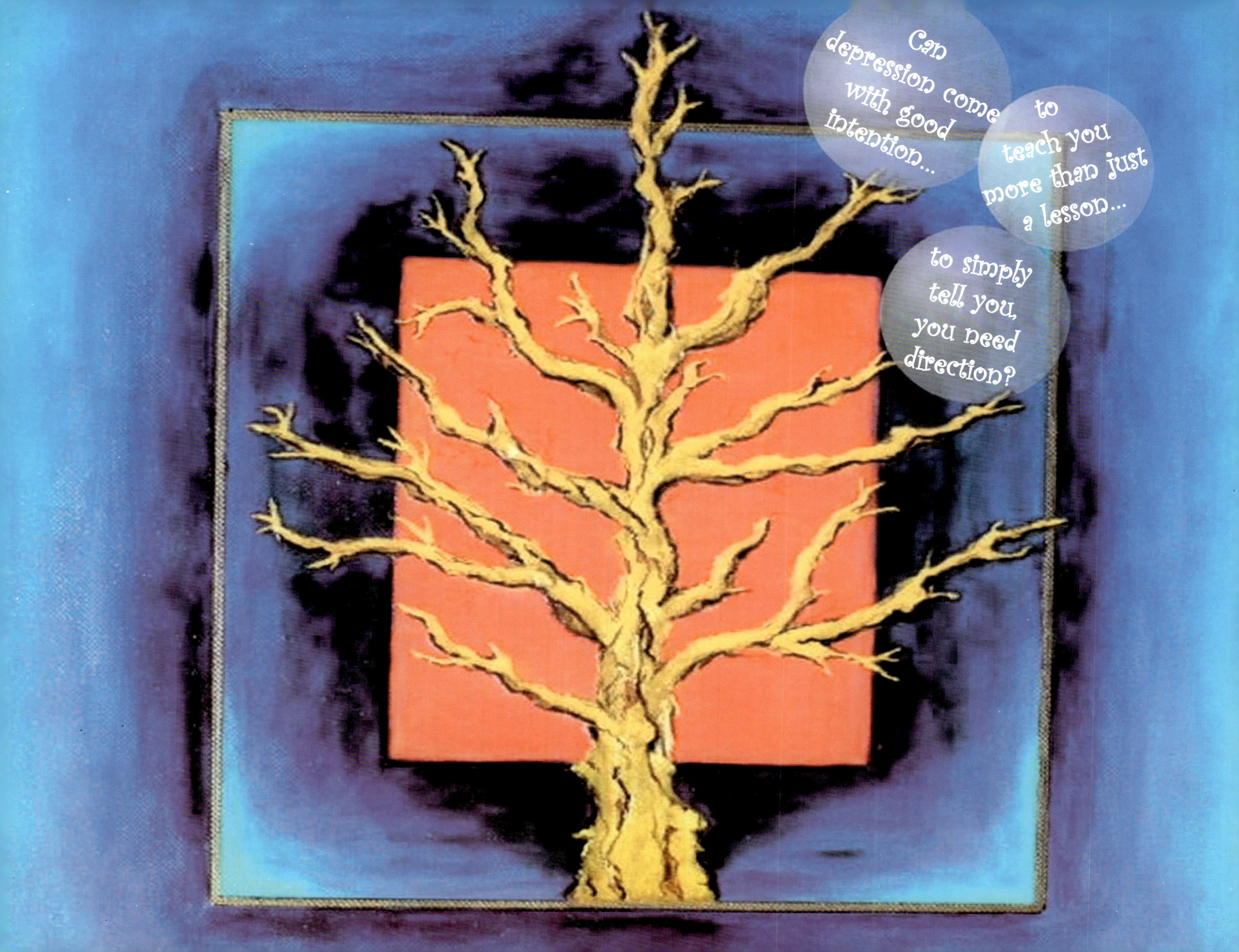
Can depression come with good intention...
to teach you more than just a lesson...
to simply tell you, you need direction?

"What are you insinuating, Merry Miss Humm? What is it Skinny should become…a tree-hugger, how fun!" Sir Grouchy Spider said as he began the web he spun.

He attempted to cover up Skinny's family tree since he judged this exercise to be nothing but bad.

This made Skinny mad,
"Let me be!
I want to be free!

I want to find the organic ingredients in me!
This has nothing to do with hugging trees!"

She shouted at the spider at the top of her lungs, blowing threw the cobwebs and making her family's photo known.

journey
noun

1. an act or instance of traveling from one place to another.

2. something suggesting travel or passage from one place to another; *the journey from youth to maturity a journey through time.*

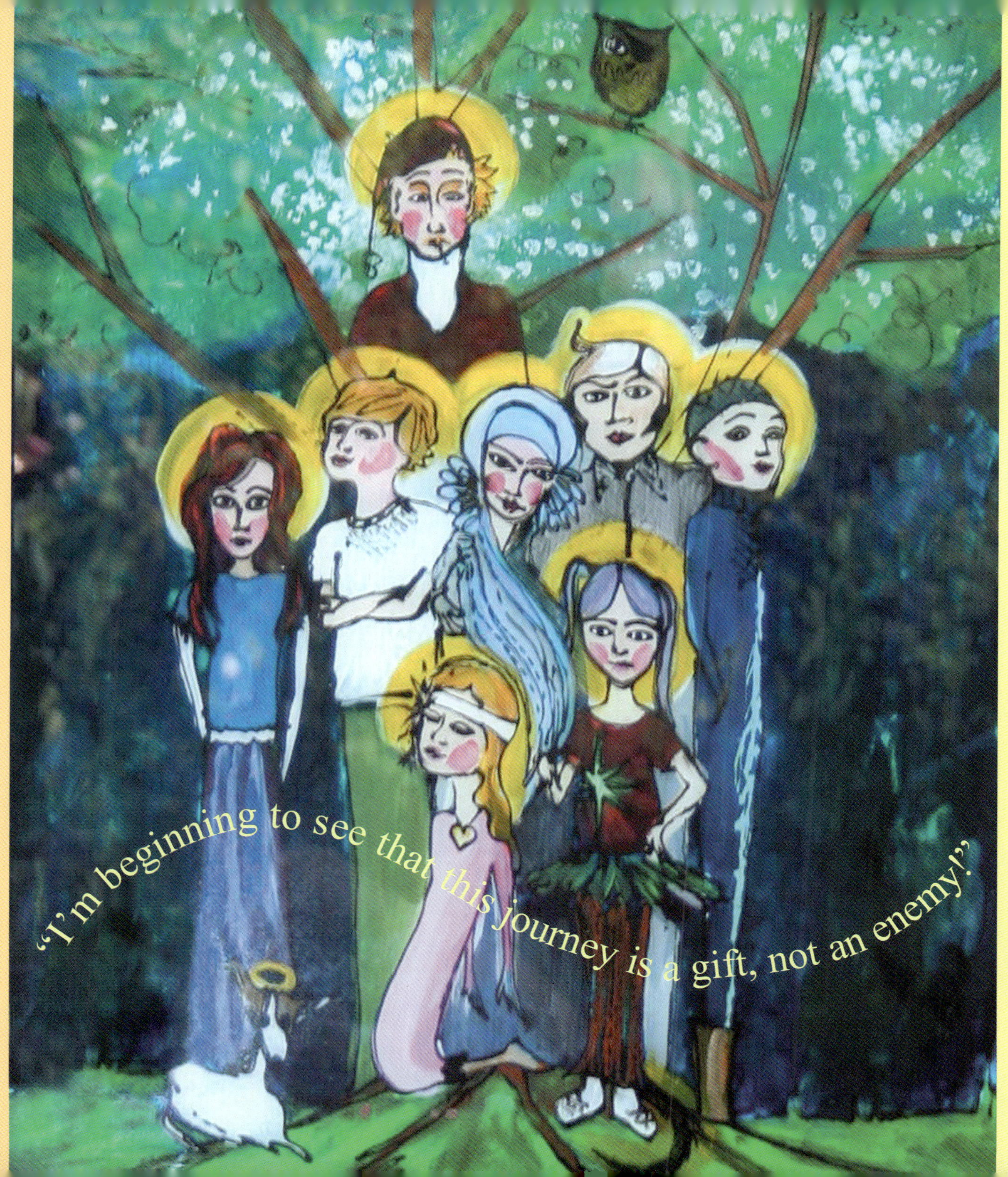
"I'm beginning to see that this journey is a gift, not an enemy!"

gift
noun

1. a notable capacity, talent, or endowment.

2. something voluntarily transferred by one person to another without compensation.

3. often implies special favor by God or nature; *the gift of singing beautifully.*

Dean Doll shoed the spider away and Merry Miss Humm continued in her objective way, "You've come so far and you must take it day by day. I will help you to let go of the sadness from which you have already learned."

"What are you saying? I should move on at last?" Skinny asked.

Merry answered, "Yes, now that you've
courageously honored your past.
We work on all sorts of things in these walls here, dear. Let's move on and I will teach you skills to help you feel less fear."

"Hmmmm, I have a thought! Let's make today a good day! Joy is a decision you make with each and every moment." Merry hummed on, "Expressing your needs, setting your boundaries are some of your new vocabulary. Allow yourself room to practice them too, now set your intention to love the
inner child in you
by knowing when to say when
and who to let in!"

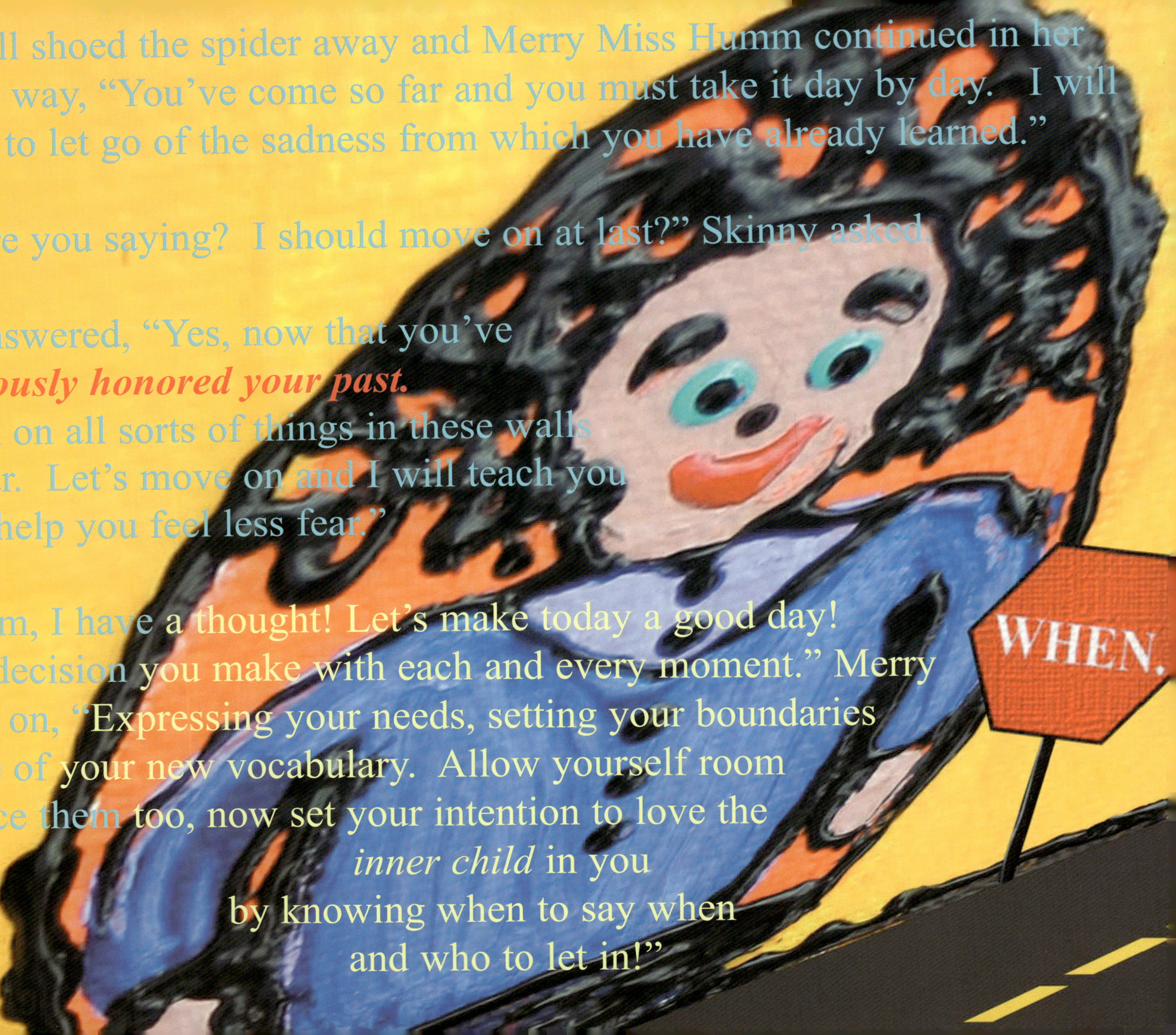

express

verb

1. to represent in words, STATE: to give or convey a true impression of, SHOW, REFLECT: to make known the opinions or feelings of (oneself), to give expression to the artistic or creative impulses or abilities of (oneself), to represent by a sign or symbol, to manifest or produce (a character, molecule, or effect) by a genetic process.

2. suggests an impulse to reveal in words, gestures, actions, or what one creates or produces; *expressed her feelings in music., an editorial voicing their concerns.*

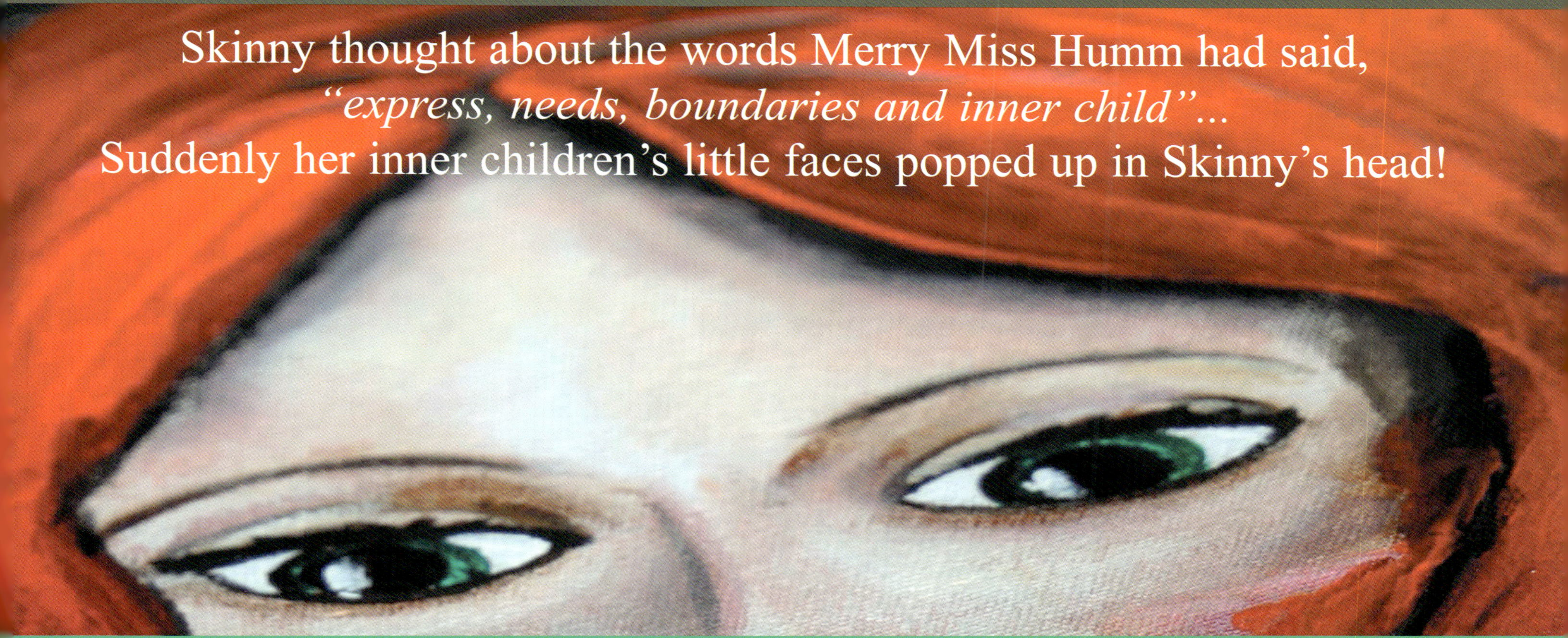

Skinny thought about the words Merry Miss Humm had said,
"express, needs, boundaries and inner child"...
Suddenly her inner children's little faces popped up in Skinny's head!

boundary

noun

1. something that indicates or fixes a limit or extent.

2. that which divides one entity or political unit from another.

She went to tell Merry Miss Humm what they looked like and what they said. She wanted to discuss all the memories in her head, but they had run out of time. Already they had talked a ton, but there was only fifty minutes a session.

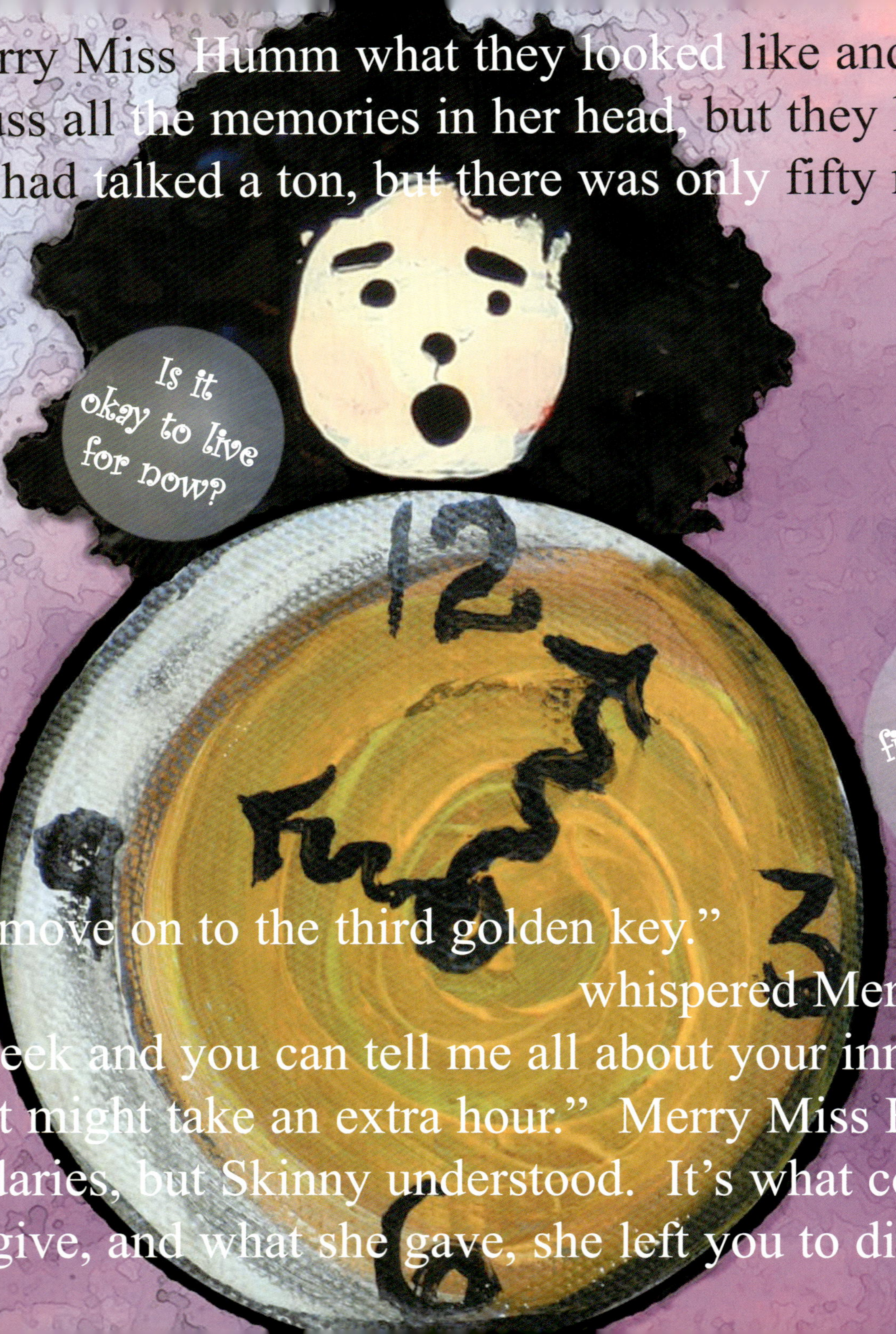
Is it okay to live for now?
Can you find your favorite child photo of you?
Talk to it too!

"Hmmm…for now move on to the third golden key."
whispered Merry Miss Humm.
"Come back next week and you can tell me all about your inner children! Two you said? That might take an extra hour." Merry Miss Humm was strict with her time boundaries, but Skinny understood. It's what contributed to how much Merry could give, and what she gave, she left you to dig.

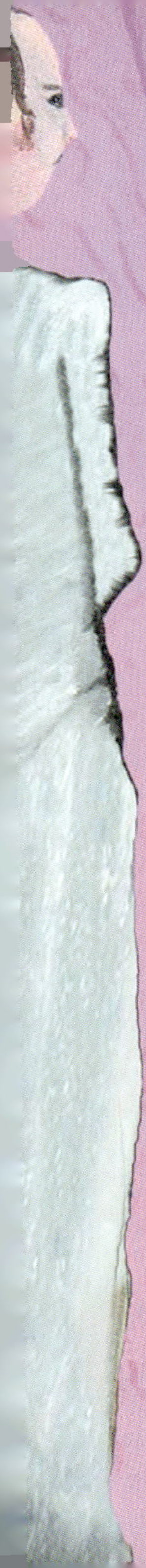

Merry Miss Humm added before Skinny and her dolls were to leave, "We'll work on Dean Doll and Father Deana Marie not being ONE! Enmeshment is never any fun." Dean Doll smiled at the thought he would be coming back too! He really just wanted to be accepted for being more *colorful* than most.

Skinny stood up for Dean Doll, "I love colorful people and that's who you are! Don't you ever think because of your differences there is something wrong with what you do! There is something wrong with everyone else if they can't appreciate the unique design of you!"

Father Deana Marie contemplated how he could sue. All this talk was now making him blue. Who was he if Dean Doll was perfect being who he was? He was so confused. His rules wouldn't mean anything anymore. On top of that he would have to learn how to have feelings of his own and face his other half head on.

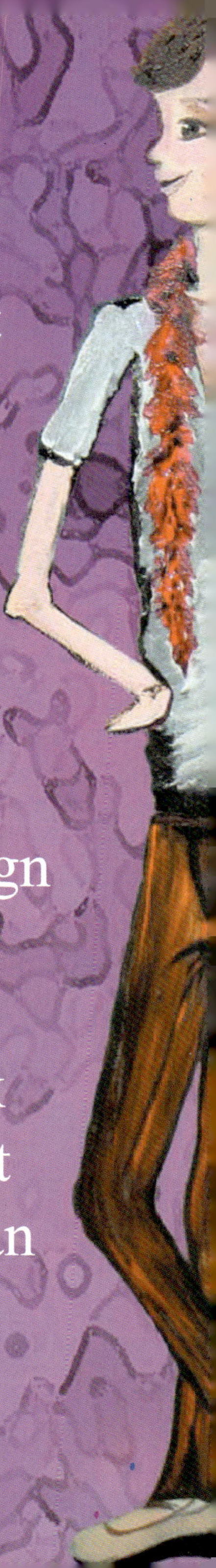

Sir Grouchy Spider was behaving himself, but still passive-aggressively spelling bad words out. Seemed it was the only way he could express without Skinny coming apart at the seams.

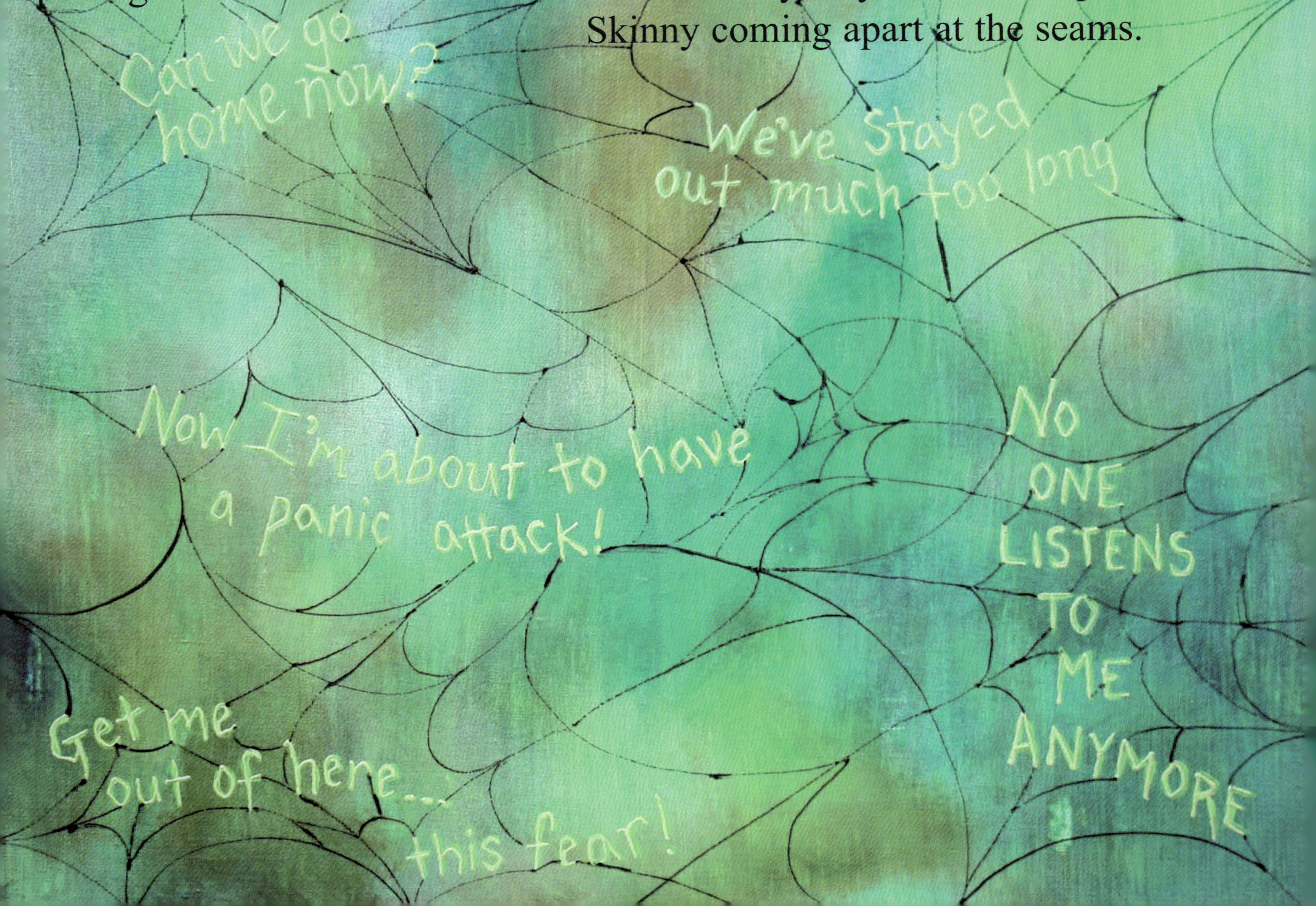
Can we go home now?
We've Stayed out much too long
Now I'm about to have a panic attack!
NO ONE LISTENS TO ME ANYMORE
Get me out of here... this fear!

Lonely Miss C. sat in awe on the couch. When Skinny said good-bye until next week, she accidentally left Lonely behind, but Lonely didn't mind. There were things for her to find in her nervous little mind that might have been too much for Skinny Miss S. to stay kind.

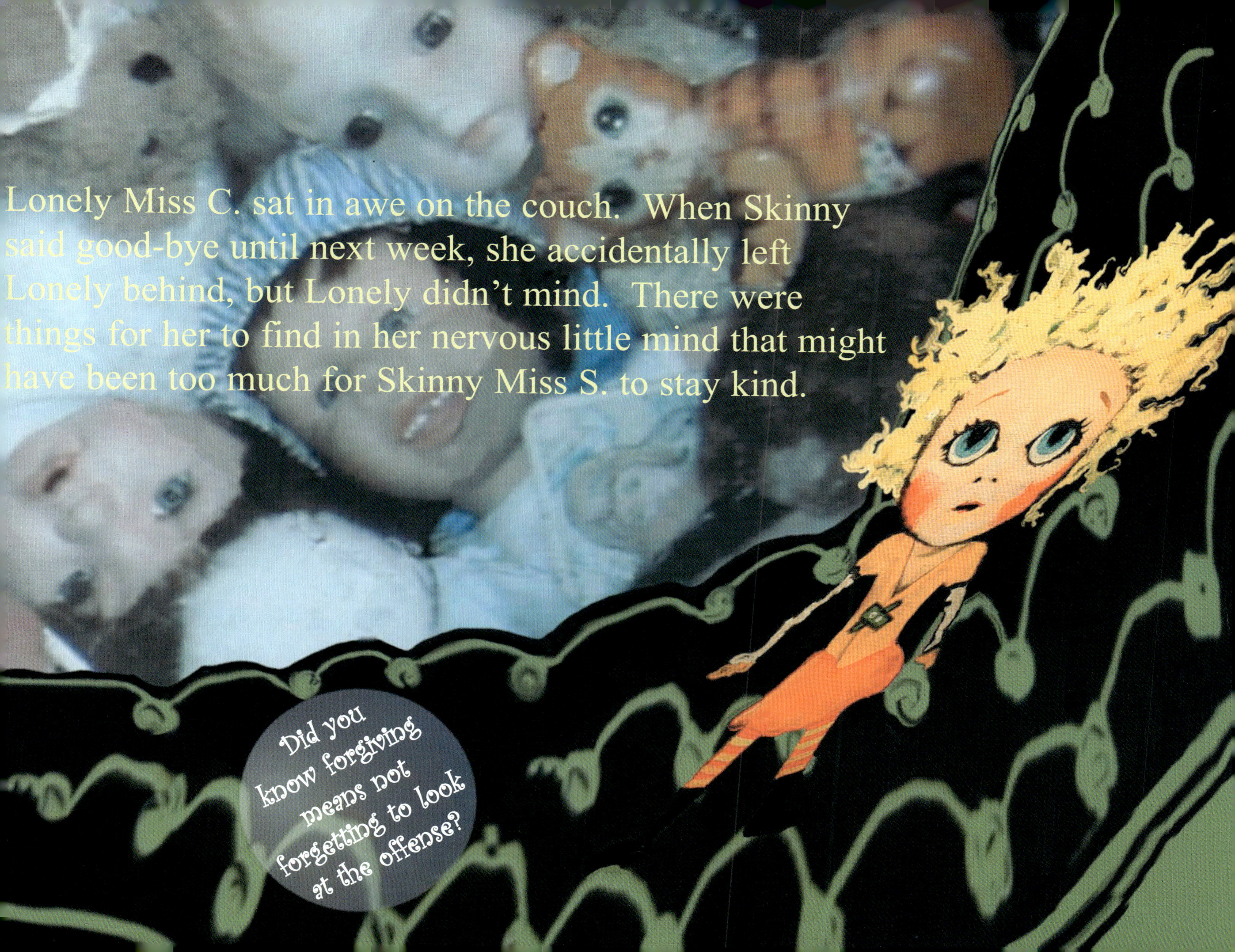
Did you know forgiving means not forgetting to look at the offense?

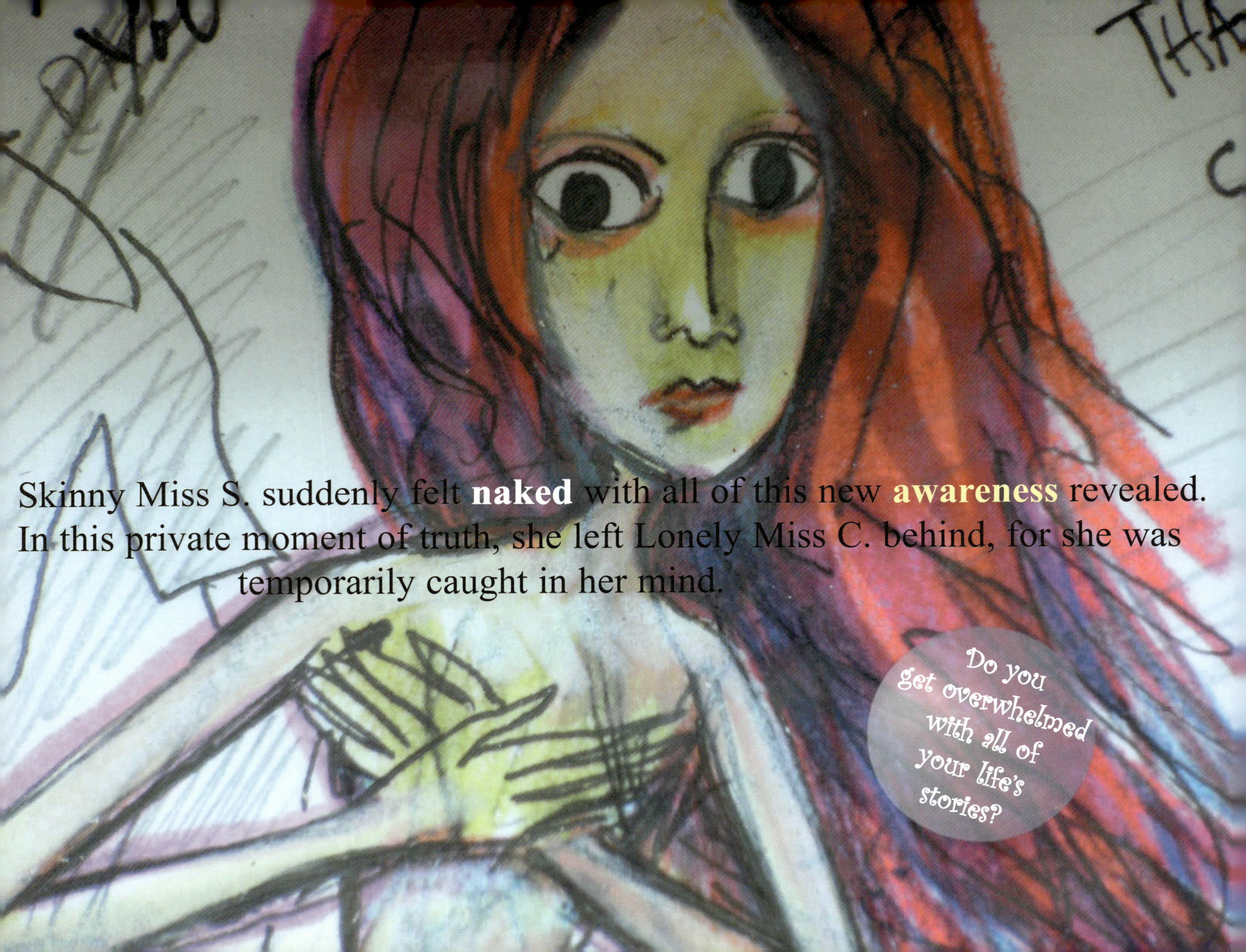

Skinny Miss S. suddenly felt **naked** with all of this new **awareness** revealed. In this private moment of truth, she left Lonely Miss C. behind, for she was temporarily caught in her mind.

Do you get overwhelmed with all of your life's stories?

dressing

noun

1. the act or process of one who dresses, an instance of such act or process.

2. a sauce for adding to a dish; *as a salad*, a seasoned mixture usually used as a stuffing; *as for poultry*.

3. material *as ointment or gauze*, applied to cover a lesion or wound

"I have a lonely voice who wants me to see everything in order to get through to the truth. I have a gay voice who wants out of the Catholic Church. I have a priest voice who believes in the powers that he thinks he has and who am I to take that away? I have a very angry voice who likes to keep me tied up in a web. I have lots to forgive. I have memories that are now out of the closet, but what am I to believe? They are a little twisted up and hard to swallow. That could be why I live in such sorrow. I have a cat I never see and an owl who stares at me. I have higher powers who came from my inside out to tell me what my deep forgotten pain is about. They are my inner children in need of a strong parent. Wow, now I'm feeling better looking at all the things I use to not be able to see."

It would take Skinny a few more books to understand this mess, but somehow she could finally hear her voice coming through. She excused herself and trusted she was on to something new. She was thinking of when she returned home, all of the kinds of dressings she would change into! First, she had one more stop.

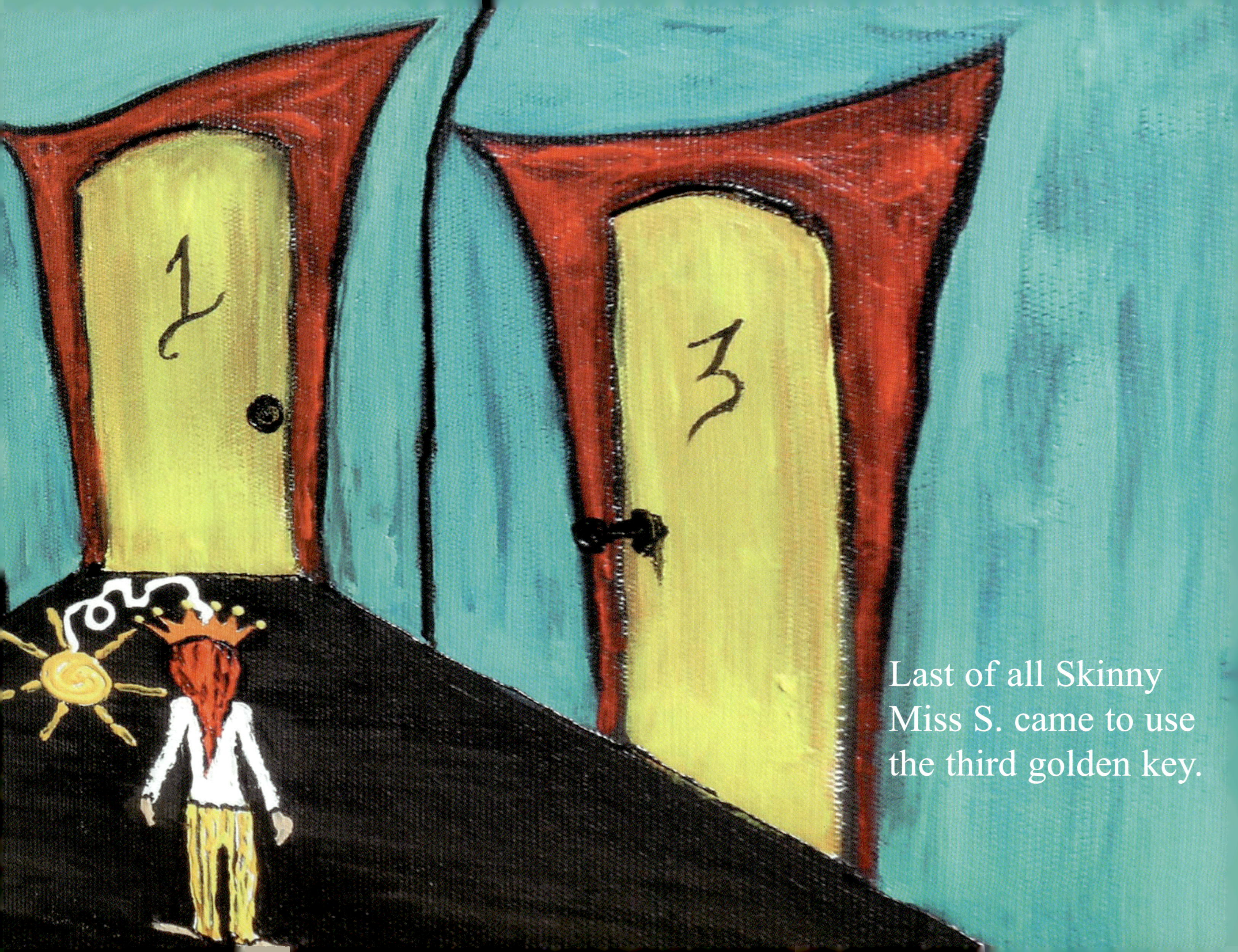

Last of all Skinny Miss S. came to use the third golden key.

golden
adjective

1. bright, metallic, or lustrous like gold; of the color of gold; *golden hair.*

2. made or consisting of gold; *golden earrings.*

3. exceptionally valuable, advantageous, or fine; *a golden opportunity.*

4. having glowing vitality; *golden youth.*

5. highly talented and favored; destined for success; *television's golden boy.*

6. richly soft and smooth; *a golden voice.*

7. indicating the fiftieth event of a series; *a golden wedding anniversary.*

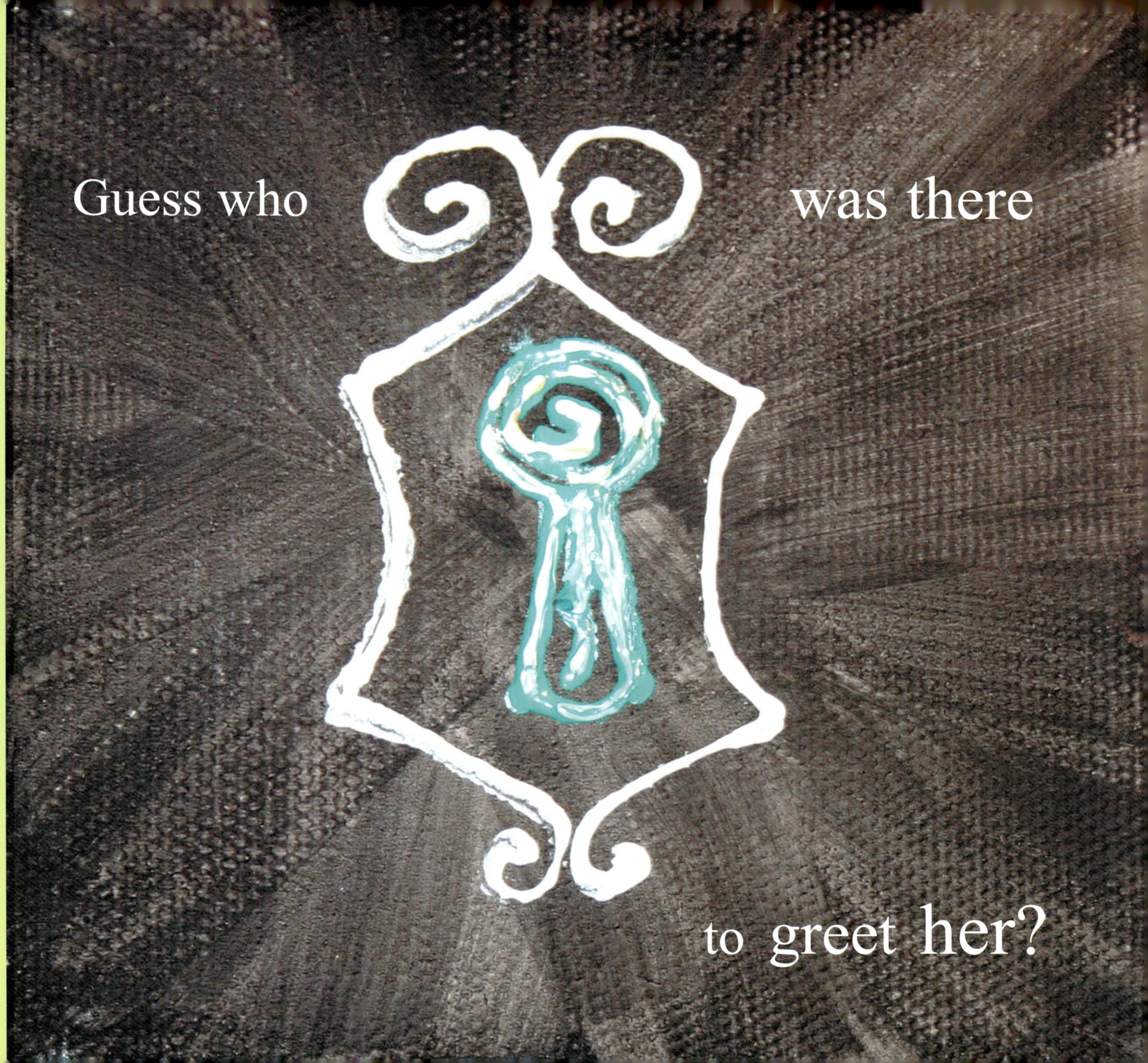

Guess who was there to greet her?

diva

noun

1. PRIMA DONNA
2. a usually glamorous and successful female performer or personality

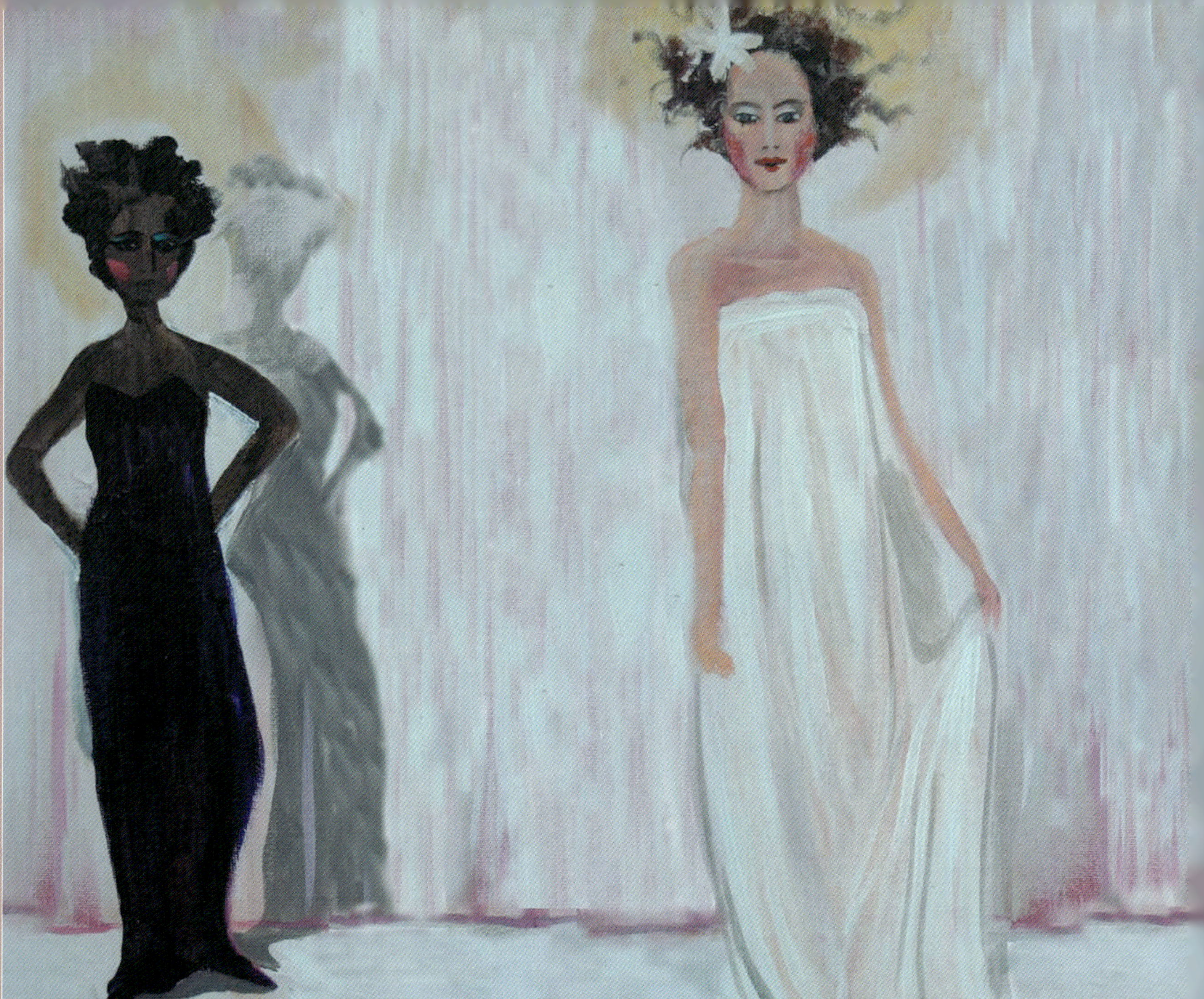

It was a friendly group of other Misses! No one asked her any
"*WHY NOT?*" and in unison!

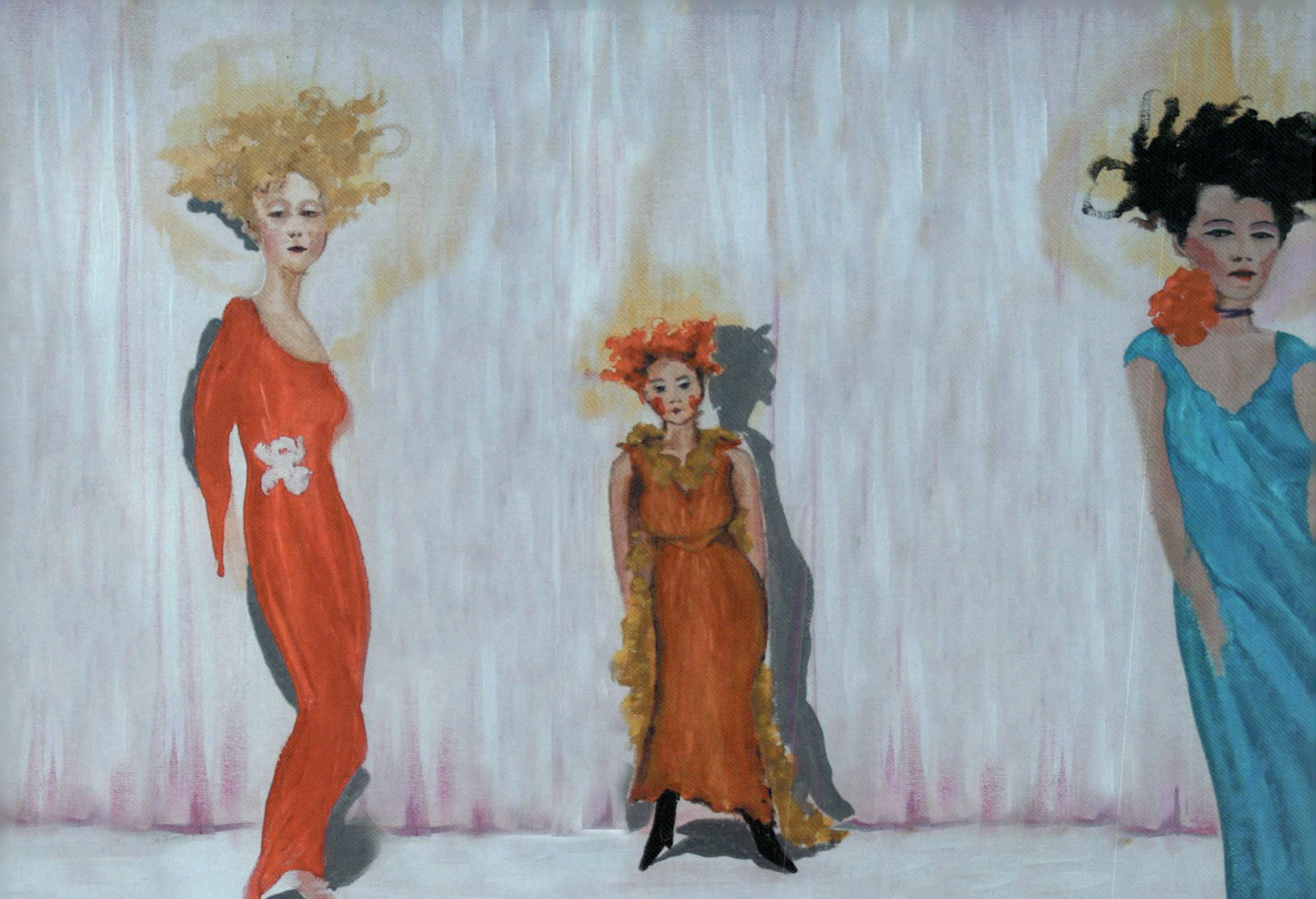

questions like Skinny was use to. Well, just one...
Dean Doll was overjoyed, “FABULOUS! Here I fit in!!”

Support Group:

In a support group, members provide each other with various types of help, usually nonprofessional and nonmaterial, for a particular shared, usually burdensome, characteristic.

The help may take the form of providing and evaluating relevant information, relating personal experiences, listening to and accepting others' experiences, providing sympathetic understanding and establishing social networks.

A support group may also work to inform the public or engage in advocacy.[20]

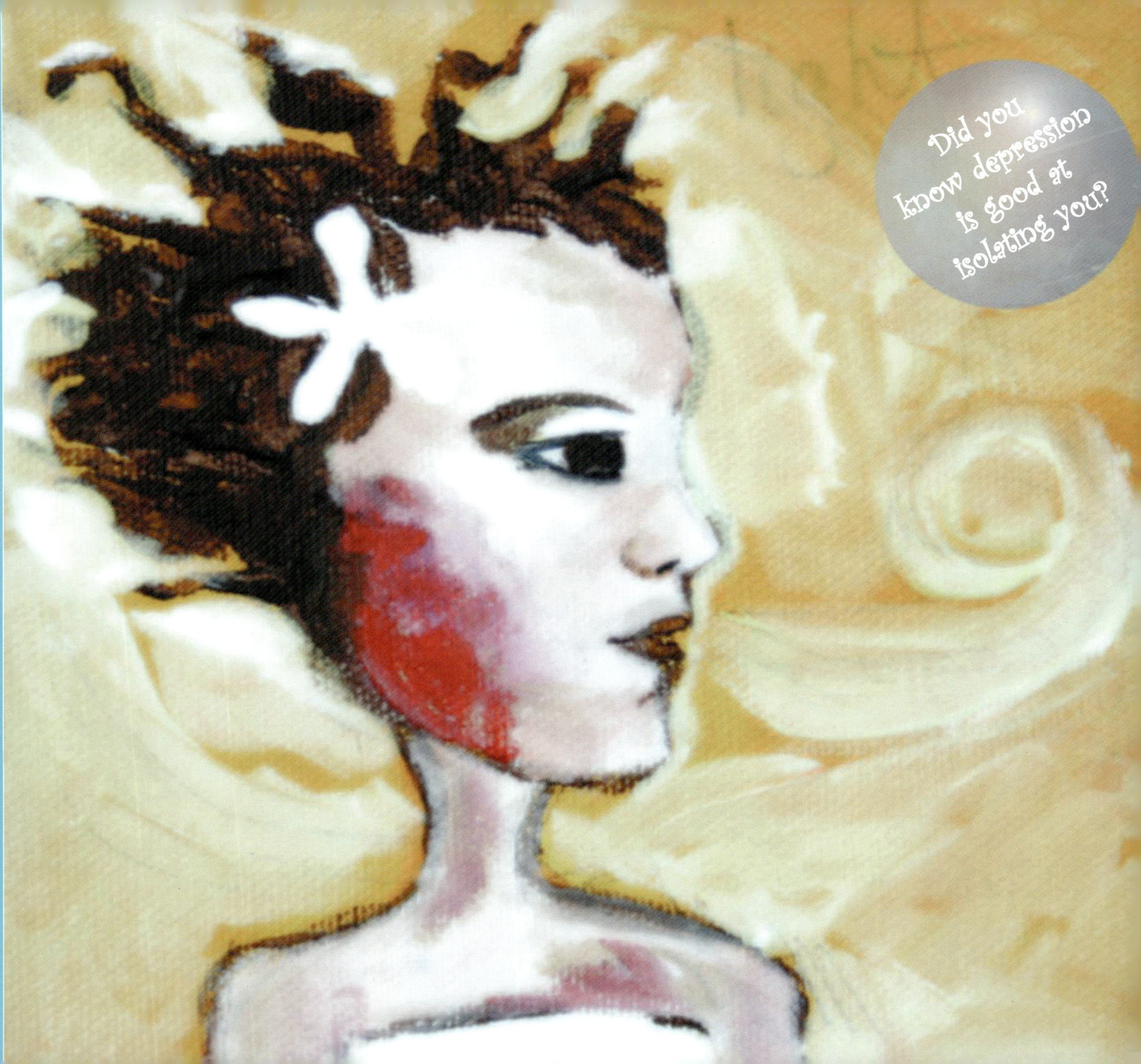

Are you humble and know it's true?

Reach out for an answer, not just a clue!

They shared their struggles and how they were conquered. They referred each other to competent doctors.

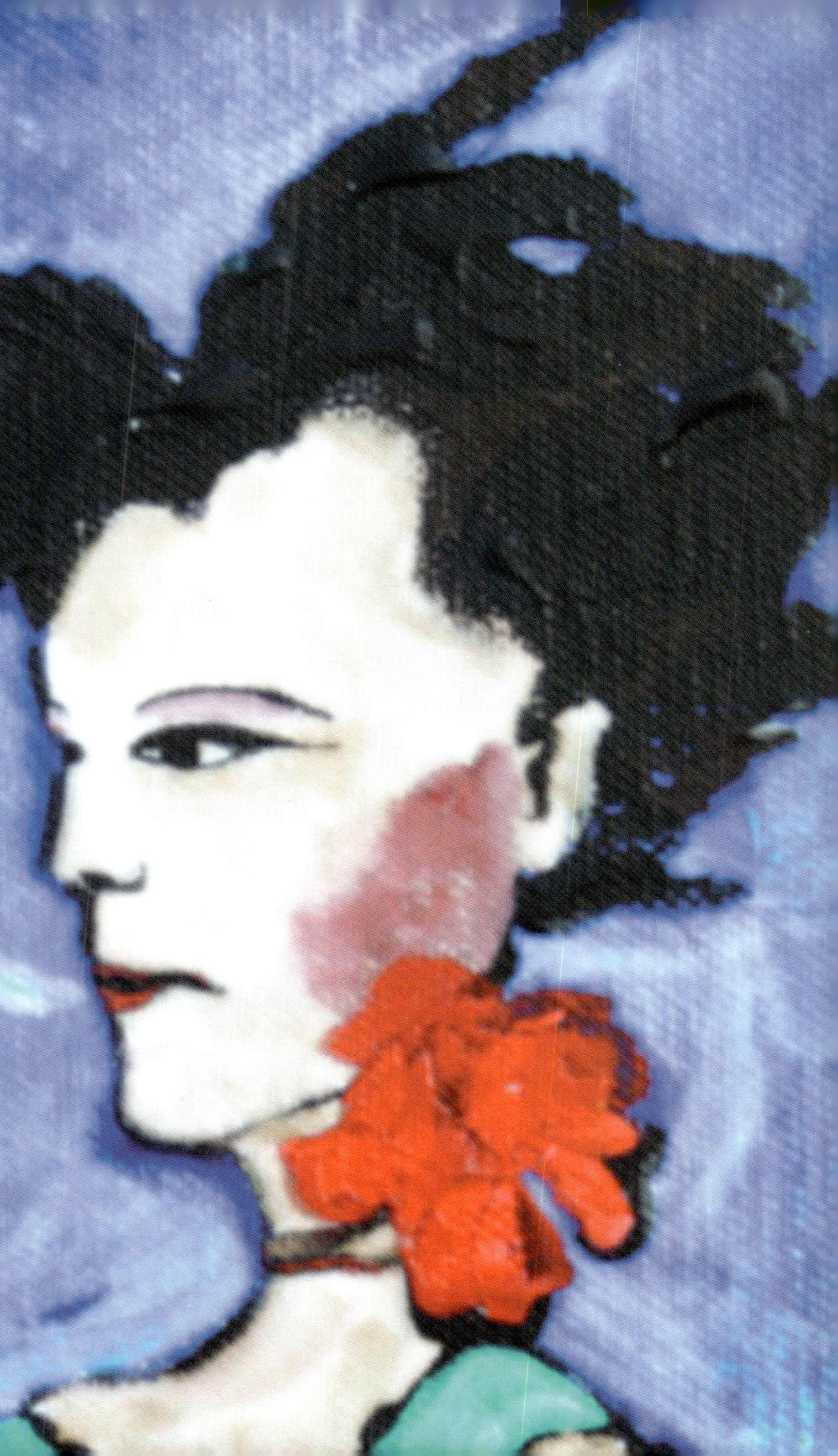

They spoke freely and honestly and listened with total confidentiality. The Misses were accepting of different mentalities and realities.

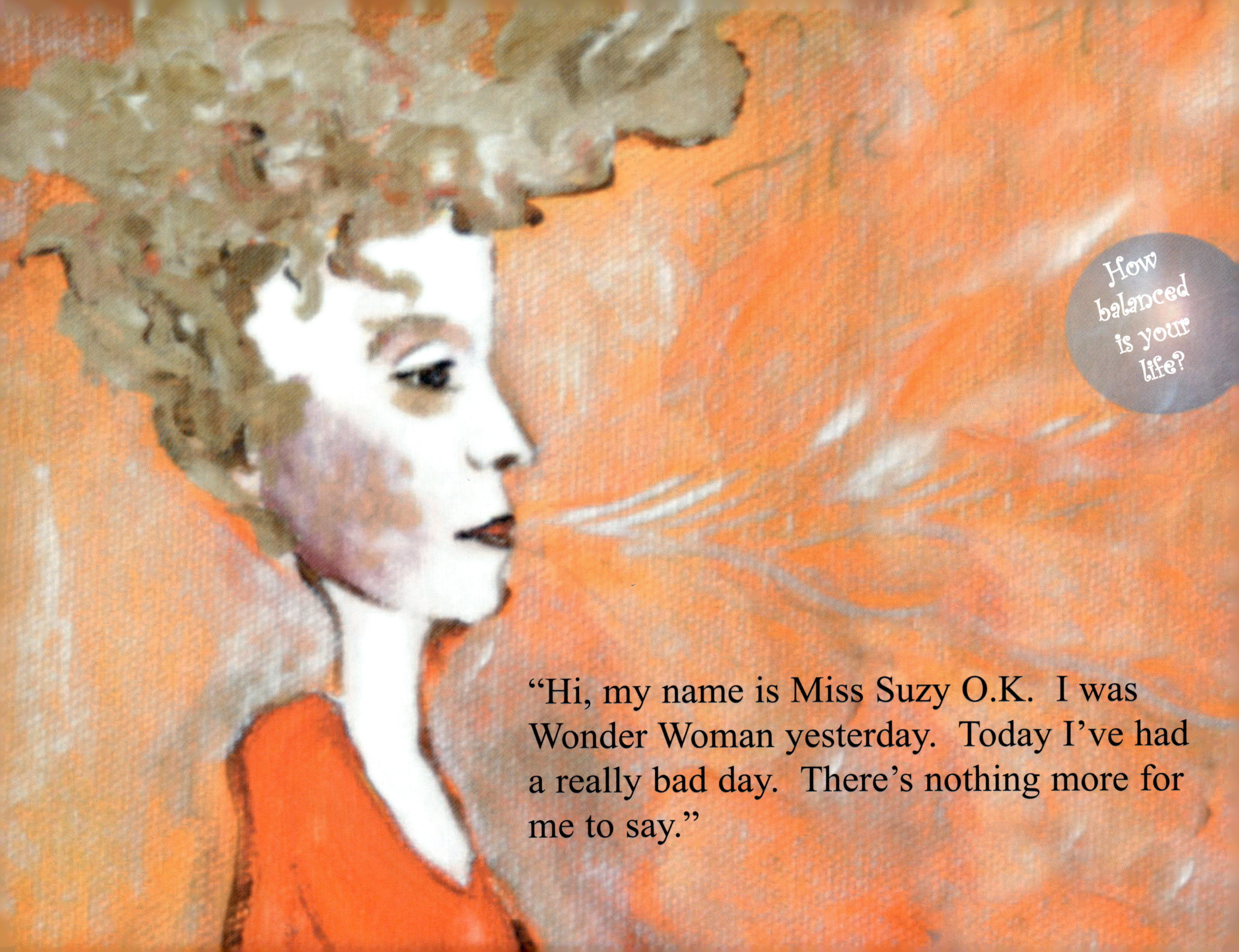

"Hi, my name is Miss Suzy O.K. I was Wonder Woman yesterday. Today I've had a really bad day. There's nothing more for me to say."

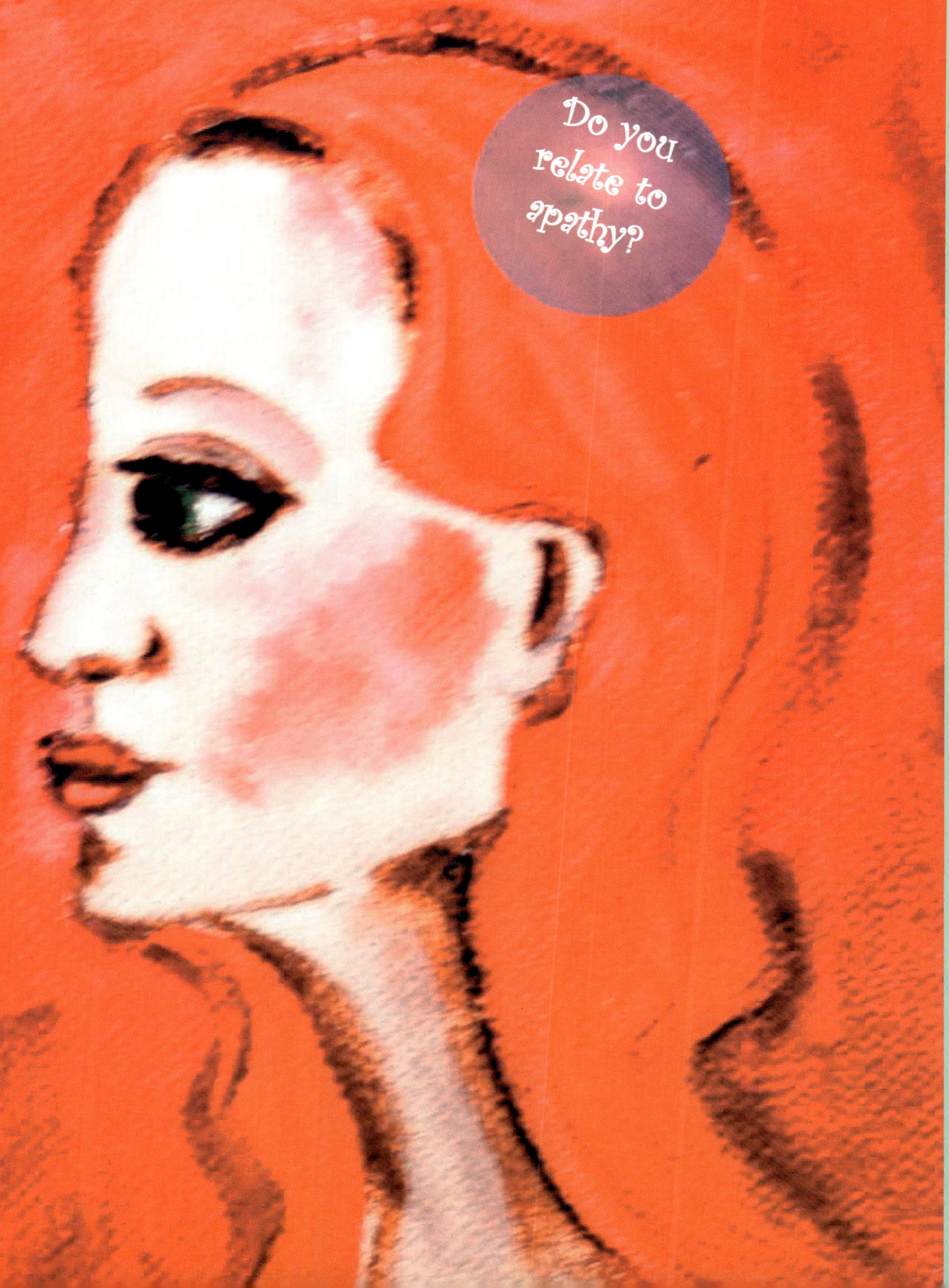

"I've felt
nothing
that much,
that I wasn't able
to stay in touch."

thought Skinny to
herself silently.

apathy
noun

1. lack of feeling or emotion: IMPASSIVENESS

2. lack of interest or concern: INDIFFERENCE

DIAGNOSTIC CRITERIA FOR:

Bipolar Disorder

[Manic Episode explained only; Major Depressive Episode explained on previous pages.]

There are six separate criteria sets for Bipolar I Disorder: Single Manic Episode, Most Recent Episode Hypomanic, Most Recent Episode Manic, Most Recent Episode Mixed, Most Recent Episode Depressed, and Most Recent Episode Unspecified. Bipolar I Disorder, Single Manic Episode, is used to describe individuals who are having a first episode of mania. The remaining criteria sets are used to specify the nature of the current (or most recent) episode in individuals who have had recurrent mood episodes.

Manic Episode A. A distinct period of abnormally and persistently elevated, expansive, or irritable mood, lasting at least 1 week (or any duration if hospitalization is necessary). B. During the period of mood disturbance, three (or more) of the following symptoms have persisted (four if the mood is only irritable) and have been present to a significant degree: (1) inflated self-esteem or grandiosity (2) decreased need for sleep (e.g., feels rested after onl 3 hours of sleep) (3) more talkative than usual or pressur to keep talking

(4) flight of ideas or subjective experience that thoughts are racing (5) distractibility(i.e., attention too easily drawn to unimportant or irrelevant external stimuli) (6) increase in goal-directed activity (either socially, at work or school, or sexually) or psychomotor agitation (7) excessive involvement in pleasurable activities that have a high potential for painful consequences (e.g., engaging in unrestrained buying sprees, sexual indiscretions, or foolish business investments) C. Thesymptoms do not meet criteria for a Mixed Episode. D. The mood disturbance is sufficiently severe to cause marked impairment in occupational functioning or in usual social activities or relationships with others, or to necessitate hospitalization to prevent harm to self or others, or there are psychotic features. E. The symptoms are not due to the direct physiological effects of a substance (e.g., a drug of abuse, a medication, or other treatment) or a general medical condition (e.g., hyperthyroidism). Note: Manic-like episodes that are clearly caused by somatic antidepressant treatment (e.g., medication, electroconvulsive therapy, light therapy) should not count toward a diagnosis of Bipolar I Disorder.[21]

alcoholism

noun

1. a chronic disorder characterized by dependence on alcohol, repeated excessive use of alcoholic beverages, the development of withdrawal symptoms on reducing or ceasing intake, morbidity that may include cirrhosis of the liver, and decreased ability to function socially and vocationally.

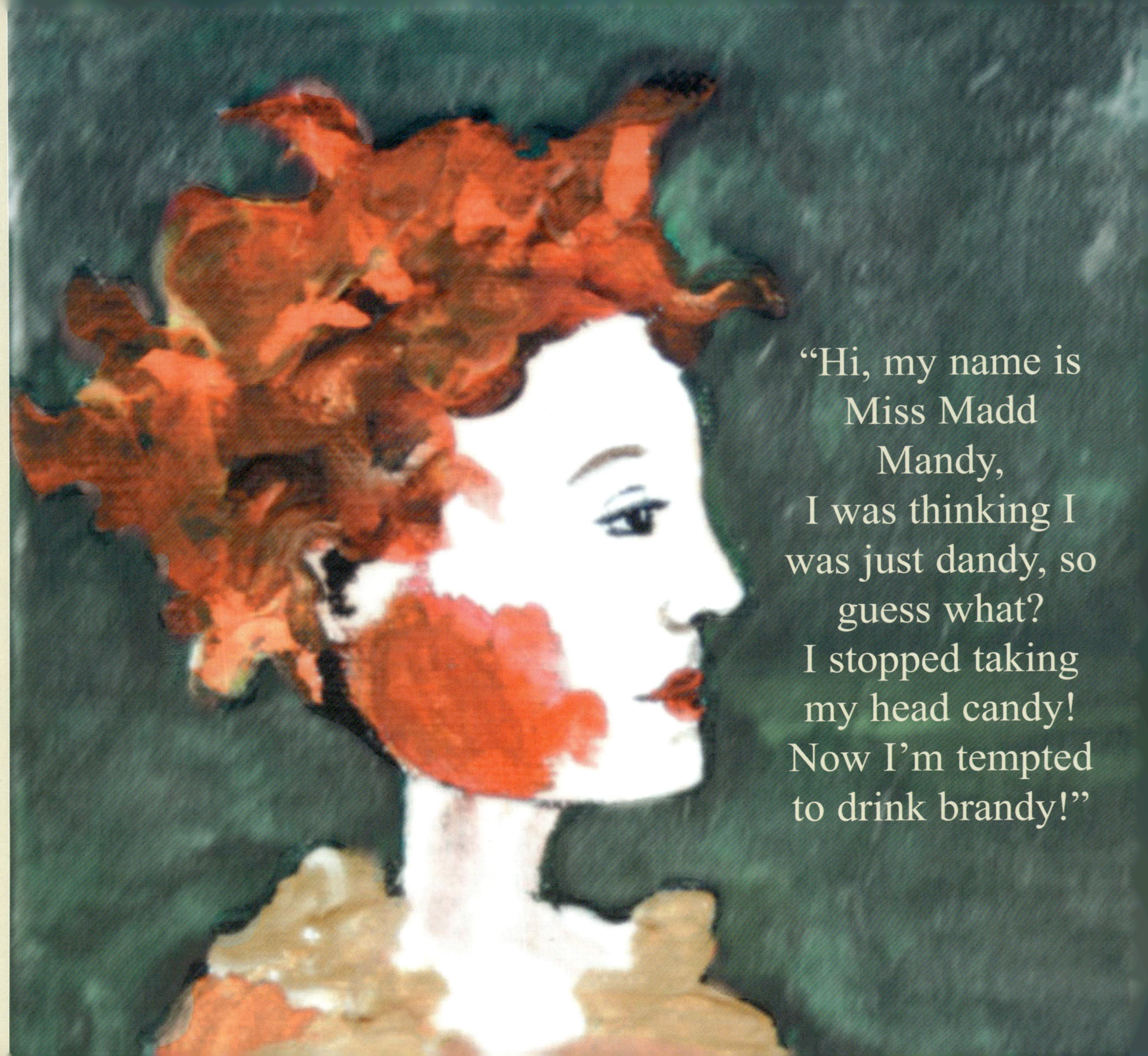

"Hi, my name is
Miss Madd
Mandy,
I was thinking I
was just dandy, so
guess what?
I stopped taking
my head candy!
Now I'm tempted
to drink brandy!"

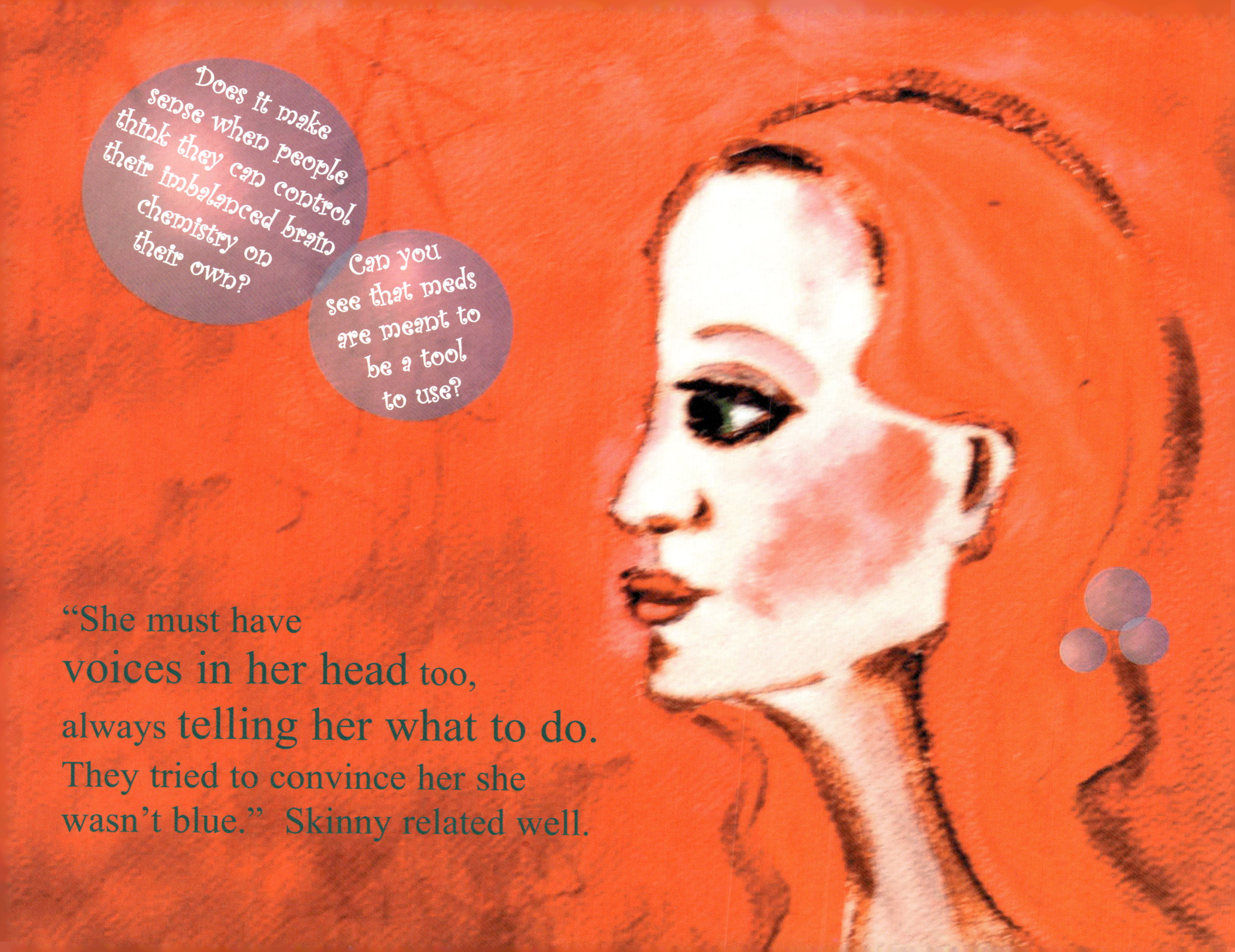
Does it make sense when people think they can control their imbalanced brain chemistry on their own?
Can you see that meds are meant to be a tool to use?

"She must have **voices in her head** too,
always **telling her what to do.**
They tried to convince her she
wasn't blue." Skinny related well.

DIAGNOSTIC CRITERIA FOR:

Substance Abuse

A. A maladaptive pattern of substance use leading to clinically significant impairment or distress, as manifested by one (or more) of the following, occurring within a 12-month period:

(1) recurrent substance use resulting in a failure to fulfill major role obligations at work, school, or home (e.g., repeated absences or poor work performance related to substance use; substance-related absences, suspensions, or expulsions from school; neglect of children or household)

(2) recurrent substance use in situations in which it is physically hazardous (e.g., driving an automobile or operating a machine when impaired by substance use)
(3) recurrent substance-related legal problems (e.g., arrests for substance-related disorderly conduct)
(4) continued substance use despite having persistent or recurrent social or interpersonal problems caused or exacerbated by the effects of the substance (e.g., arguments with spouse about consequences of intoxication, physical fights)

B. The symptoms have never met the criteria for Substance Dependence for this class of substance.[22]

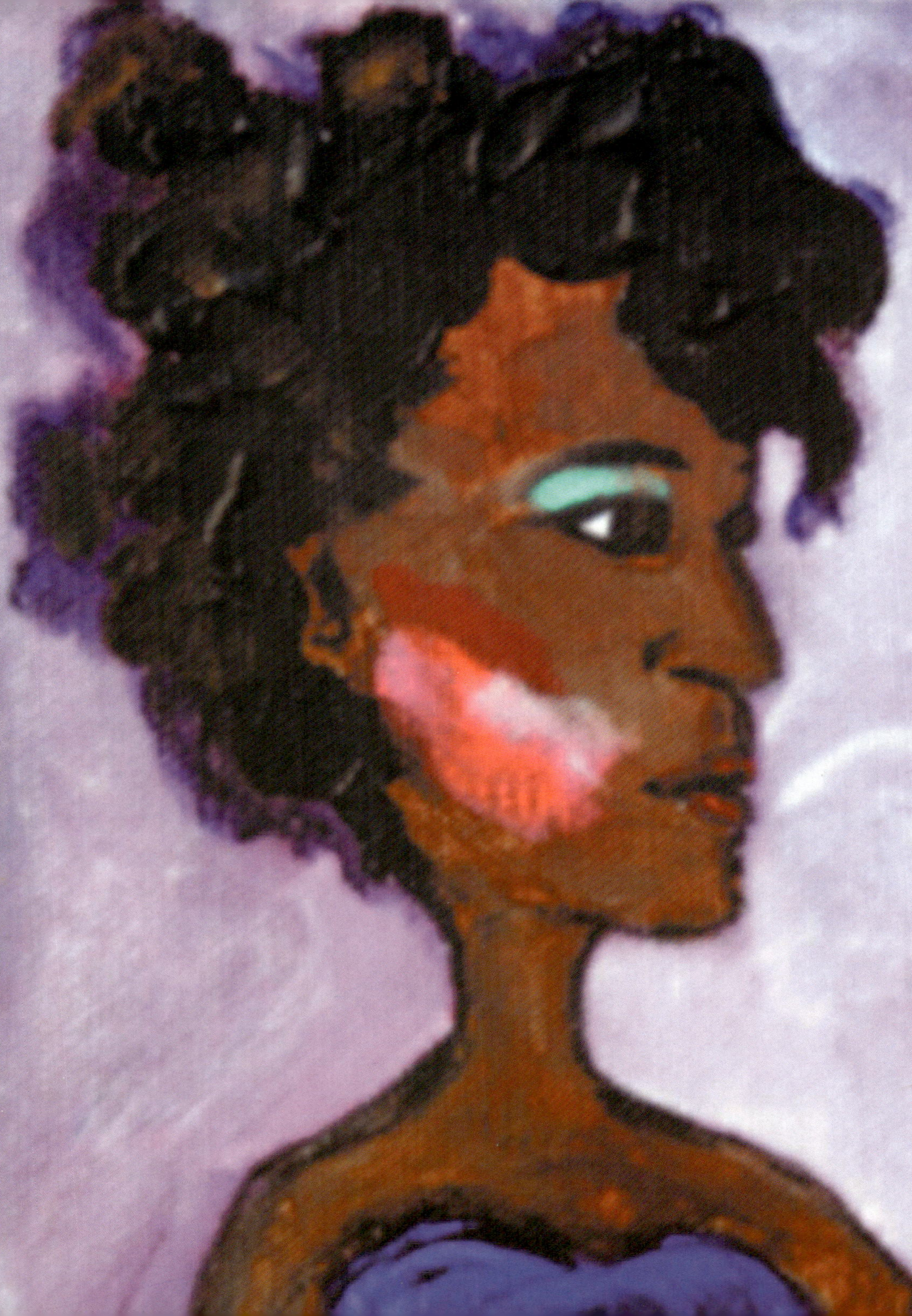

“Hi, my name is
Miss Betty Lee D.

For months now I’ve been
using all the golden keys.

Because of them, I’ve found
the person I used to be!”

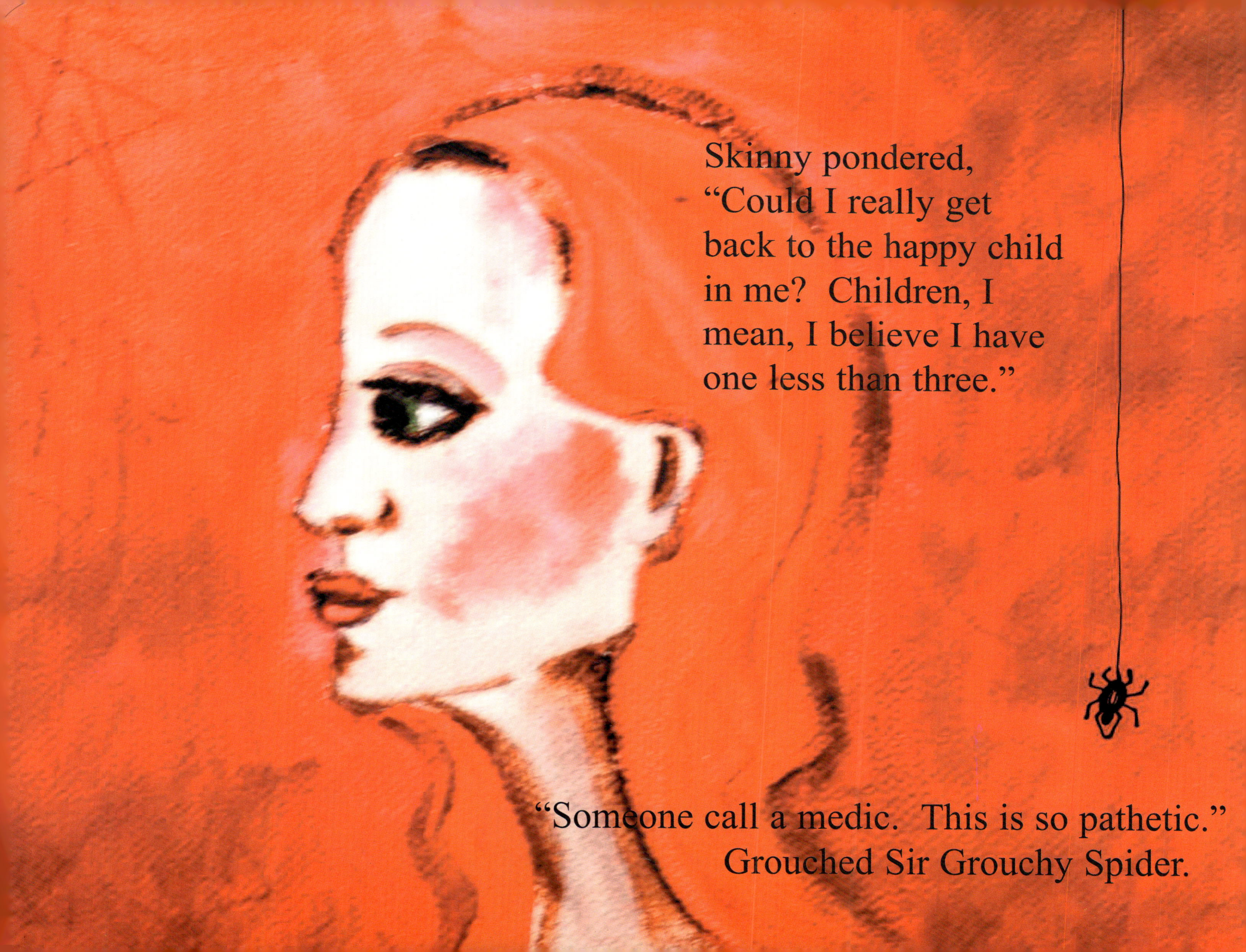

Skinny pondered, "Could I really get back to the happy child in me? Children, I mean, I believe I have one less than three."

"Someone call a medic. This is so pathetic."
Grouched Sir Grouchy Spider.

The hour was up and it was time for all of the Misses to leave. They gave to Skinny Miss S. a glass heart vase and told her it would glow when her heart was filled with her ***inner truth.***

"Oh, my lucky stars! There it is! It's glowed before! Let it glow again!" Skinny's heart was racing as she recognized what it was the Misses were so kind to give. It was the very same glass heart vase from the mysterious book of mysteriously written words that Skinny read in the well! "How could this be! How did you know to give this back to me!?" Skinny asked.

"Oh, Skinny! You are such a trip! From what bottle did you sip?" The Misses looked at her and smiled having no idea they gave her something she had already mystically had at one time in her two little hands.

"This time around I will give my glass heart vase a happy home! I won't take it into anymore dark wells!" Skinny felt secure for the moment even without anything currently in it. Emptiness was not such a bad thing. It meant detachment from all things. To Skinny this thought caused her to carry on joyfully. She had hope that her inner children would return to their heart's home on their own, now that she would take care of it for life.

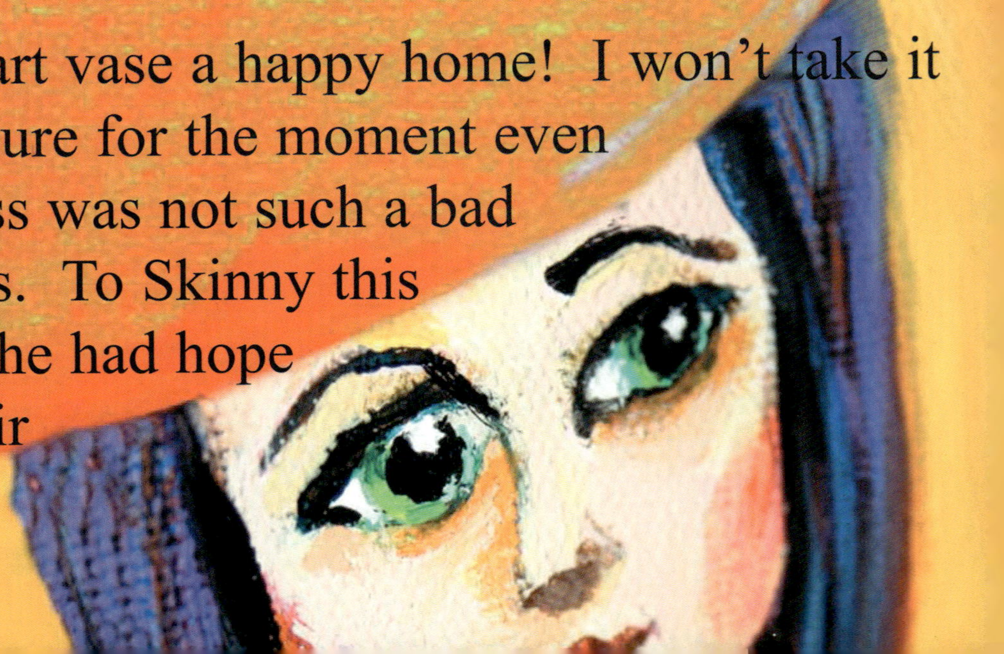

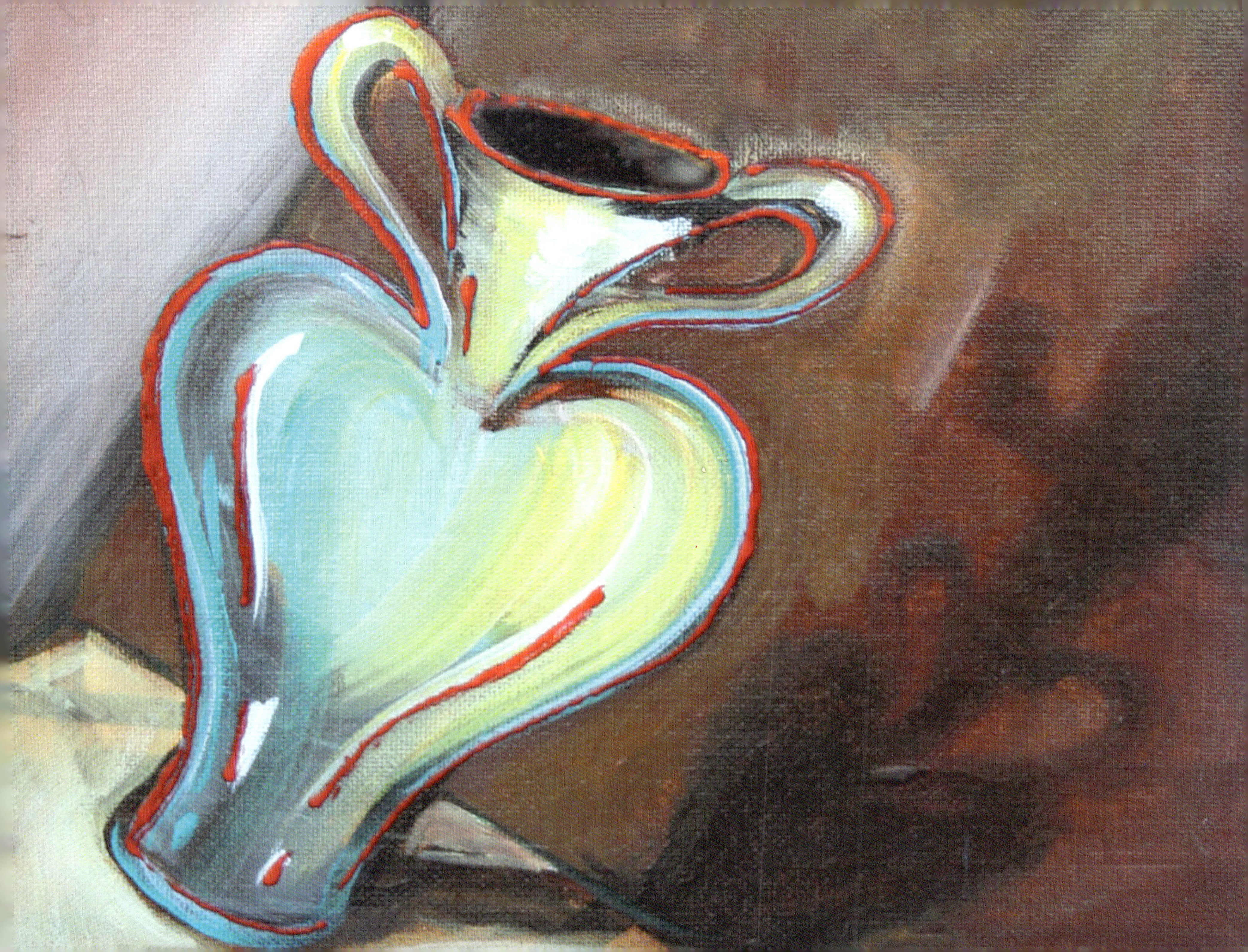

Finally, the Misses all joined in and wrapped up with the

Magical Intelligence Prayer.

"Now I too fit in!" shouted Father Deana Marie.

"Let us lead together." He was learning too.

"May our mentality be strong enough to change the things we are in control of, medicate the things we think we can't control, and the wisdom to follow those directions."

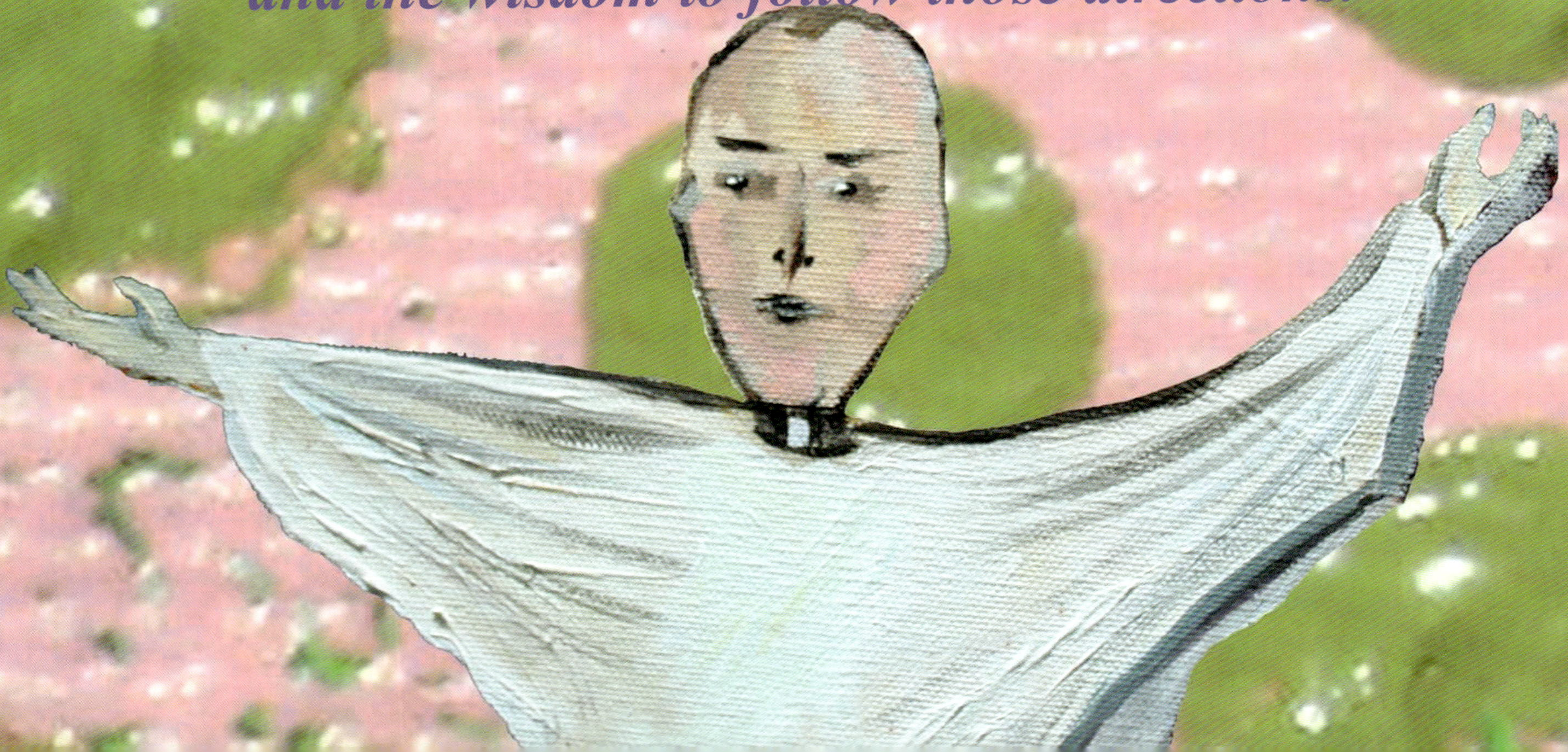

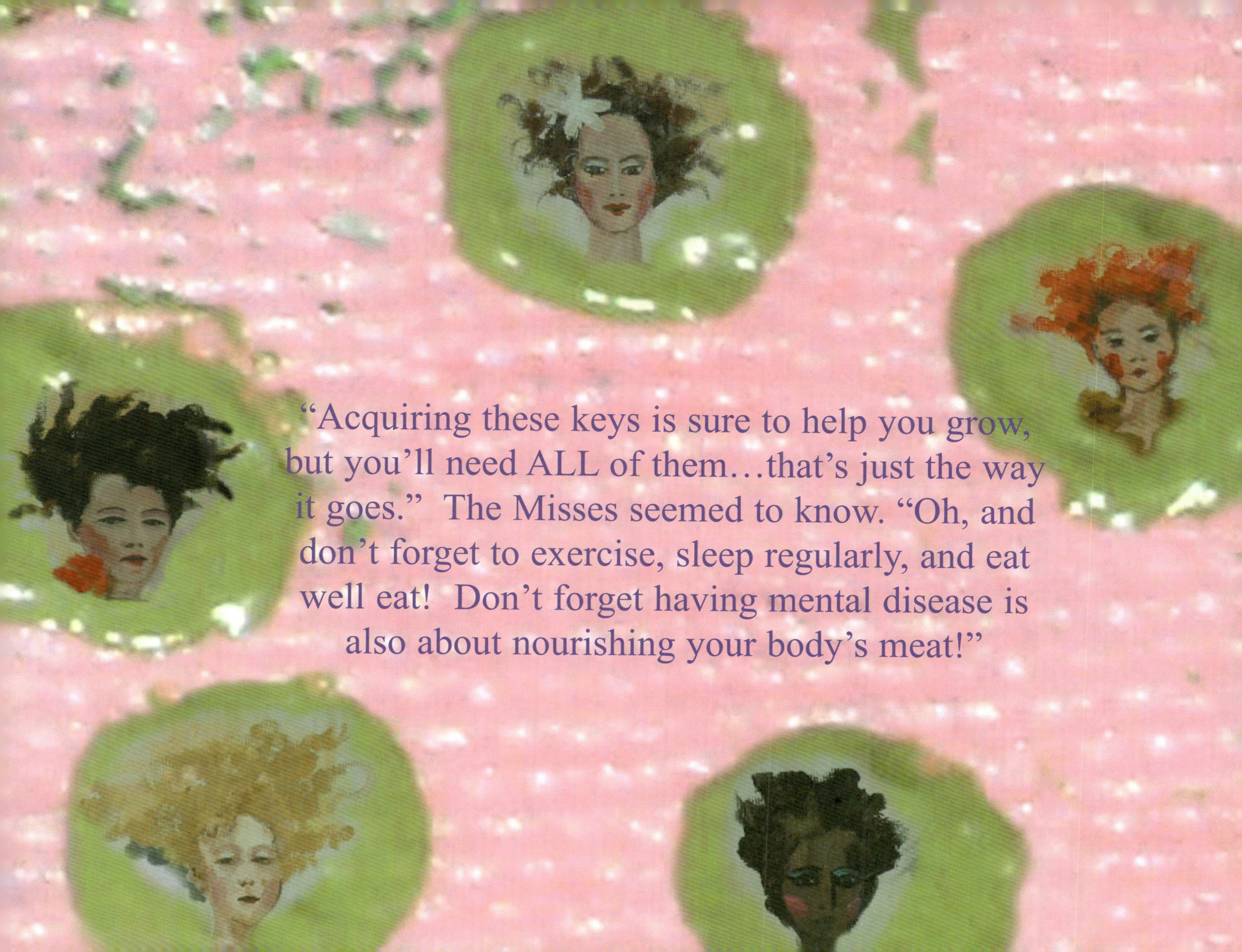

"Acquiring these keys is sure to help you grow, but you'll need ALL of them…that's just the way it goes." The Misses seemed to know. "Oh, and don't forget to exercise, sleep regularly, and eat well eat! Don't forget having mental disease is also about nourishing your body's meat!"

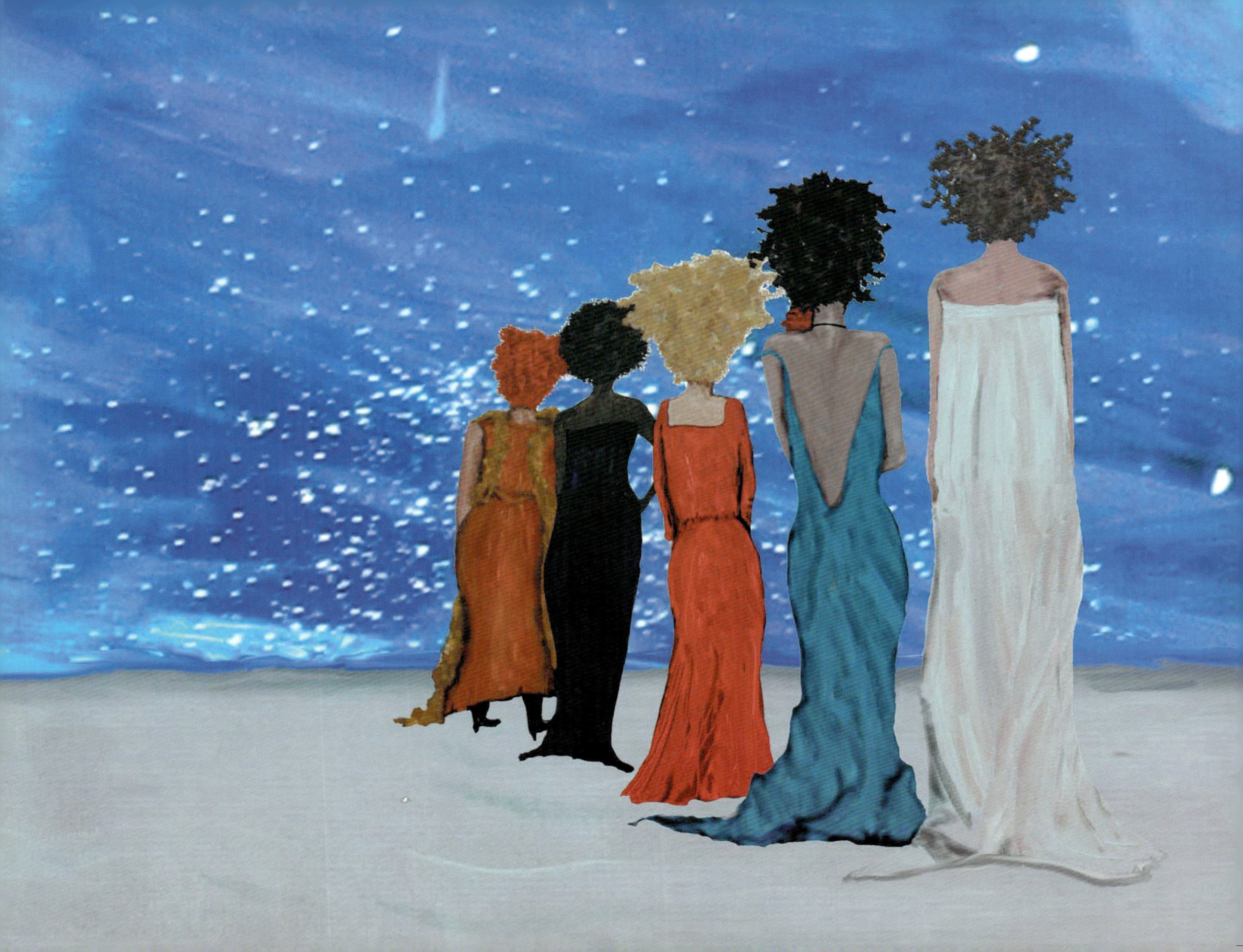

There's always a time in any style of therapy, and this time…time was up. All the Misses hugged each other as they turned to leave. They would be brave and go out into the world practicing what they knew to be their truth without judgment or blame on any other dame.

Skinny Miss S. felt encouraged that she had safe places to visit with her three golden keys.

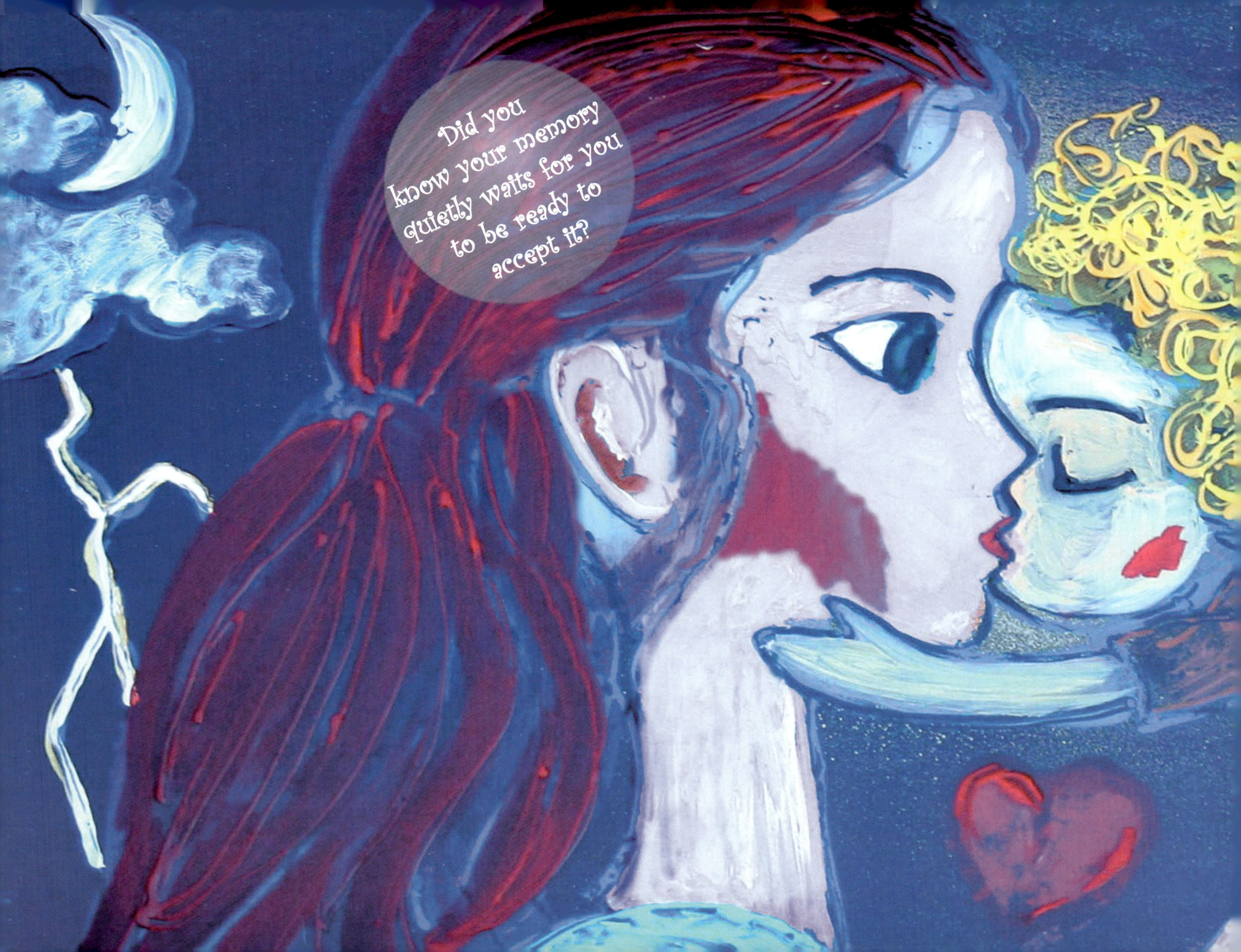
Did you
know your memory
quietly waits for you
to be ready to
accept it?

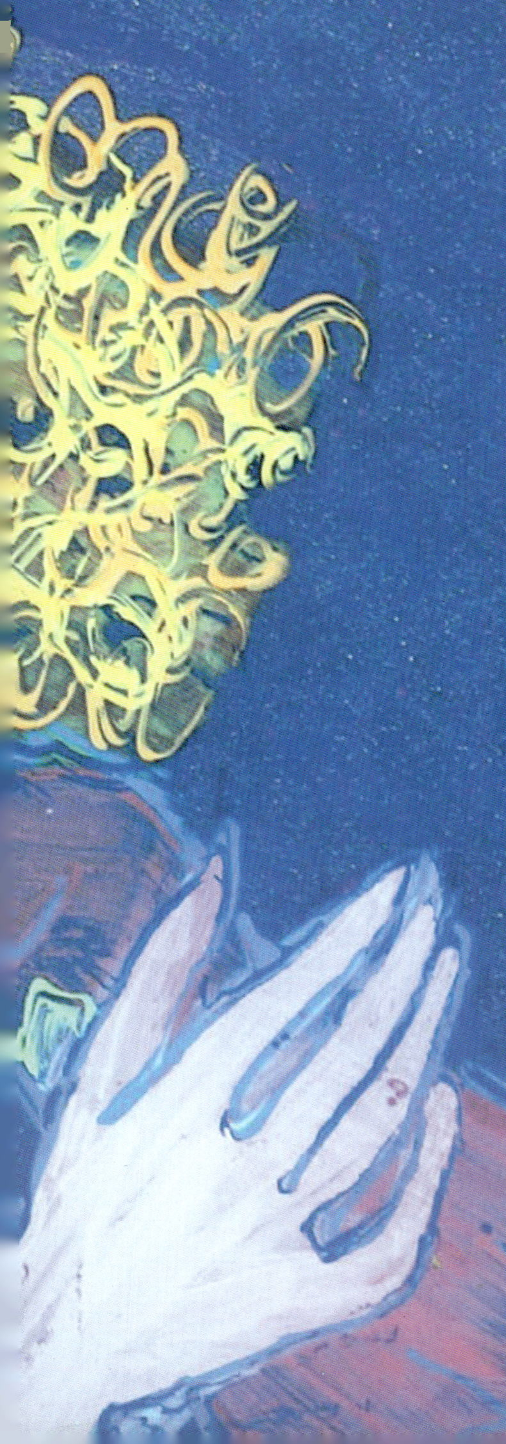

When Skinny Miss S. was all through going through the three golden doors with the three golden keys, she found herself in the great outdoors again. She realized she had forgotten Lonely Miss C. back in therapy. Just then Lonely came out of Merry Miss Humm's door. She was gleaming from ear to ear, but was quiet as a mouse.

Skinny picked Lonely up and gave her a big hug, "Miss Lonely! How was your therapy? Why haven't you said a word?"

"Because I really wasn't being heard." answered Lonely Miss C. "I figure we will talk about your pain when you are fit, not because I have made you do it. I know now that isn't my place. You have to go through your process at your own pace."

doll
noun

1. a small-scale figure of a human being used especially as a child's plaything.

2. a pretty but often empty-headed young woman.

3. an attractive person.

"Thank you, Lonely, for really listening. I'm so very sorry I wasn't ready to face all of those repressed memories that you have had to see alone. In the well I looked at them and they looked at me.

My inner children made it possible for me to feel. We can now talk about them and really heal!

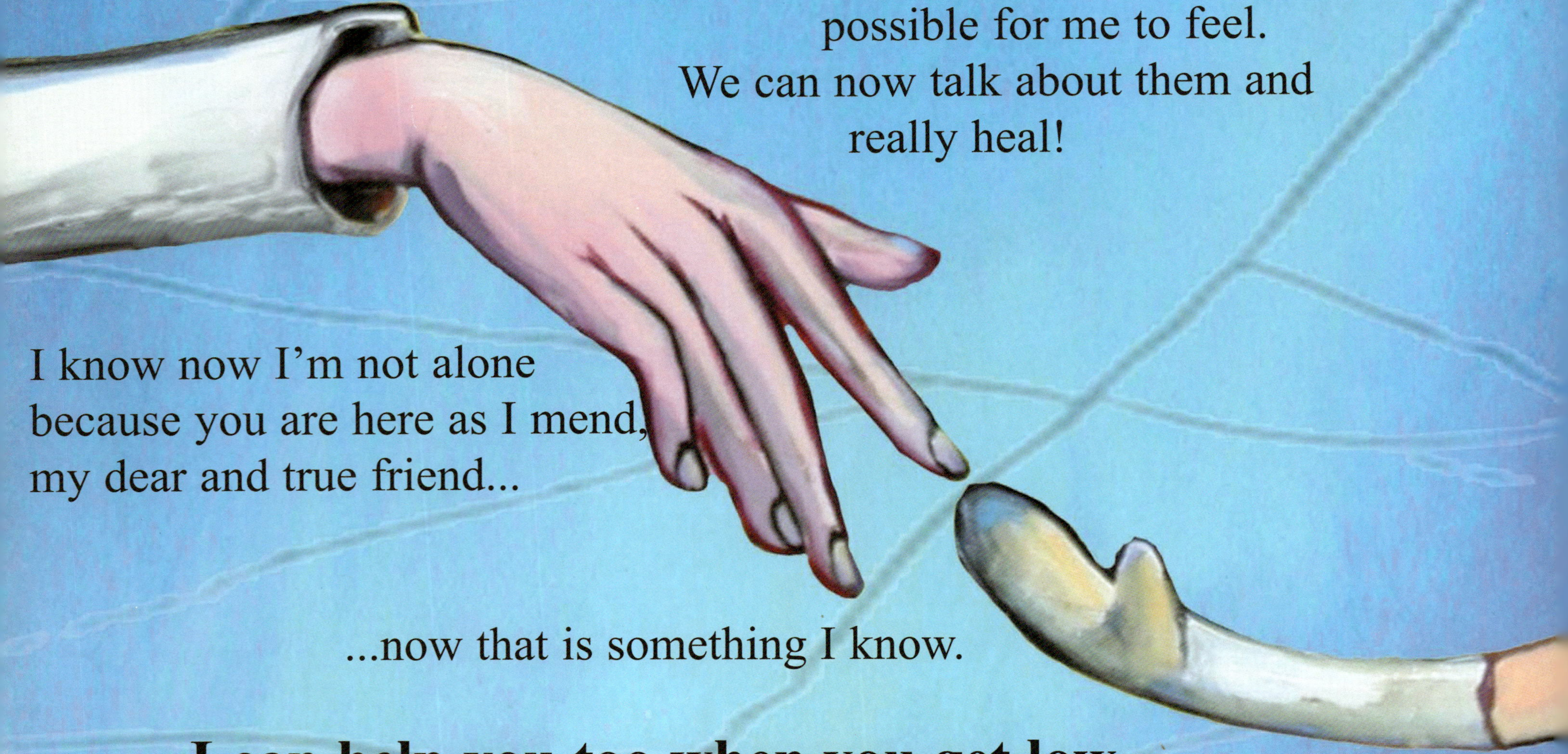

I know now I'm not alone because you are here as I mend, my dear and true friend...

...now that is something I know.

I can help you too when you get low.

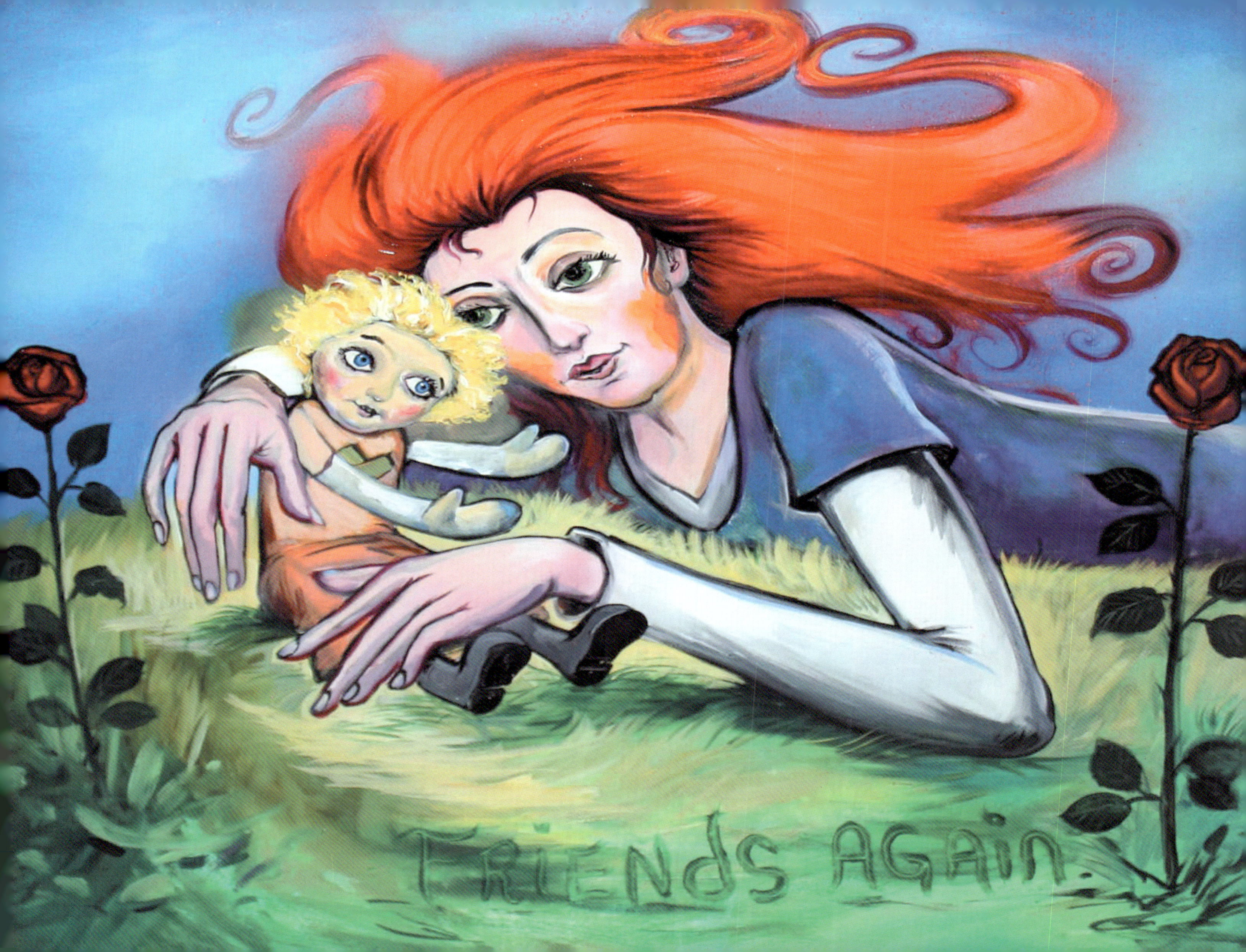
FRIENDS AGAIN.

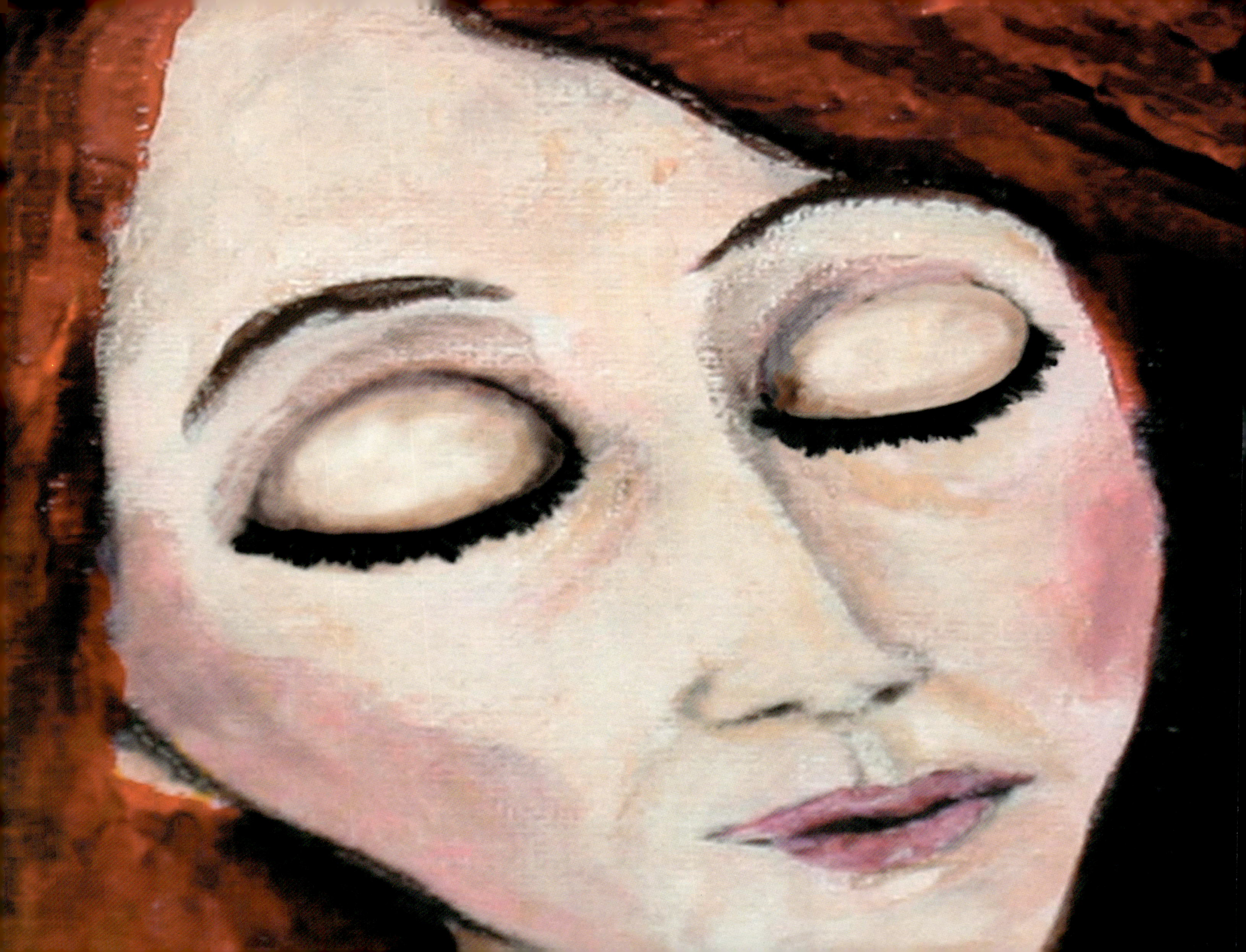

She closed her eyes

to thank whoever was listening

for getting her this far.

She was **grateful**

that she had **friends**

who cared for her so.

Did you know your future can be your favorite plan?

When she was finished she opened her eyes...

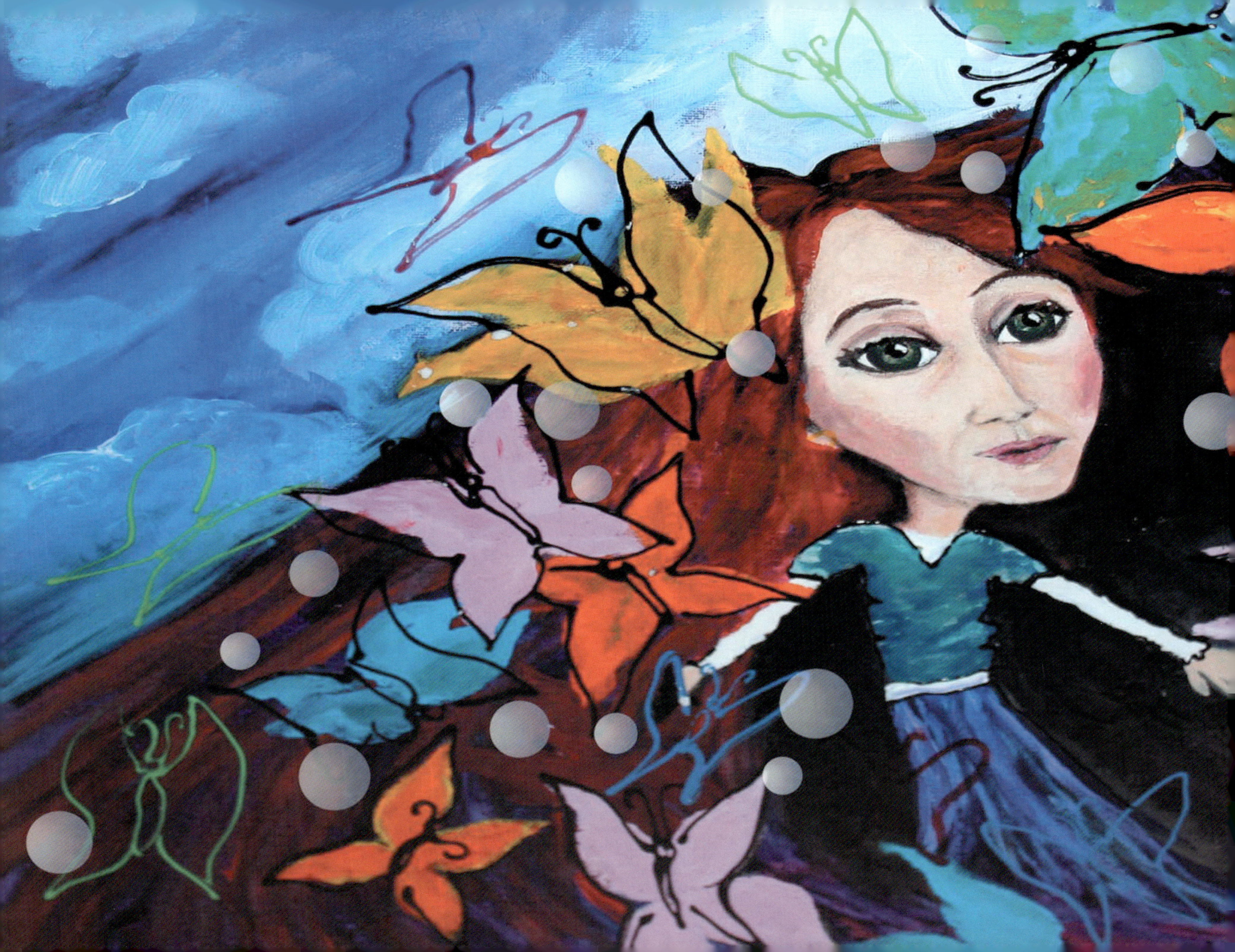

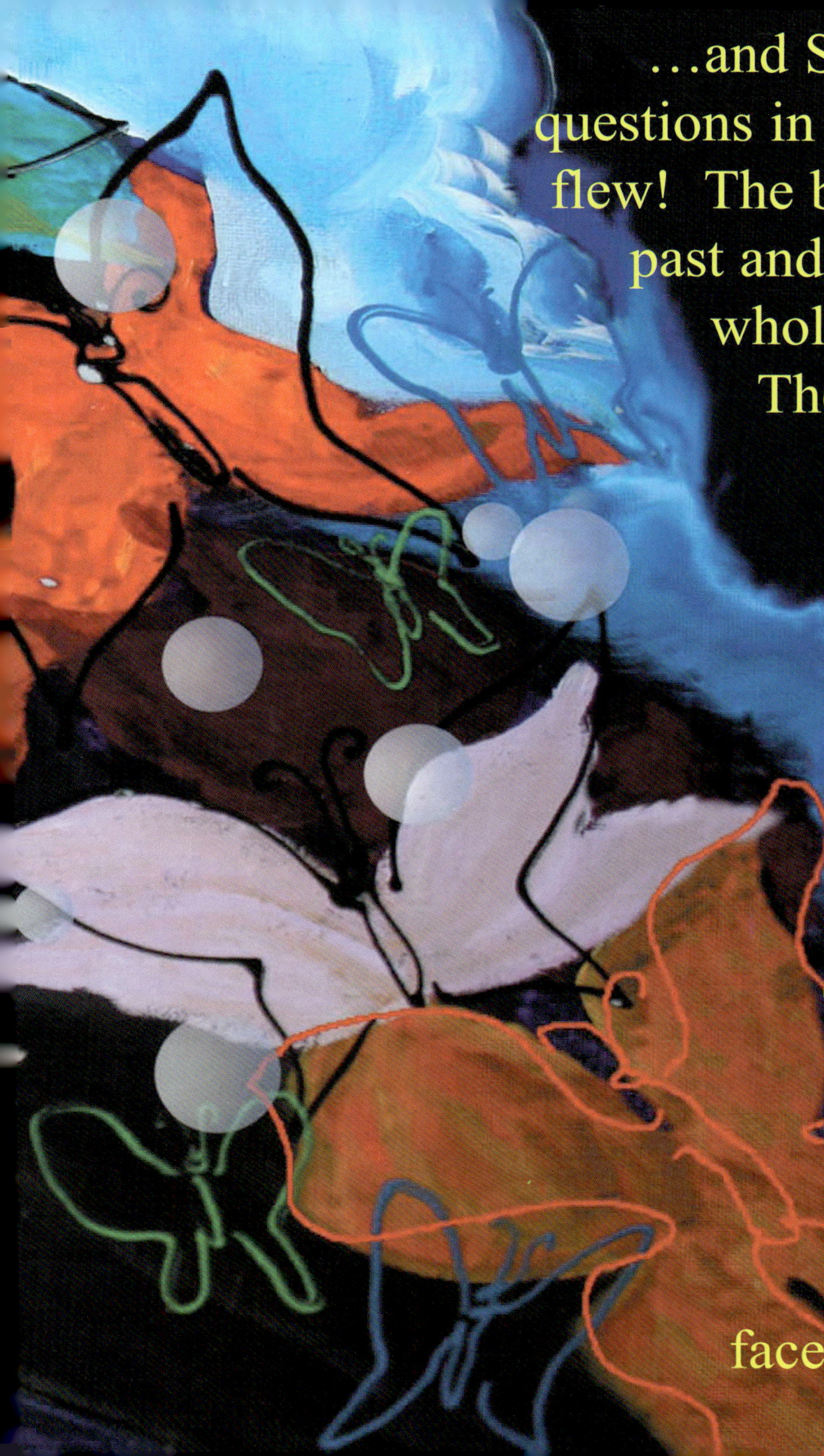

…and SAW THE BUTTERFLIES! Surrounded by questions in bubbles, yes, they were! Free as ideas they flew! The bubbles traveled throughout the pages of her past and she began to remember they were there the whole way, just not as clear and helpful as today. They must have come clear from her gratitude which shifted her attitude.

The butterflies flew around her head as she admired their colors…
colors she remembered a long time ago.
Each one swooped down to kiss
her on her eyes, nose and toes.

They continued to flutter and Skinny looked up as Lonely's true mother, "Look at the colors, Lonely Miss C. Pinch me and tell me this is not just a tease!" Lonely picked her chin up and her face lit up bright. Her eyes danced with delight.

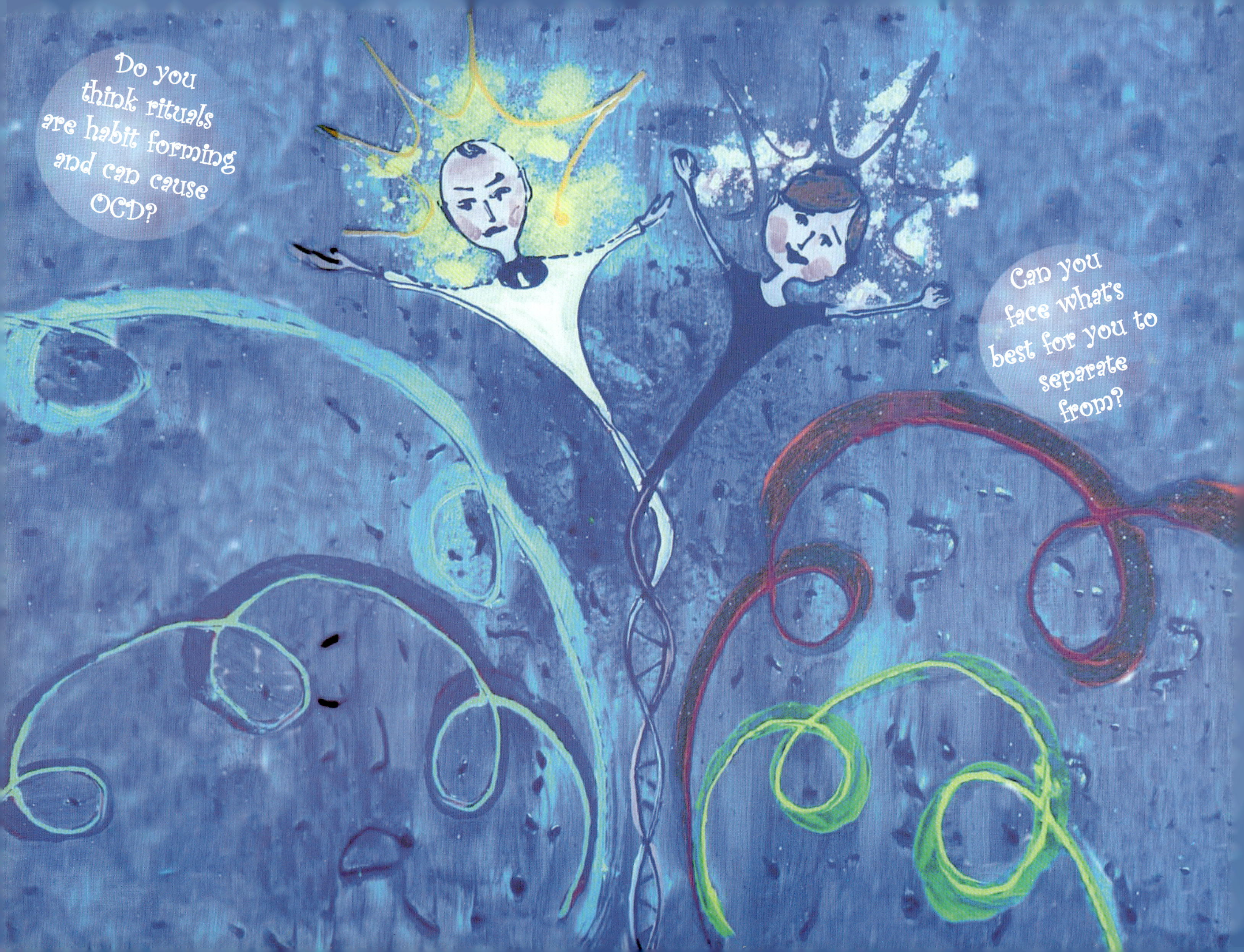
Do you think rituals are habit forming and can cause OCD?
Can you face what's best for you to separate from?

Dean Doll was ecstatic and Skinny yelled out, "Color me **TRUE!** I no longer want the lie in you!" and Skinny promised to separate the two. Like a division of a knife between Dean Doll and Father Deana Marie, the colors ran through.

"I've never imagined such fabulous hues-
Oranges and yellows, purples and blues!"
... and the ONE became TWO!!

Did you know you can wish and dream of colors unseen?

The colors were powerful and even came over Father Dean Marie's black and white robed costume. He was now as colorful a person as everyone else. Dean Doll kept what was under their skirt, and Father Dean Marie decided the doctrine of the Church didn't let him be the woman he truly wanted to always be.

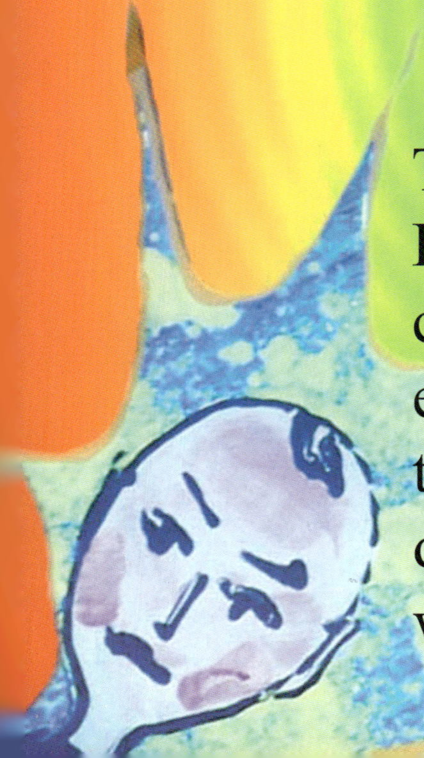

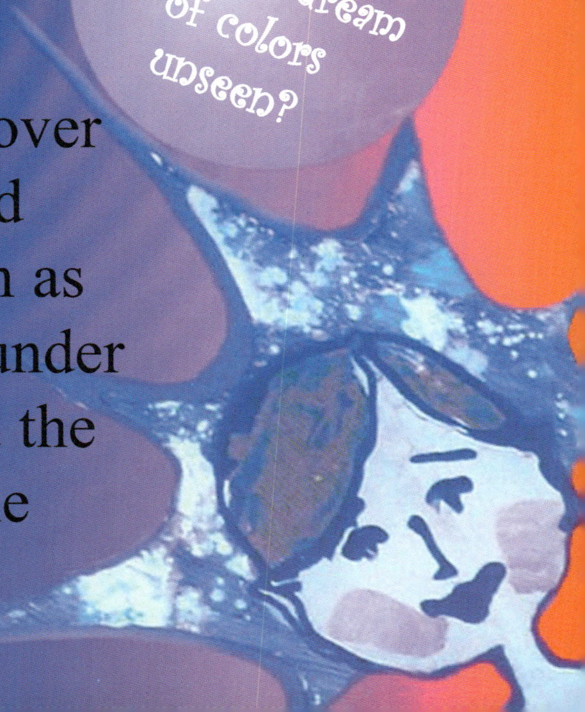

"Should we consult the tarot cards to see why the butterflies are here?" asked Father Deana Marie filled with fear. He thought maybe who he wanted to be wasn't **right.**

"There is no reason to fear Father Deana Marie. It just means we are all finally free! We are free because we have taken responsibility to be the **change** we want to see."

Because of the colors even Skinny's tarot readings weren't as important as before. She wasn't as insecure to have to know all that much more.

Did you know that a religion that is not true to YOU will not suit you?

While Father watched the butterflies go by, Dean Doll accepted every color in the sky.

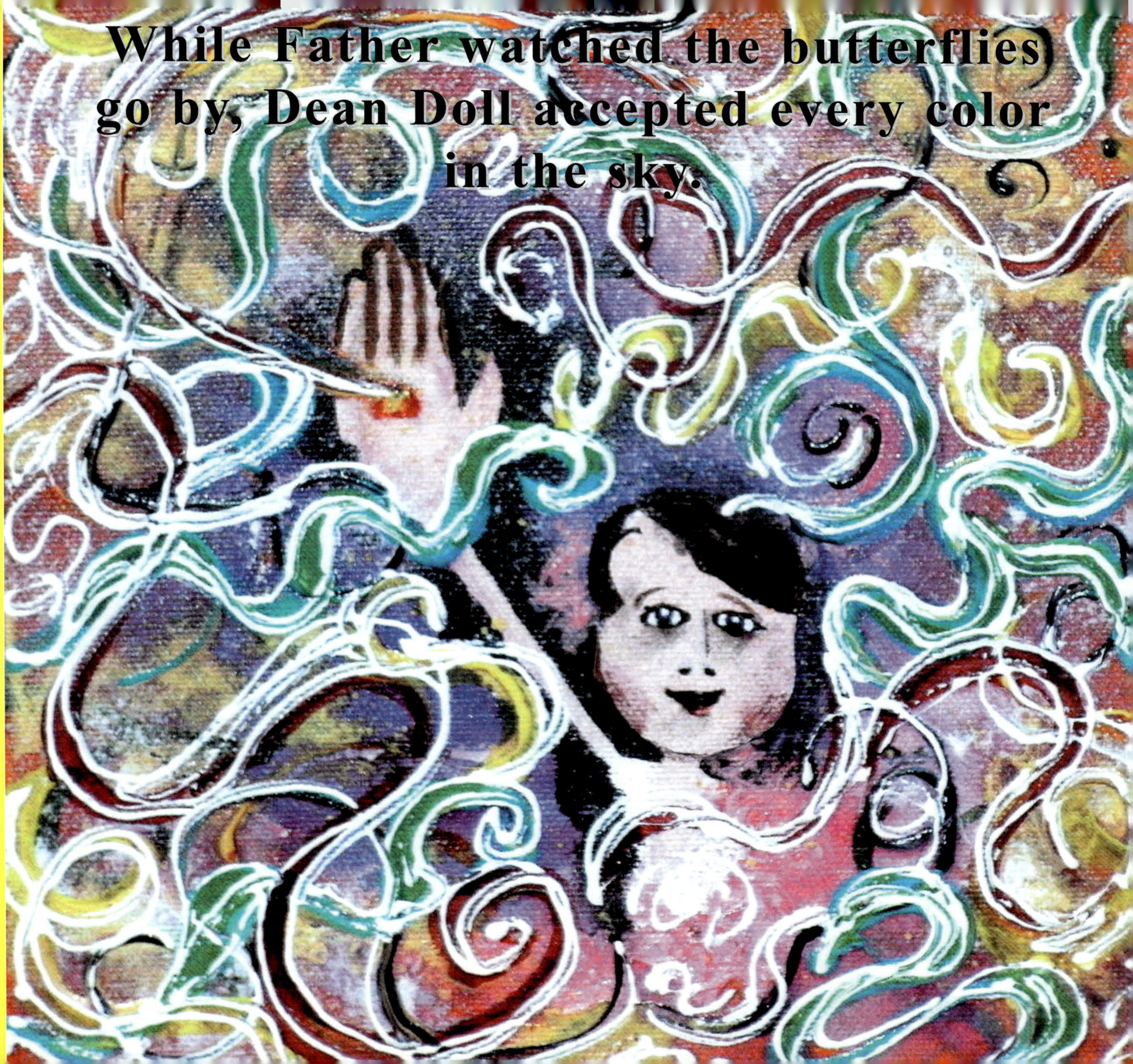

individuality

noun

1. total character peculiar to and distinguishing an individual from others.

2. the quality or state of being indivisible.

3. separate or distinct existence.

4. INDIVIDUAL.

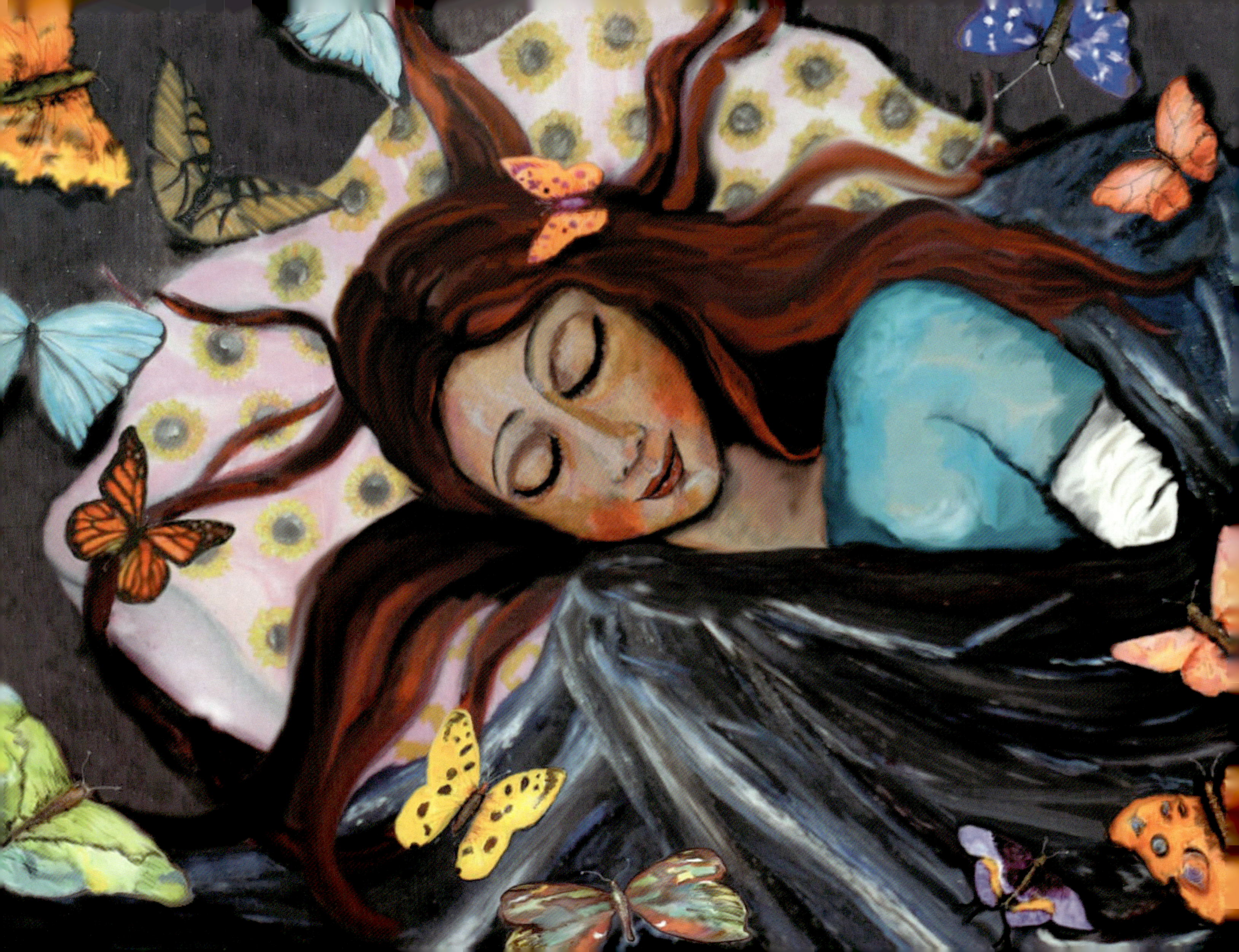

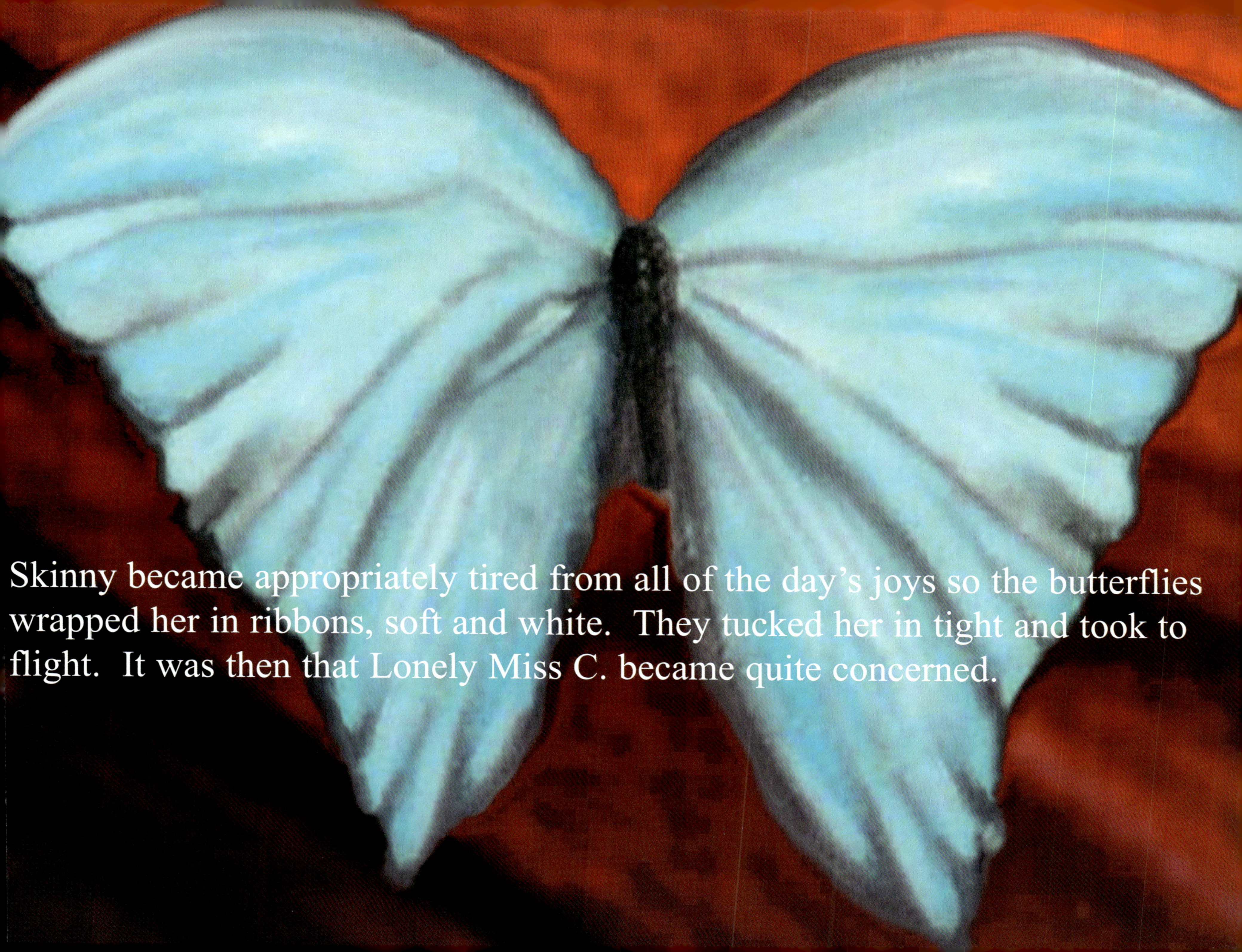

Skinny became appropriately tired from all of the day's joys so the butterflies wrapped her in ribbons, soft and white. They tucked her in tight and took to flight. It was then that Lonely Miss C. became quite concerned.

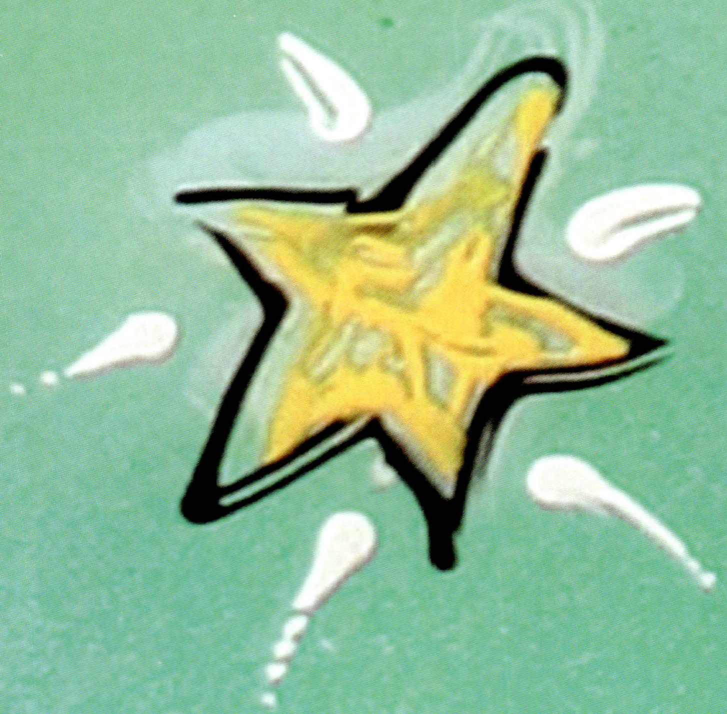

"Don't go to sleep like yesterday.
I like you much better as you are today.

What if the colors fade or take a holiday?
It's your responsibility to not run away!

Why, why, why,

my Skinny Miss S. were you oh so gray
having no colors inside until today?"

Lonely Miss C. was frightened again.
She didn't think Skinny's joy would sustain.

joy

noun

1. the emotion evoked by well-being, success, or good fortune or by the prospect of possessing what one desires.

2. delight, the expression or exhibition of such emotion.

3. gaiety, a state of happiness or felicity.

4. bliss, a source or cause of delight.

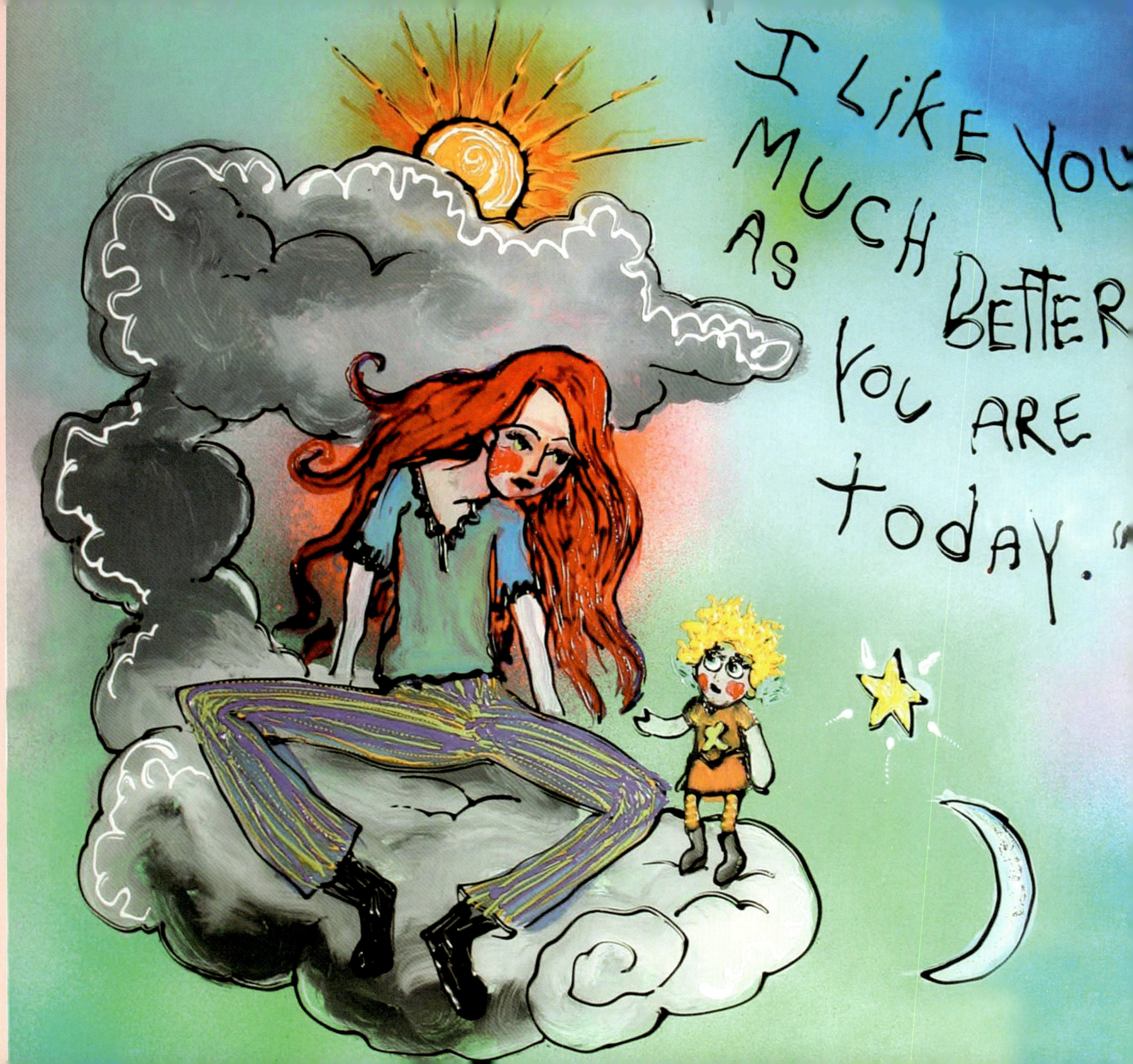

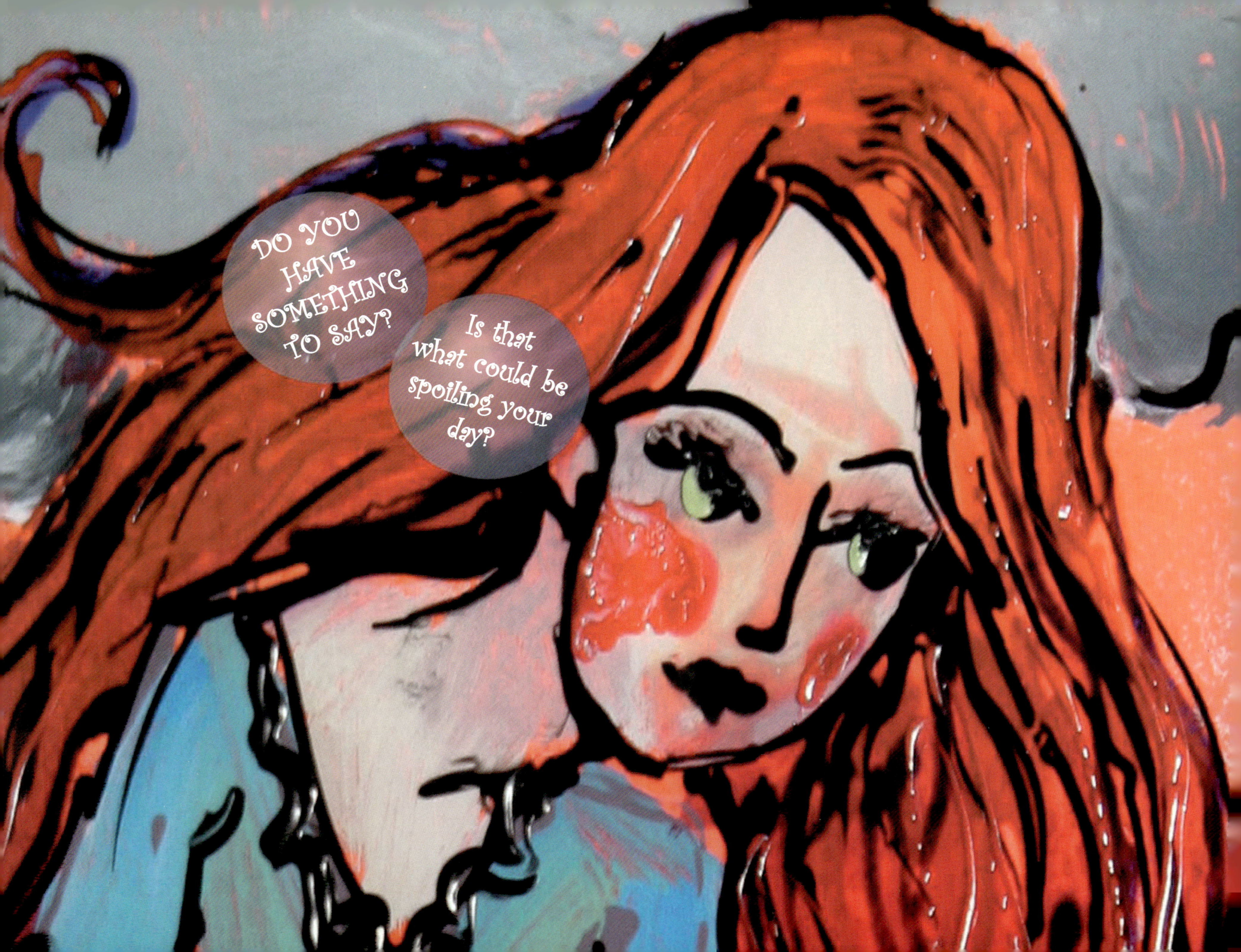
DO YOU HAVE SOMETHING TO SAY?
Is that what could be spoiling your day?

dream
noun

1. a series of thoughts, images, or emotions occurring during sleep.

2. an experience of waking life having the characteristics of a dream; *as a visionary creation of the imagination, a state of mind marked by abstraction or release from reality.*

3. something notable for its beauty, excellence, or enjoyable quality; *the new car is a dream to operate.*

4. a strongly desired goal or purpose; *a dream of becoming president.*

5. something that fully satisfies a wish; *a meal that was a gourmet's dream.*

"I'm not really sure. I don't think there is just one cure. I mostly had anger that needed to be expressed and explored. It made me sick, took over my brain and made this dress a mess!

I must have had **something to say,** and that's okay. It comes to using my voice each and every day…"

Skinny was so happy that Lonely and she were friends again, although she still needed to be heard. "Now Lonely Miss C., excuse me.

I know we are a team, but it's high time I sleep, not to escape, but to dream!" Lonely felt better after hearing the strength in Skinny's reply.

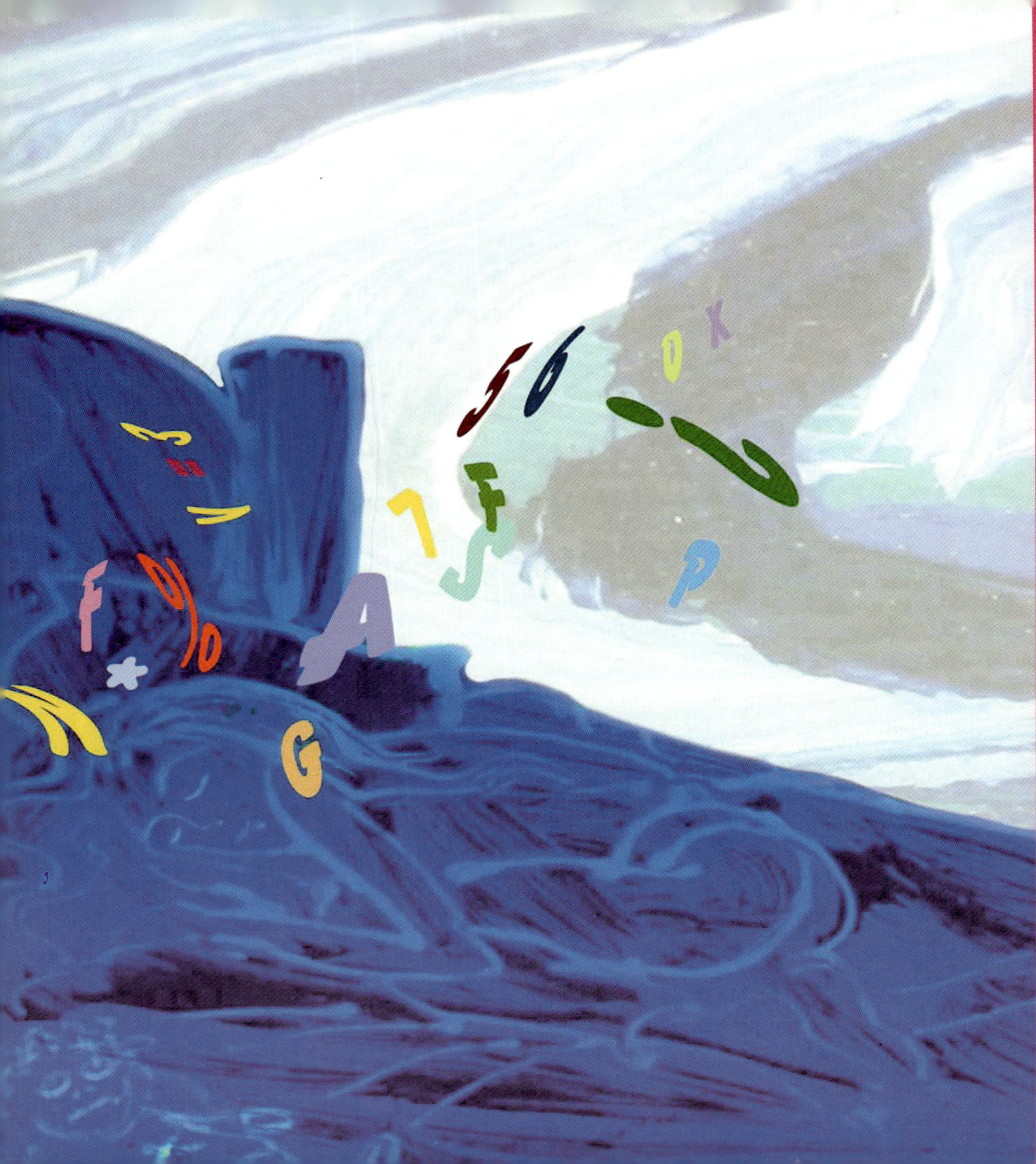

formula

noun

1. a set form of words for use in a ceremony or ritual, a conventionalized statement intended to express some fundamental truth or principle especially as a basis for negotiation or action.

2. RECIPE, PRESCRIPTION: a milk mixture or substitute for feeding an infant.

3. a general fact, rule, or principle expressed in usually mathematical symbols, a symbolic expression of the chemical composition or constitution of a substance, a group of symbols (as letters and numbers) associated to express facts or data (as the number and kinds of teeth in the jaw), a combination of signs in a logical calculus.

4. a customary or set form or method allowing little room for originality.

Skinny Miss S. fell fast asleep. In her dream she was surrounded by letters, numbers, and symbols of some sort. She began to add things up in her head, then suddenly woke up and said, "There is a formula for beating depression:

Doctor + Therapist + Support Group = DTS

(Depression Treated Successfully)!

All of her dolls agreed and knew the three golden keys had planted a seed.

What is your formula which solves the problem in you?

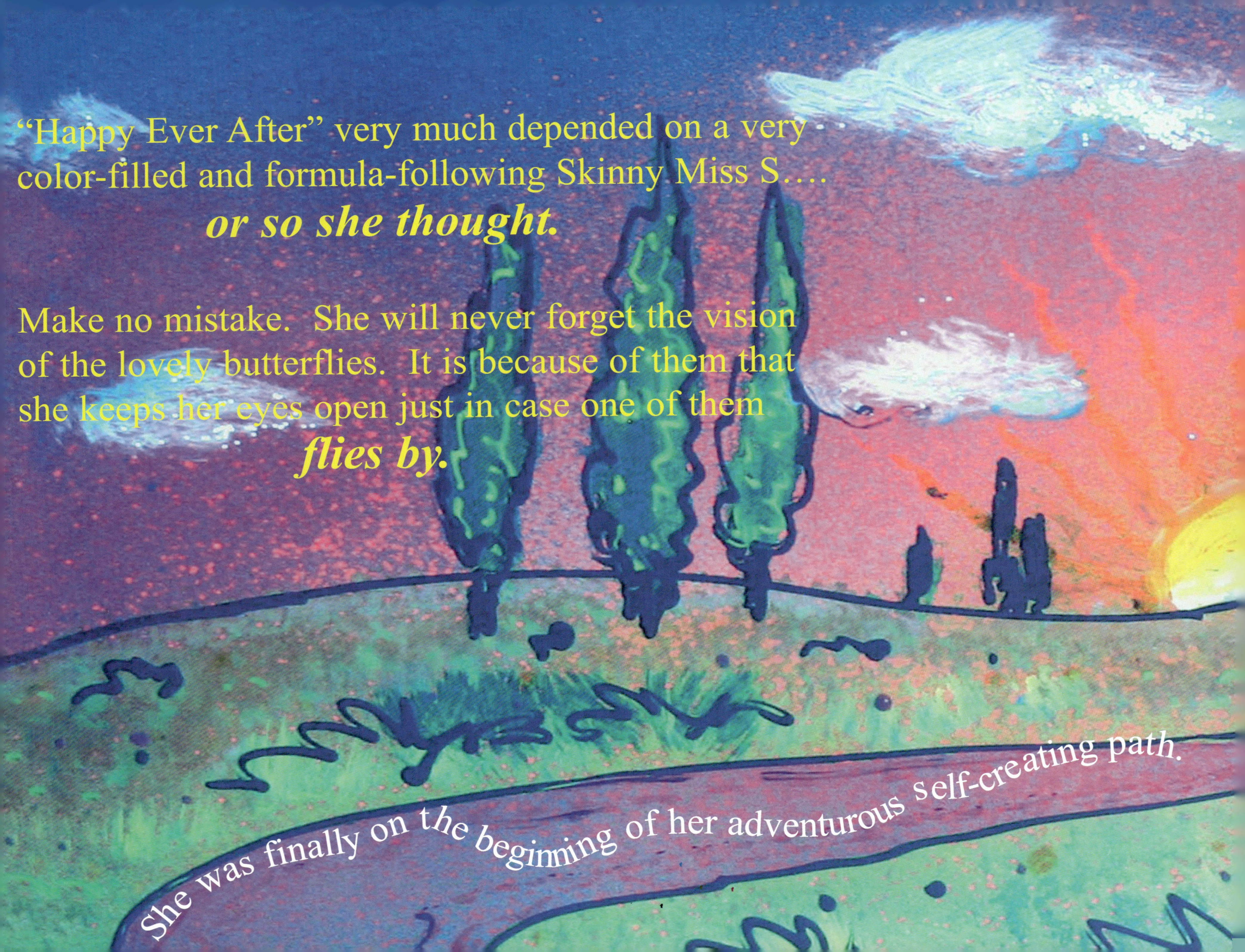

"Happy Ever After" very much depended on a very color-filled and formula-following Skinny Miss S….

or so she thought.

Make no mistake. She will never forget the vision of the lovely butterflies. It is because of them that she keeps her eyes open just in case one of them

flies by.

She was finally on the beginning of her adventurous self-creating path.

It was also because of them she had to send
Sir Grouchy Spider away.
She feared his webs would catch one and this
she could not have bared.

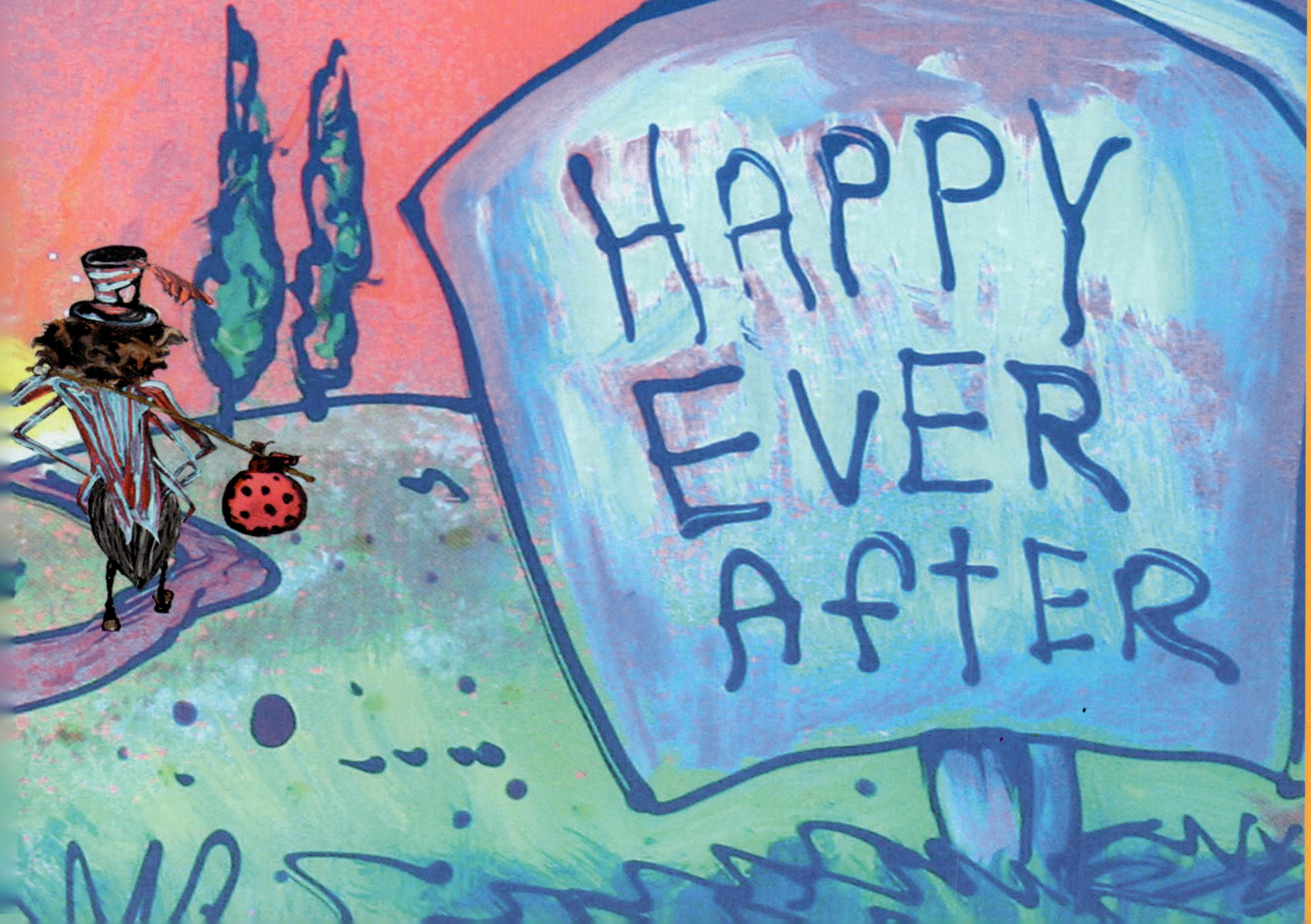

adventure
noun

1. an undertaking usually involving danger and unknown risks, the encountering of risks; *the spirit of adventure.*
2. an exciting or remarkable experience; *an adventure in exotic dining.*

hyporcrisy
noun

1. a pretense of having a virtuous character, moral or religious beliefs or principles, etc., that one does not really possess.

2. a pretense of having some desirable or publicly approved attitude.

3. an act or instance of hypocrisy.

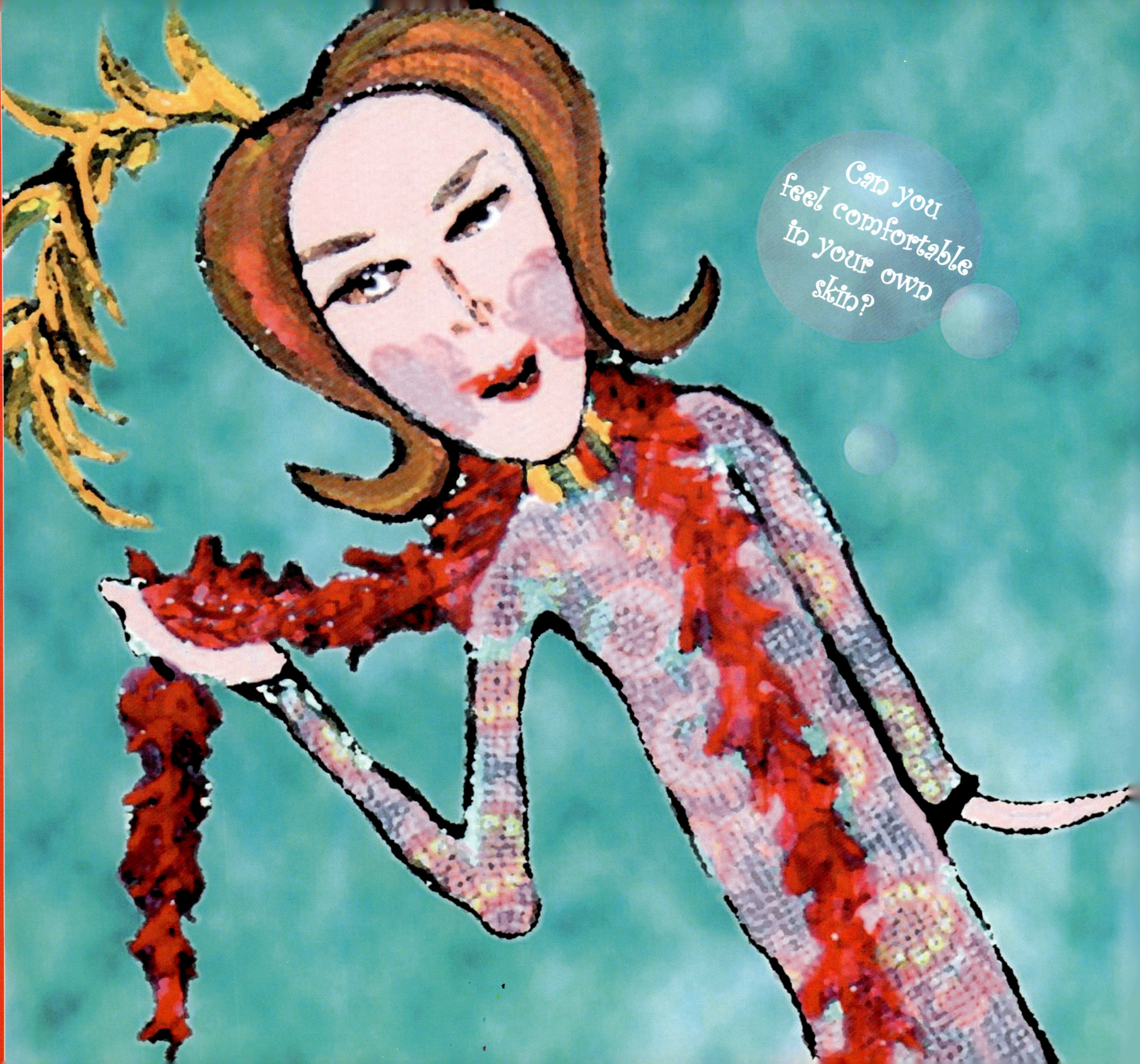

It was Dean Doll who placed the dare and Father Deana Marie who accepted as he dropped the 'Father' and removed his collar; the hypocrisy was something greater than just a bother. He grabbed Dean Doll's boa feather instead and stuck on a fabulous feather in the wig on his head and wisely said, "Never let anyone say you're different, Skinny Miss S., just because you aren't cookie cutter like them! When you go to get dressed, do it for yourself. Put something on that expresses your mood or better yet stand in the nude!

Consider yourself blessed.

You've
come out
of
your
mess!"

DIAGNOSTIC CRITERIA FOR:

Gender Identity ~~Disorder~~

A. A strong and persistent cross-gender identification (not merely a desire for any perceived cultural advantages of being the other sex). In children, the disturbance is manifested by four (or more) of the following: (1) repeatedly stated desire to be, or insistence that he or she is, the other sex (2) in boys, preference for cross-dressing or simulating female attire; in girls, insistence on wearing only stereotypical masculine clothing (3) strong and persistent preferences for cross-sex roles in make-believe play or persistent fantasies of being the other sex (4) intense desire to participate in the stereotypical games and pastimes of the other sex (5) strong preference for playmates of the other sex. In adolescents and adults, the disturbance is manifested by symptoms such as a stated desire to be the other sex, frequent passing as the other sex, desire to live or be treated as the other sex, or the conviction that he or she has the typical feelings and reactions of the other sex. B. Persistent discomfort with his or her sex or sense of inappropriateness in the gender role of that sex. In children, the disturbance is manifested by any of the following: in boys, assertion that his penis or testes are disgusting or will disappear or assertion that it would be better not to have a penis, or aversion toward rough-and-tumble play and rejection of male stereotypical toys, games, and activities; in girls, rejection of urinating in a sitting position, assertion that she has or will grow a penis, or assertion that she does not want to grow breasts or menstruate, or marked aversion toward normative feminine clothing.

In adolescents and adults, the disturbance is manifested by symptoms such as preoccupation with getting rid of primary and secondary sex characteristics (e.g., request for hormones, surgery, or other procedures to physically alter sexual characteristics to simulate the other sex) or belief that he or she was born the wrong sex. C. The disturbance is not concurrent with a physical intersex condition. D. The disturbance causes clinically significant distress or impairment in social, occupational, or other important areas of functioning.[23]

Why is "Transgender" in the DSM-IV-R?

transgender (from Latin) derivatives [trans-combination form meaning across, beyond, through] and [gender- meaning kind or sort] is a general term applied to a variety of individuals, behaviors, and groups involving tendencies that diverge from the normative gender role (woman or man) commonly, but not always, assigned at birth, as well as the role traditionally held by society.

Transgender is the state of one's "gender identity" (self-identification as woman, man, or neither) not matching one's "assigned sex" (identification by others as male or female based on physical/genetic sex). "Transgender" does not imply any specific form of sexual orientation; transgender people may identify as heterosexual, homosexual, bisexual, pansexual, polysexual, or asexual. The precise definition for transgender remains in flux, but includes:

- "Of, relating to, or designating a person whose identity does not conform unambiguously to conventional notions of male or female gender roles, but combines or moves between these."
- "People who were assigned a sex, usually at birth and based on their genitals, but who feel that this is a false or incomplete description of themselves."
- "Non-identification with, or non-presentation as, the sex (and assumed gender) one was assigned at birth."[24]

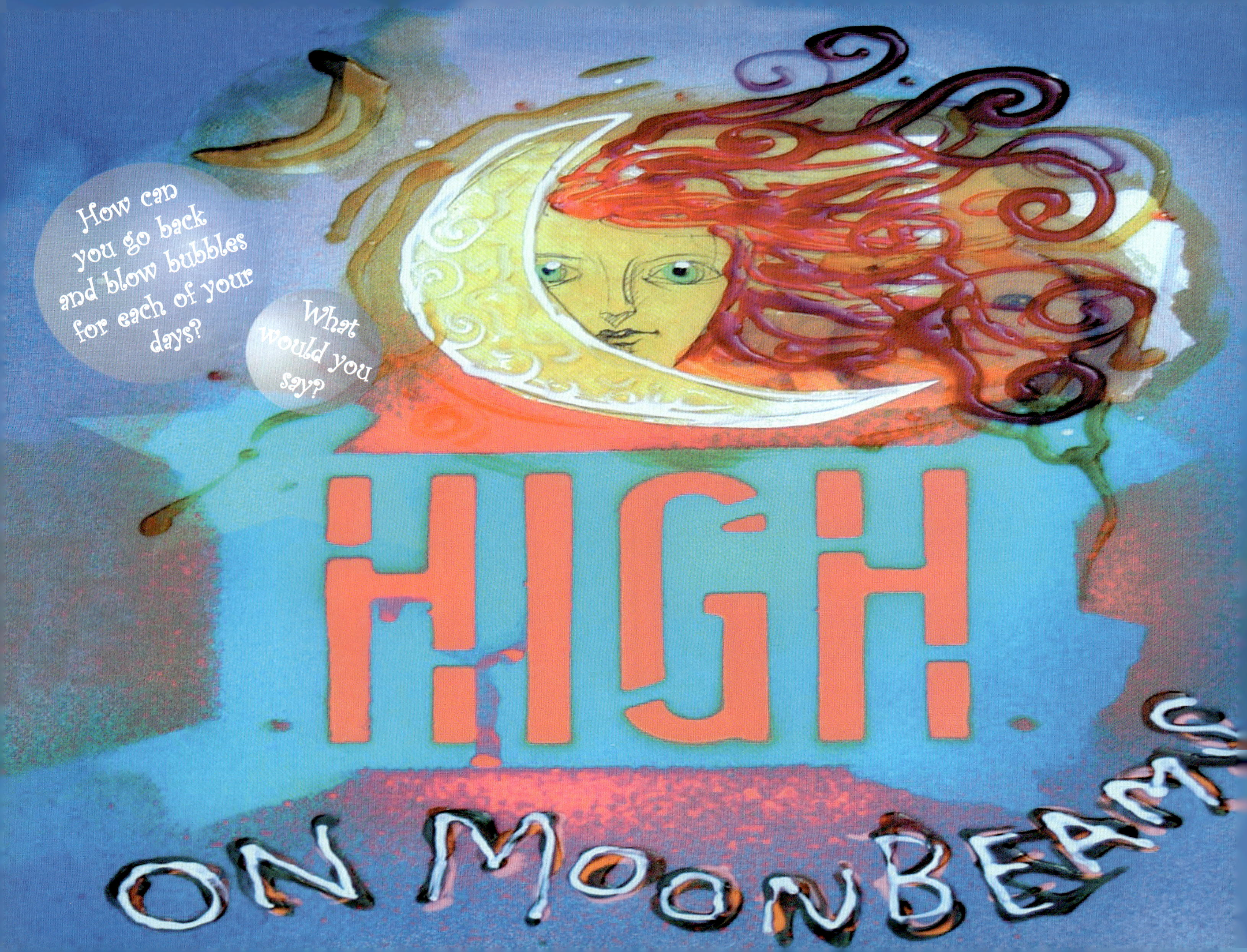
How can you go back and blow bubbles for each of your days?
What would you say?
HIGH
ON MOONBEAMS

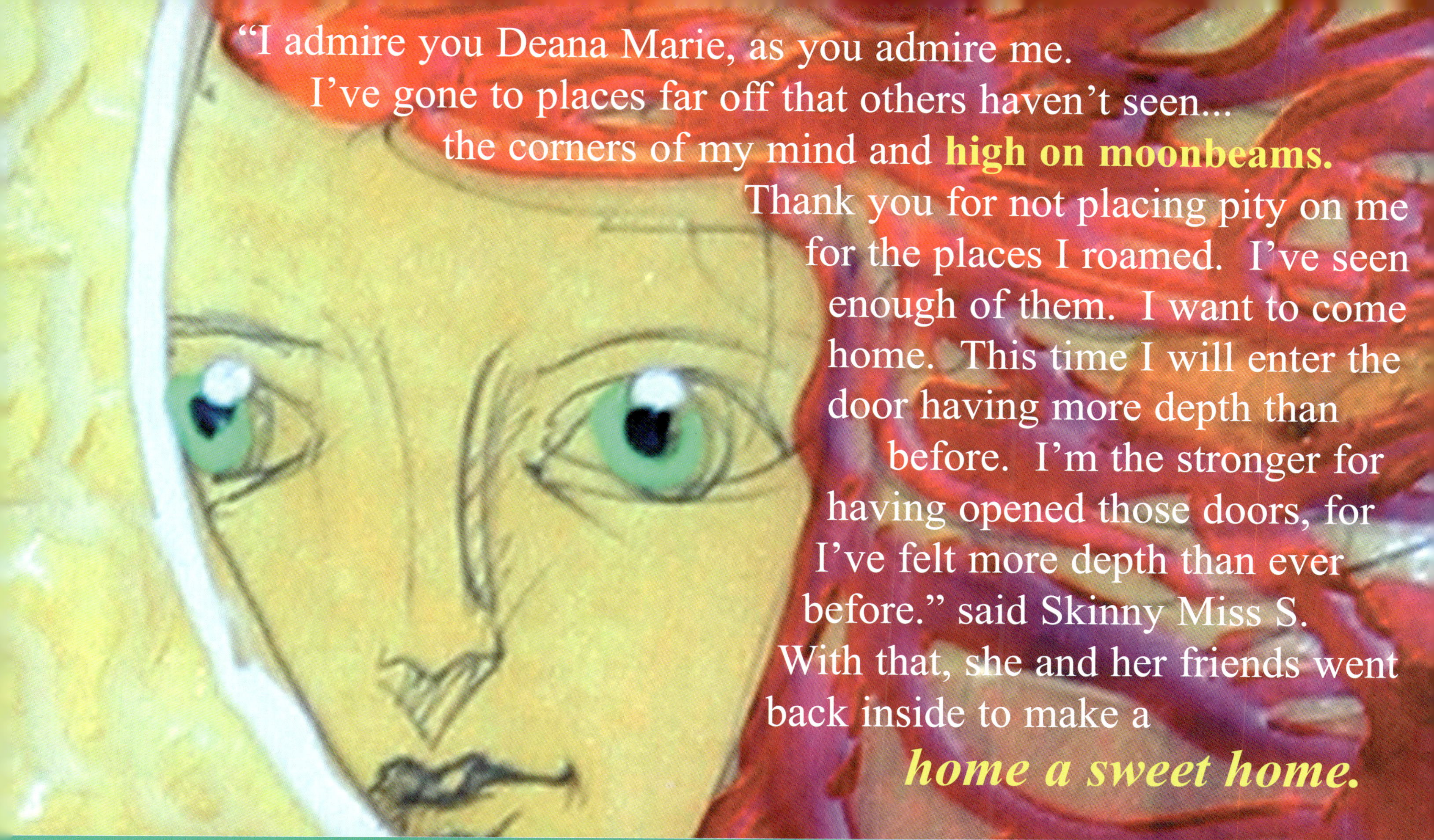

"I admire you Deana Marie, as you admire me.
I've gone to places far off that others haven't seen...
the corners of my mind and **high on moonbeams.**
Thank you for not placing pity on me for the places I roamed. I've seen enough of them. I want to come home. This time I will enter the door having more depth than before. I'm the stronger for having opened those doors, for I've felt more depth than ever before." said Skinny Miss S. With that, she and her friends went back inside to make a

home a sweet home.

home
noun

1. a house, apartment, or other shelter that is the usual residence of a person, family, or household.

2. an institution for the homeless, sick, etc.; *a nursing home.*

3. any place of residence or refuge; *a heavenly home.*

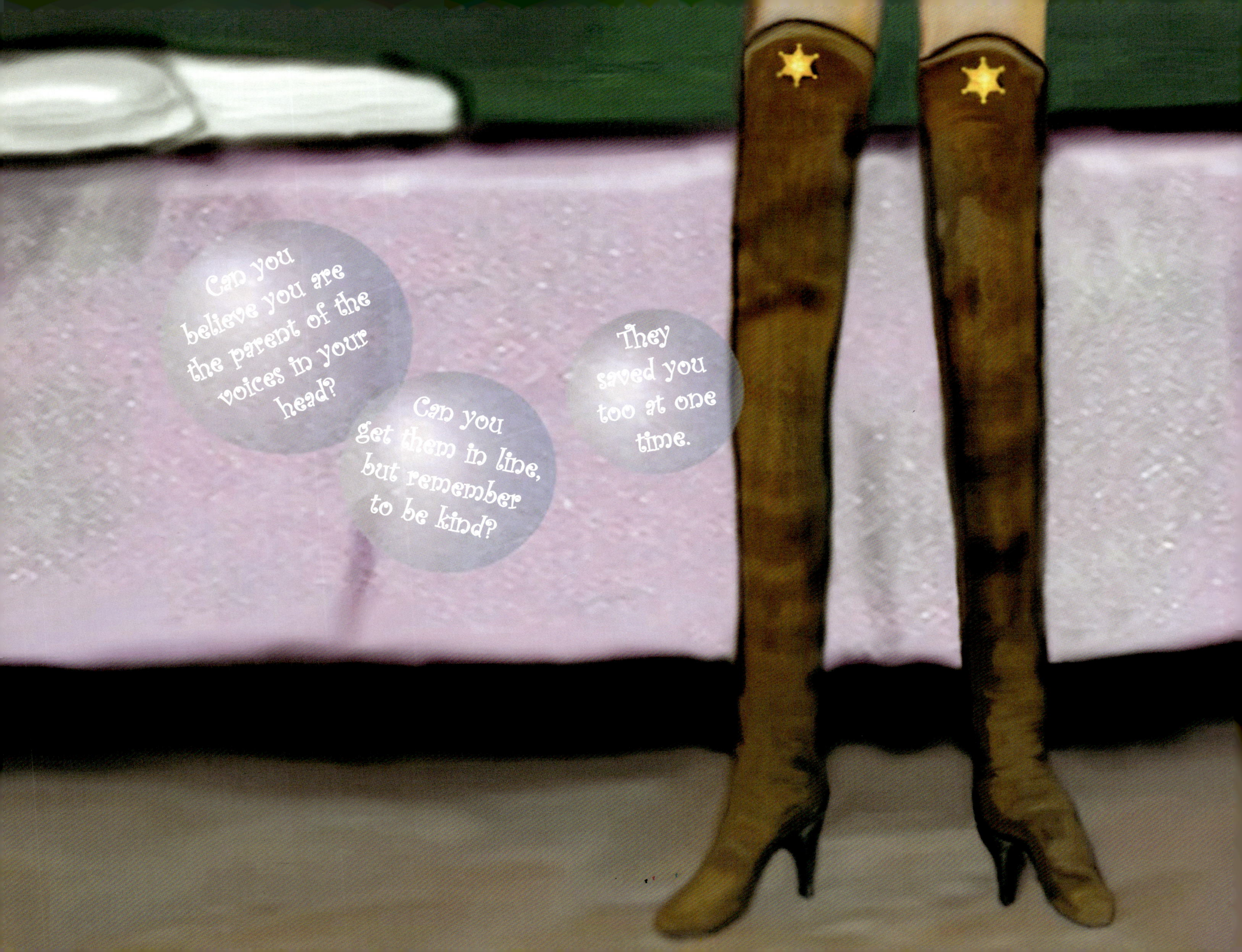
Can you believe you are the parent of the voices in your head?
Can you get them in line, but remember to be kind?
They saved you too at one time.

"Now I'm going to get dressed in a saucy little outfit, but it won't be complete without a dog at my boot's heel. It's time I get that

big black cat

out from hiding and a dog is just the trick. It's not healthy to have a cat living this way. It causes me great pain! What better way than to bring in an apartment-sized Great Dane!"

Did you know animals are good for depression?

Adopt a pet...

they need love too!

Skinny did just that, got dressed that is and picked a beautiful red for her lips. I thought what a kick! She reached for the door, opened it a lick, she turned to me like never before and candidly said, "Mister Will O. Owl, what are you here for?"

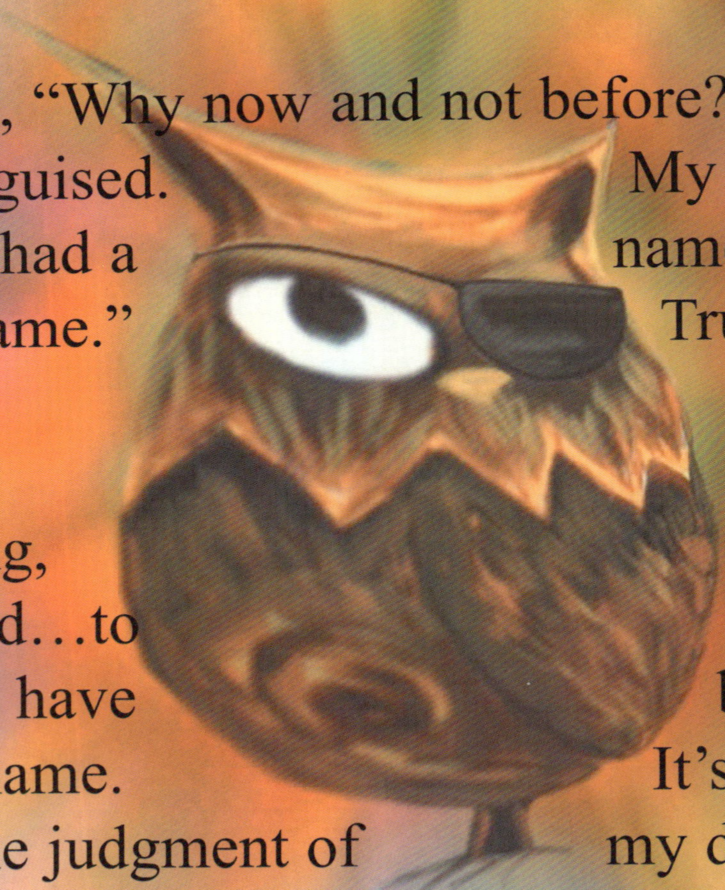

"You see me?" I asked, "Why now and not before?" I was surprised to be caught when I was disguised. My unpatched eye turned big in size. "I didn't know I had a name! Huh, somewhat like your depression…just the same." Truly we never formally introduced ourselves.

"I've seen you all along, but was too tired, blue, depressed and confused…to thank you for looking out for me and what could have been slipped into my cup of tea! Yes, you have a name. It's Mister Will O. Owl and you are in charge of the judgment of my day. Am I having a good one and am I allowed to play?" Now Skinny was letting me, her stuffed owl, play God! She wondered how I would handle her questions.

I wondered how she would handle my suggestions.

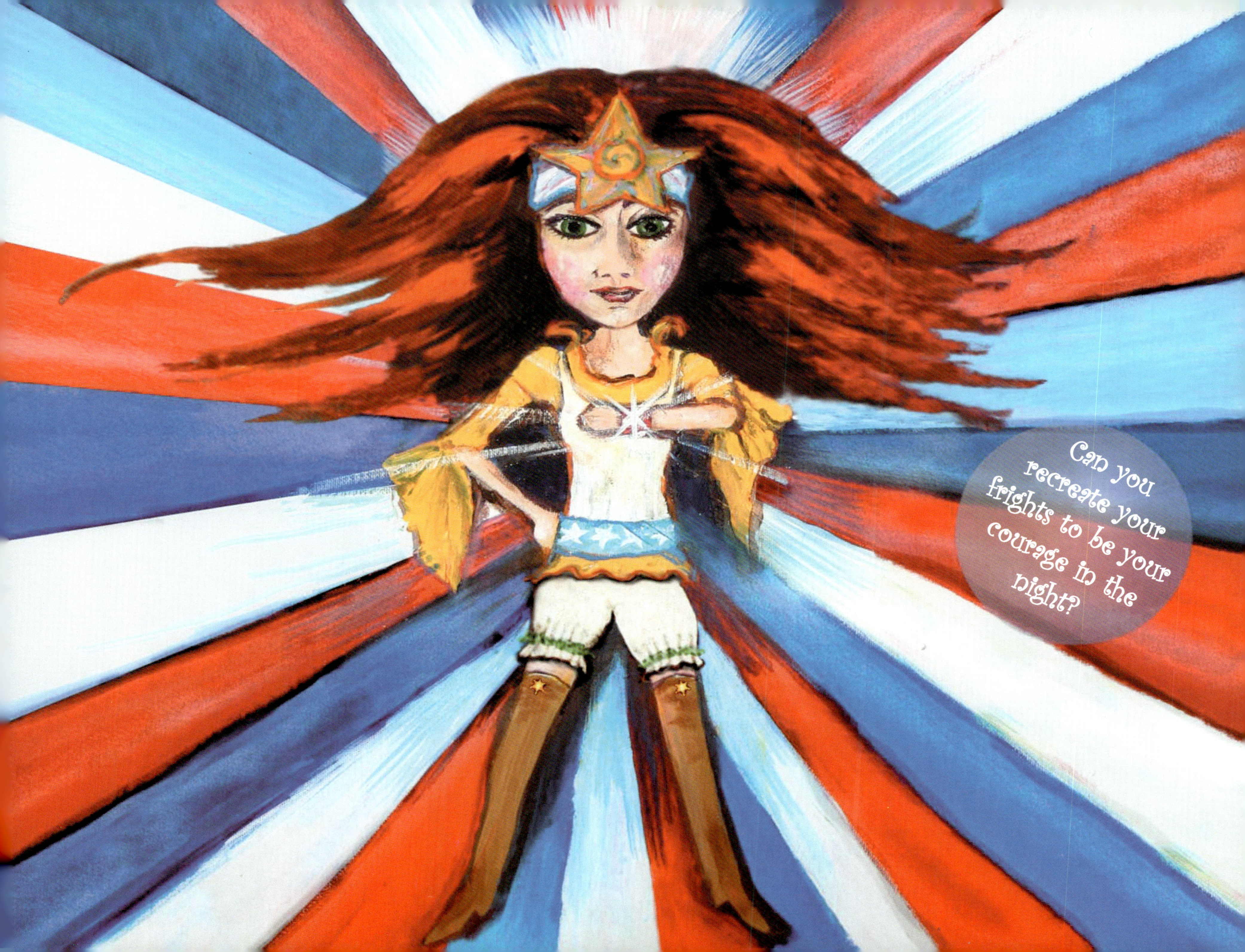

Can you recreate your frights to be your courage in the night?

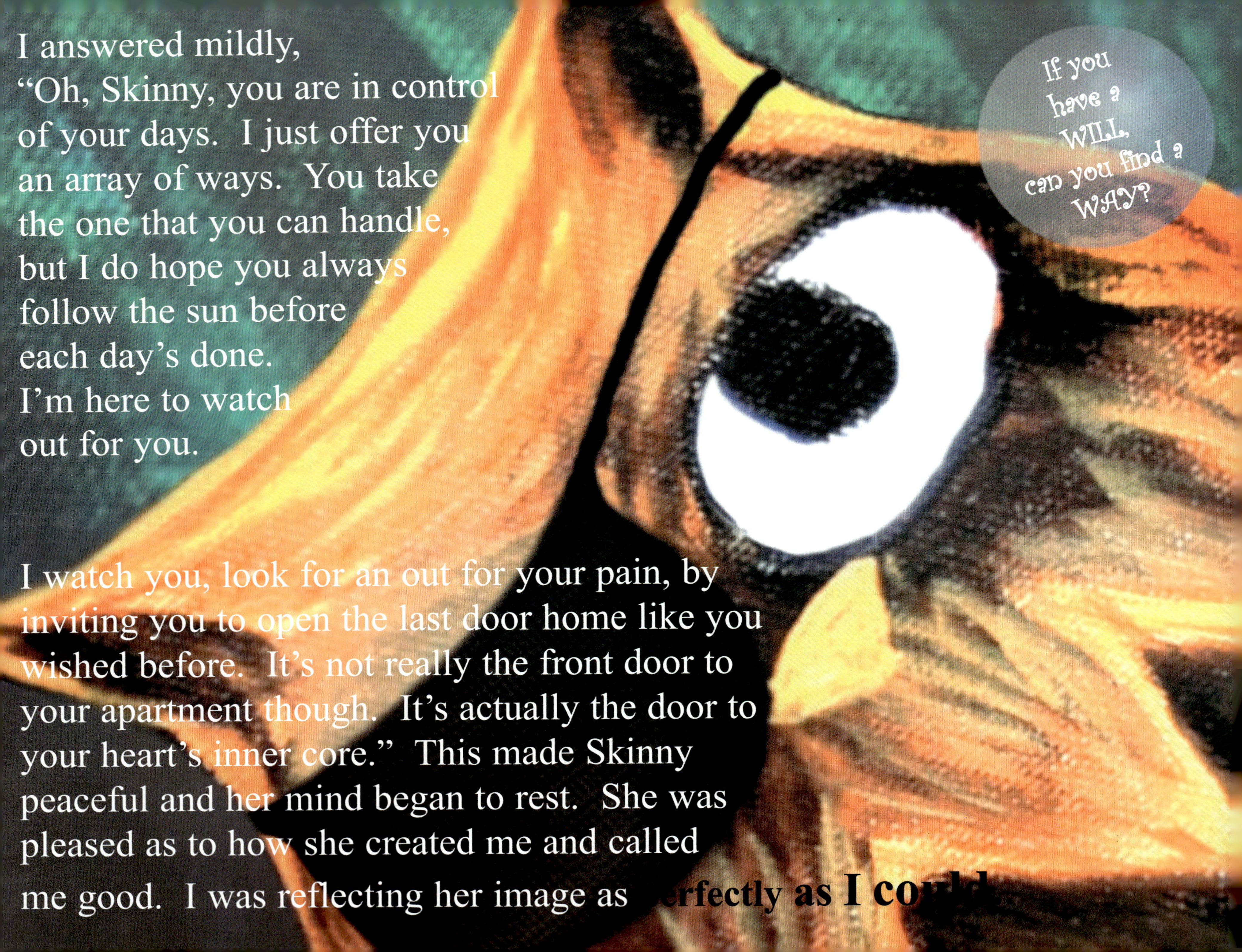

I answered mildly,
"Oh, Skinny, you are in control of your days. I just offer you an array of ways. You take the one that you can handle, but I do hope you always follow the sun before each day's done. I'm here to watch out for you.

If you have a WILL, can you find a WAY?

I watch you, look for an out for your pain, by inviting you to open the last door home like you wished before. It's not really the front door to your apartment though. It's actually the door to your heart's inner core." This made Skinny peaceful and her mind began to rest. She was pleased as to how she created me and called me good. I was reflecting her image as **perfectly as I could.**

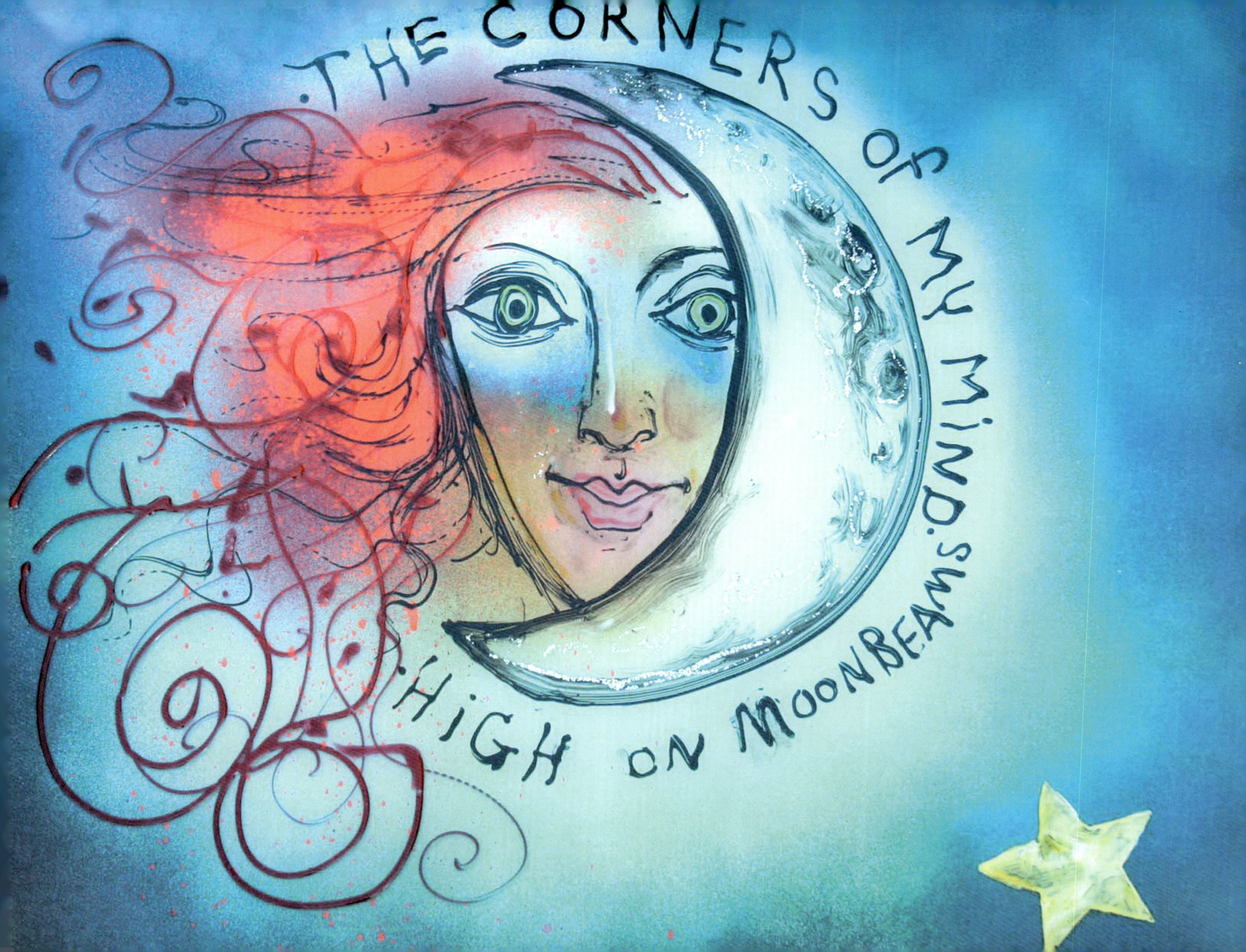
THE CORNERS OF MY MIND.
HIGH ON MOONBEAMS

heart

noun

1. a hollow muscular organ of vertebrate animals that by its rhythmic contraction acts as a force pump maintaining the circulation of the blood

2. a stylized representation of a heart.

3. the emotional or moral as distinguished from the intellectual nature: as a generous disposition.

4. COMPASSION; *a leader with heart,* LOVE, AFFECTIONS *won her heart,* COURAGE, ARDOR; *never lost heart.*

5. one's innermost character, feelings, or inclinations; *knew it in his heart, a man after my own heart.*

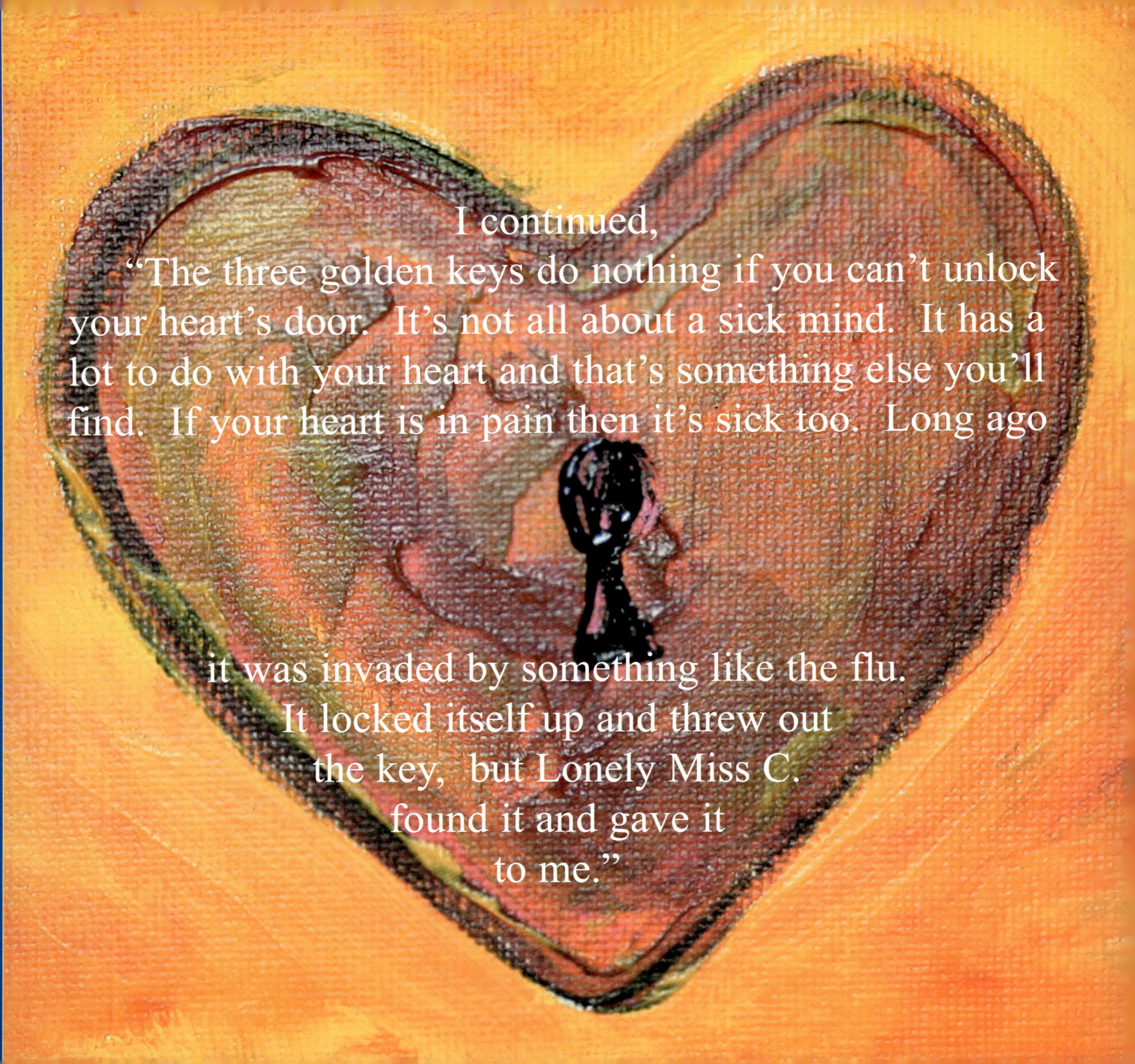

I continued,

"The three golden keys do nothing if you can't unlock your heart's door. It's not all about a sick mind. It has a lot to do with your heart and that's something else you'll find. If your heart is in pain then it's sick too. Long ago

it was invaded by something like the flu.
It locked itself up and threw out
the key, but Lonely Miss C.
found it and gave it
to me."

Skinny looked down at her doll in bewilderment.
Lonely began to explain, "I couldn't let you throw the key to your heart away!

I knew you would want it back someday."

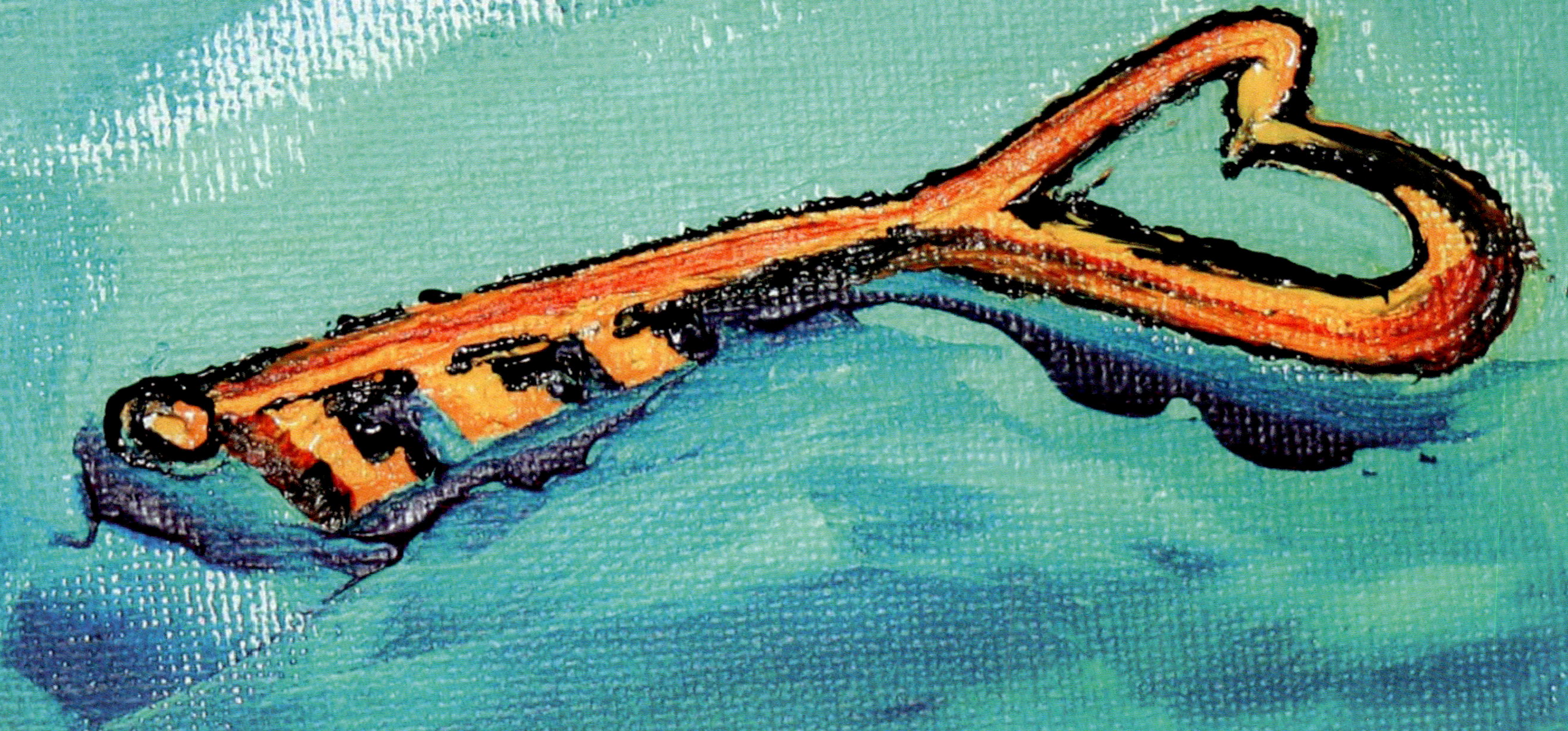

Skinny felt betrayed in a way, but accepted Lonely because of all she'd had to see. "Lonely, I know your best interest has always been for me.

I think I am ready now for the key."

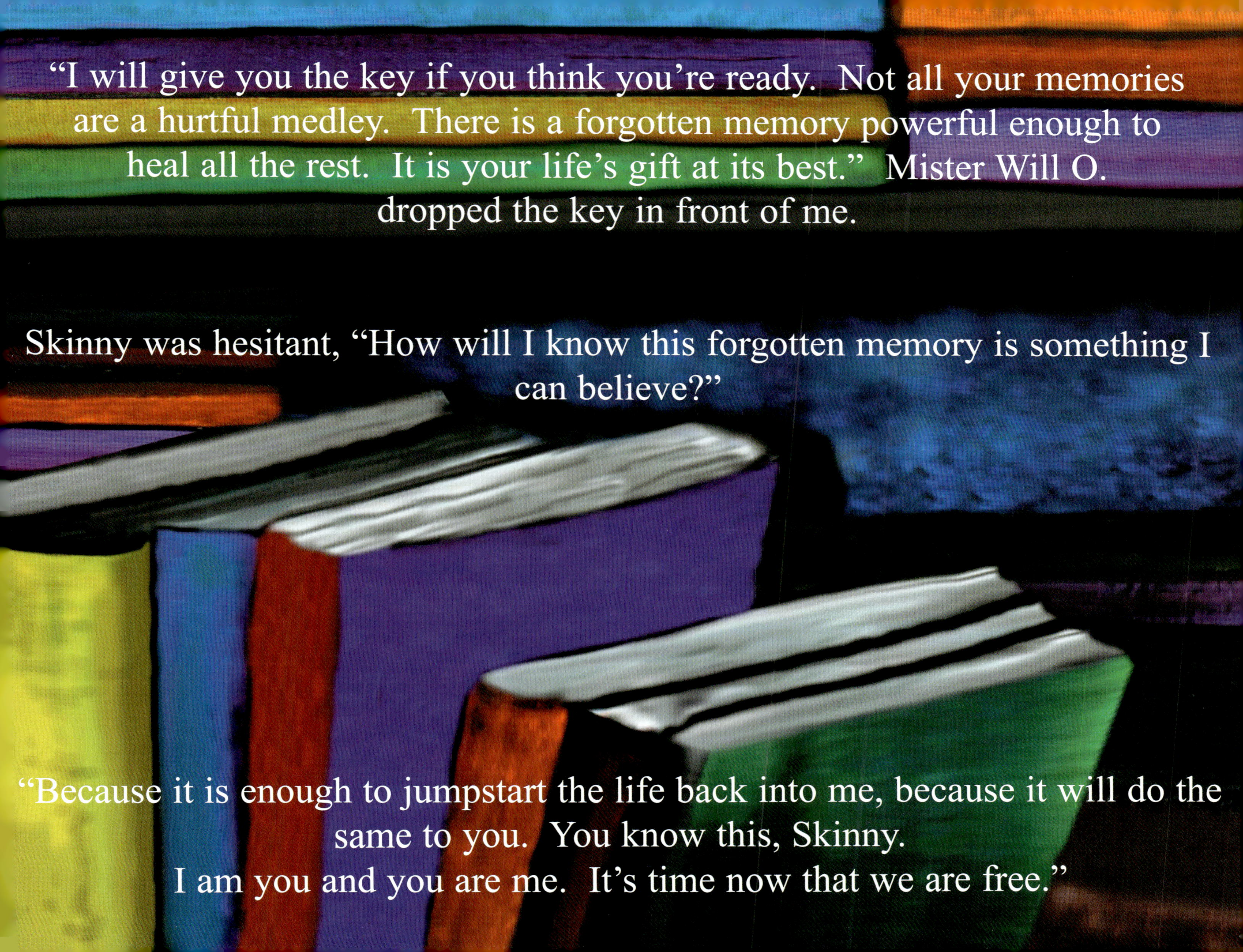

"I will give you the key if you think you're ready. Not all your memories are a hurtful medley. There is a forgotten memory powerful enough to heal all the rest. It is your life's gift at its best." Mister Will O. dropped the key in front of me.

Skinny was hesitant, "How will I know this forgotten memory is something I can believe?"

"Because it is enough to jumpstart the life back into me, because it will do the same to you. You know this, Skinny.
I am you and you are me. It's time now that we are free."

free

adjective

1. enjoying personal rights or liberty, as a person who is not in slavery; *a land of free people.*

2. exempt from external authority, interference, restriction, etc., as a person or one's will, thought, choice, action, etc.; independent; unrestricted.

3. able to do something at will; *free to choose.*

4. having immunity or being safe; *free from danger.*

5. given without consideration of a return or reward; *a free offer of legal advice.*

6. not held fast; loose; unattached; *to get one's arm free.*

7. acting without self-restraint or reserve; *to be too free with one's tongue.*

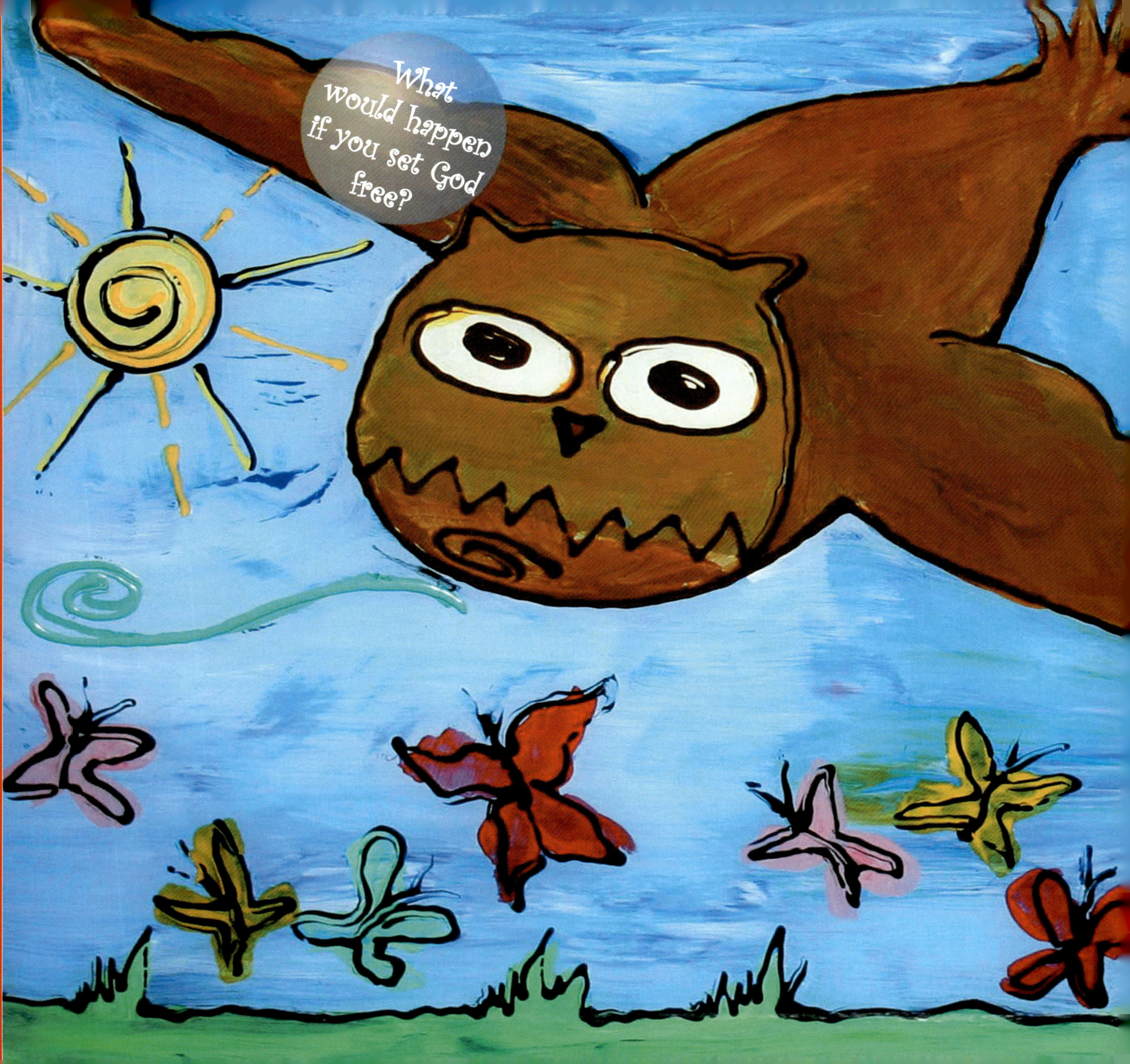

I felt a breeze that came to carry me away.
I told Skinny, "Do all that you can today to
create memories that in future days will **resonate.**
Have a wonder-full day
thus your tomorrows will be

wonder-filled."

Skinny's front door opened wide from the wind
that suddenly blew inside,
and my narrating owl... **flew away!**

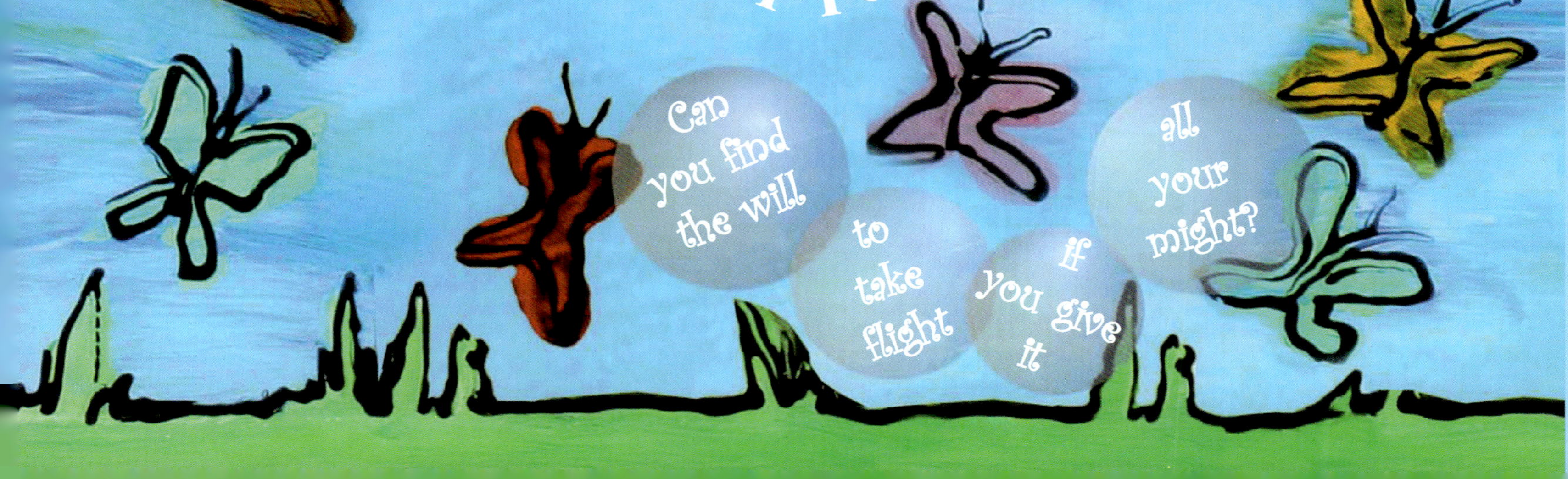
Can you find the will
to take flight
if you give it
all your might?

will
noun

1. the faculty of conscious and especially of deliberate action; the power of control the mind has over its own actions; *the freedom of the will.*

2. power of choosing one's own actions; *to have a strong or a weak will.*

3. the act or process of using or asserting one's choice; volition; *My hands are obedient to my will.*

4. wish or desire; *to submit against one's will.*

5. purpose or determination, often hearty or stubborn determination; willfulness; *to have the will to succeed.*

6. the wish or purpose as carried out, or to be carried out; *to work one's will.*

7. a male given name, form of Willis.

turn
verb

1. to cause to move around on an axis or about a center; rotate: *to turn a wheel.*

2. to cause to move around or partly around, for the purpose of opening, or closing; *to turn a key.*

3. to reverse the position or placement of; *to turn a page, to turn an egg, to turn a person around.*

4. to bring the lower layers of soil to the surface, as in plowing; *turn the menure over.*

5. to change the position of, by or as if by rotating; *to turn the handle one notch.*

6. to change or alter the course of, divert, deflect; *He turned the blow with his arm.*

Lonely Miss C.
looked at me.
"Skinny Miss S.,
that is the key to
even what I can't
see. That is the
key to the back of me."

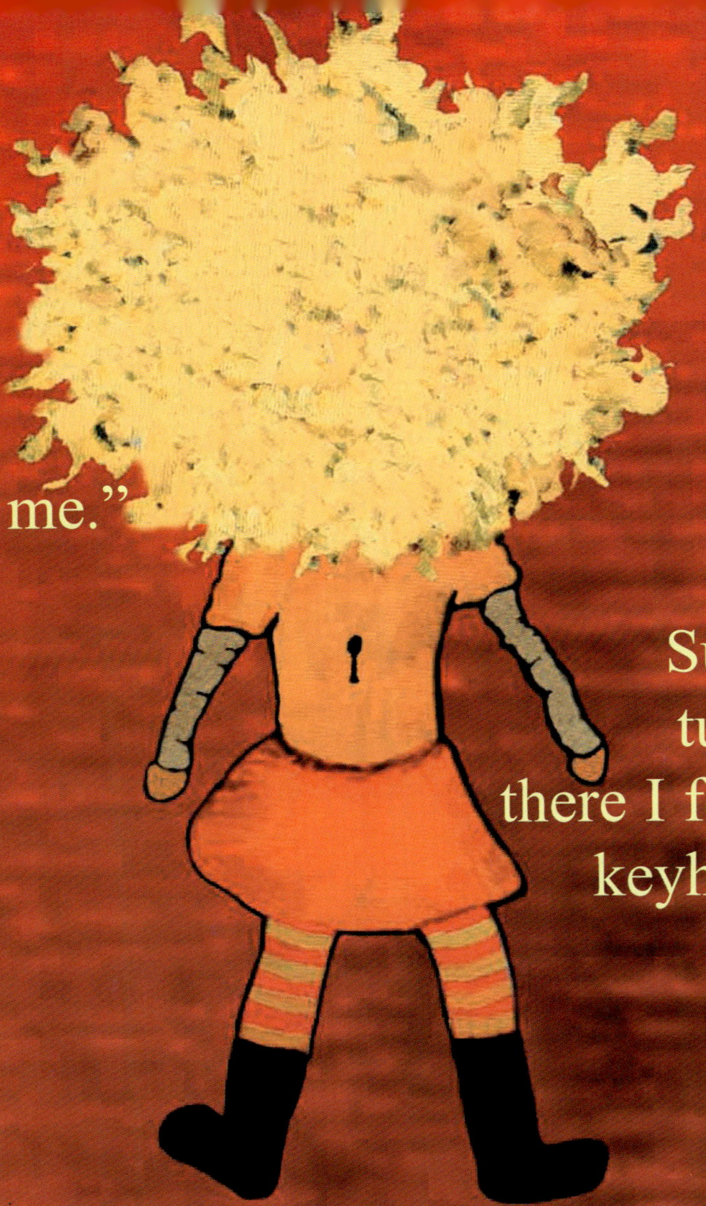

Sure enough when I
turned Lonely over,
there I found an old rusted
keyhole. I had no clue
that Lonely had a
song to play!

right
adjective

1 in accordance with what is just, good, or proper; *right conduct.*

2. conforming to facts or truth; *the right answer.*

3. of, relating to, situated on, or being the side of the body which is away from the side on which the heart is mostly located, done with the right hand; *a right hook to the jaw.*

left

adjective

1. of, relating to, situated on, or being the side of the body in which the heart is mostly located, done with the left hand; *a left hook to the jaw.*

2. of or belonging to the political Left; having liberal or radical views in politics.

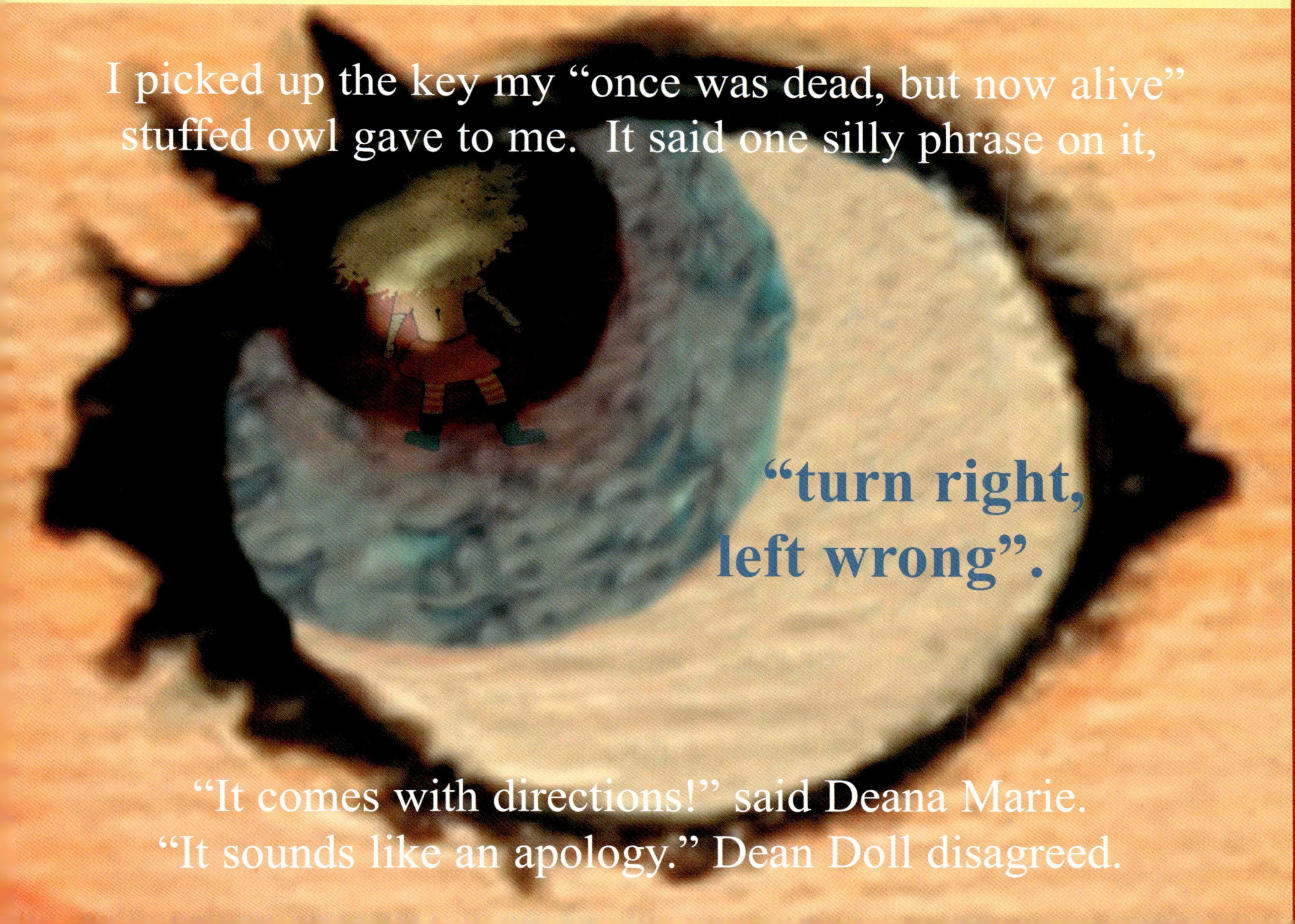

I picked up the key my "once was dead, but now alive" stuffed owl gave to me. It said one silly phrase on it,

"turn right, left wrong".

"It comes with directions!" said Deana Marie. "It sounds like an apology." Dean Doll disagreed.

wrong

adjective

1. not in accordance with what is morally right or good; *a wrong deed.*

2. deviating from truth or fact; *a wrong answer.*

3. not correct in action, judgment, opinion, method, etc., as a person, in error; *You are wrong to blame him.*

4. not proper or usual, not in accordance with requirements or recommended practice; *the wrong way to hold a golf club.*

5. not suitable or appropriate; *He always says the wrong thing.*

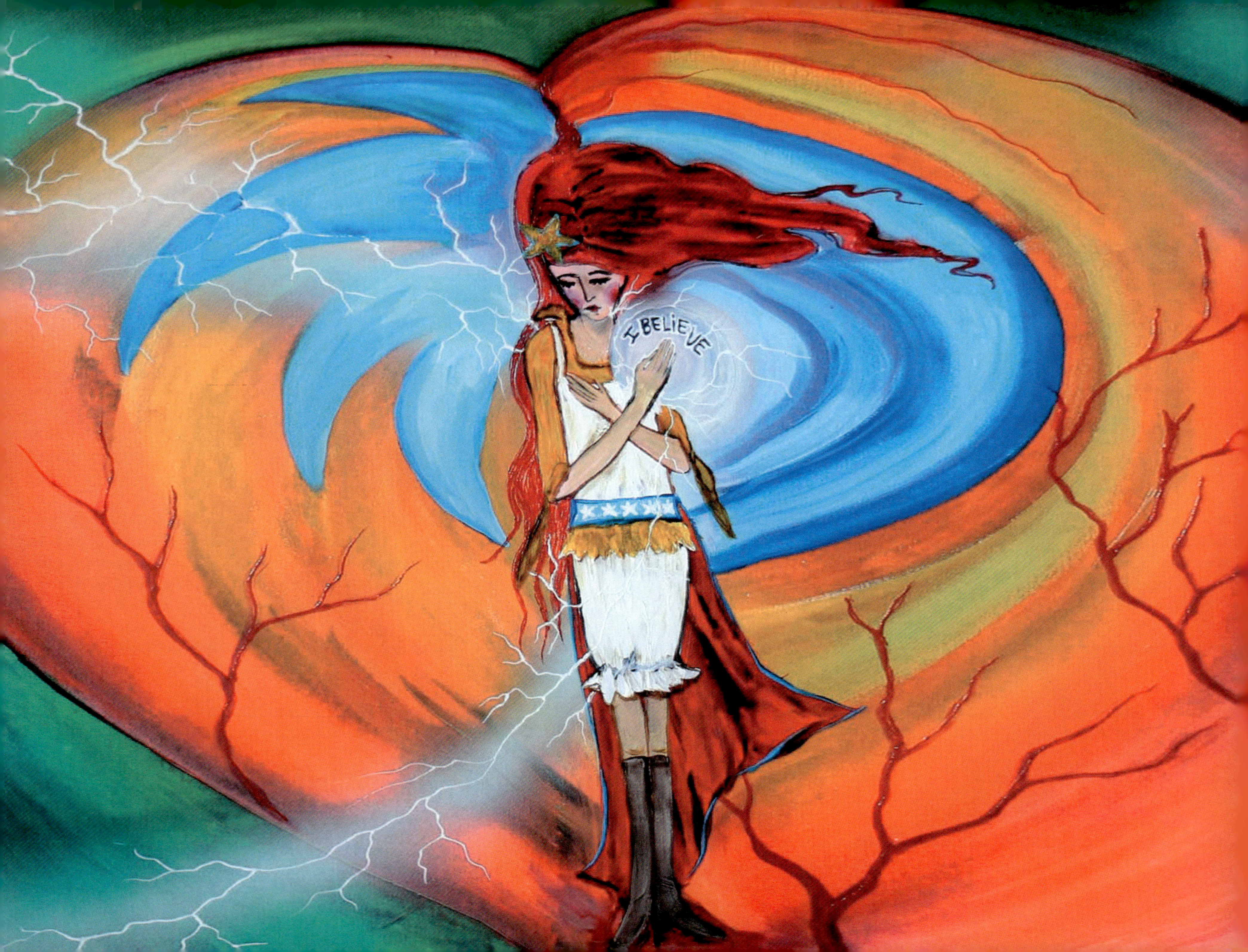
I BELIEVE

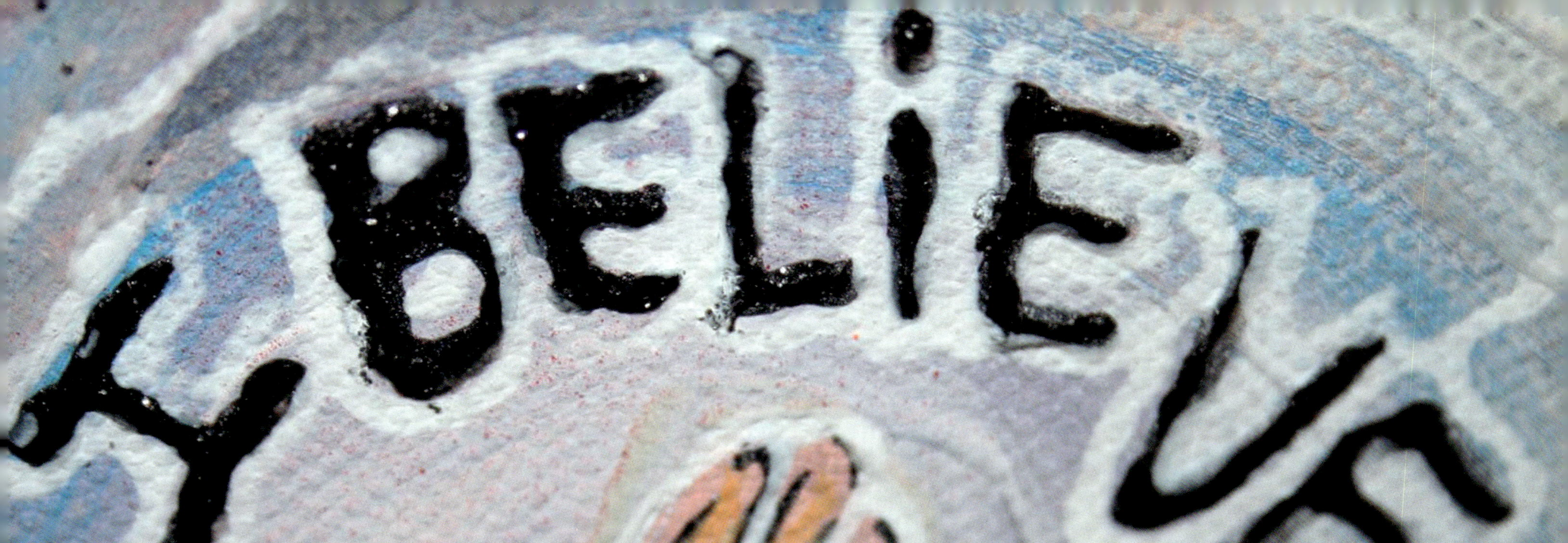

Lonely asked me if I was ready. I answered with a nod knowing this key was greater than stirring my mind, for it would stir my heart like Mister Will O. had said. I placed the key carefully in Lonely's back and turned the key to hear the song. My mind heard the tune carried by piano keys and in remembering, the pianist came rightfully back to me. He had left…wrongly. Now how could it be that it was coming through Lonely Miss C.? This was something I could not conceive, but I did believe.

It was the hardest memory to face because of the honest love the music's vibration graced. I suppose I had been most afraid this whole time to receive such a loving memory too. Accepting this gift was tough to do.

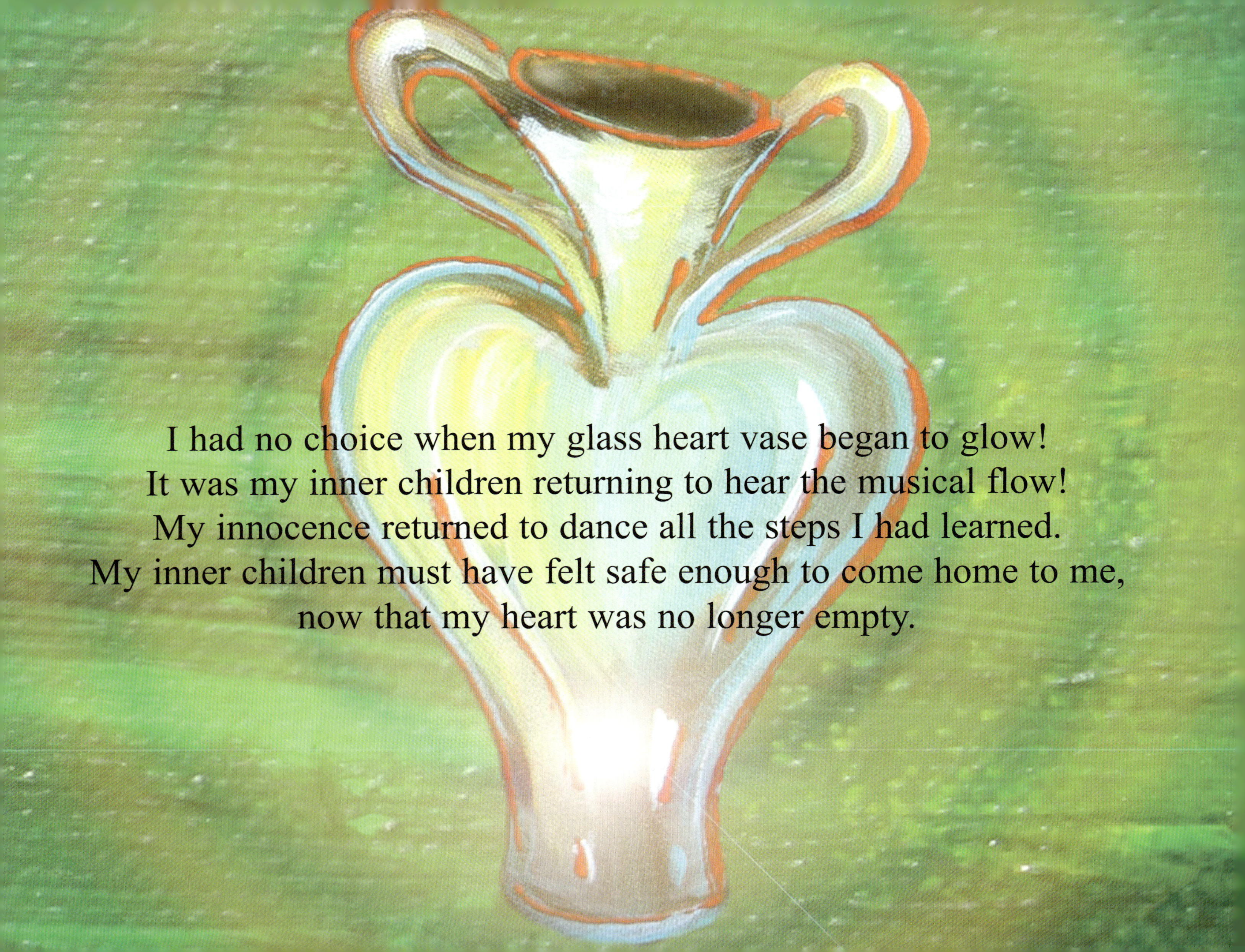

I had no choice when my glass heart vase began to glow!
It was my inner children returning to hear the musical flow!
My innocence returned to dance all the steps I had learned.
My inner children must have felt safe enough to come home to me,
now that my heart was no longer empty.

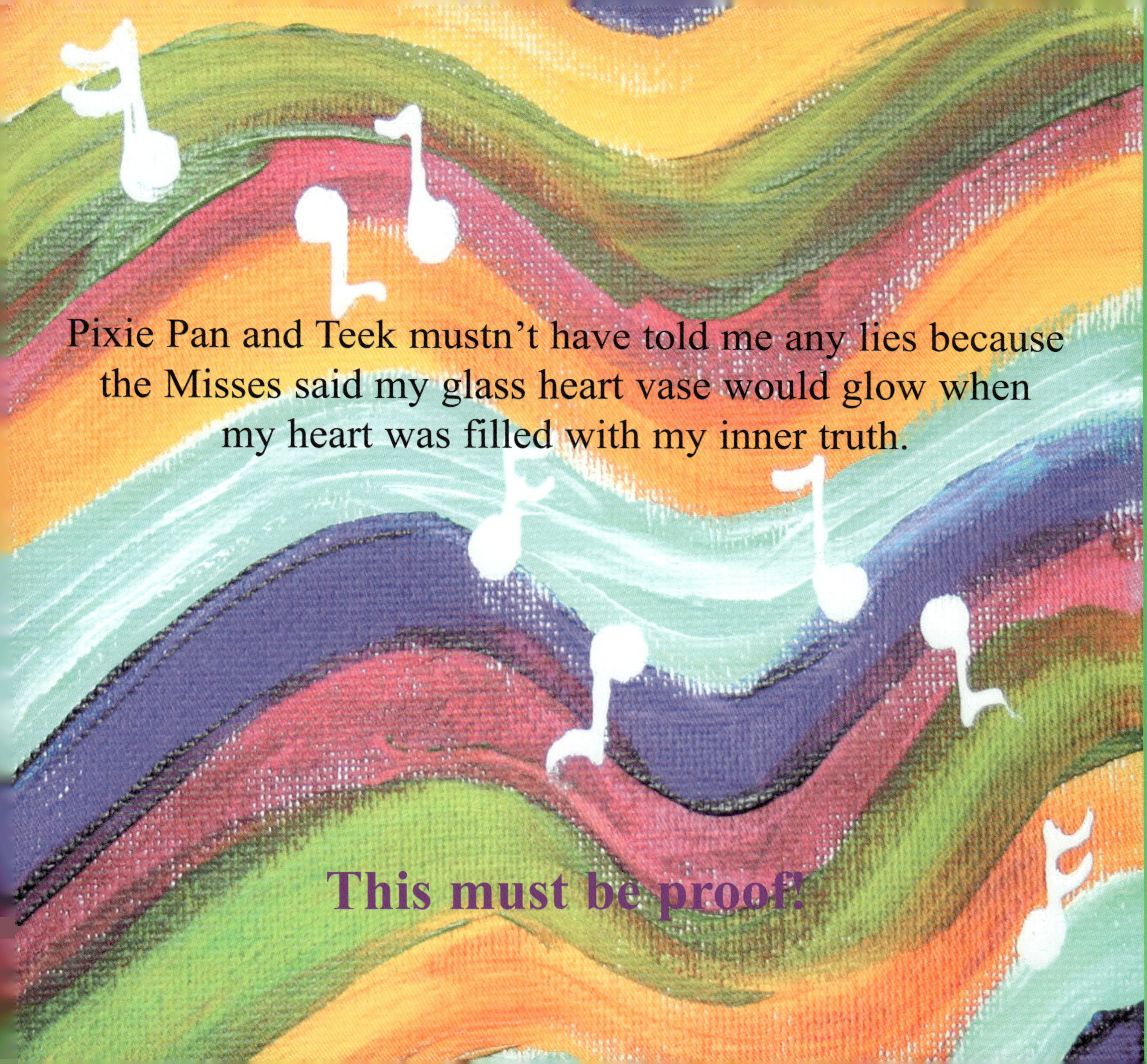

Pixie Pan and Teek mustn't have told me any lies because the Misses said my glass heart vase would glow when my heart was filled with my inner truth.

This must be proof!

truth
noun

1. the true or actual state of a matter; He *tried to find out the truth.*

2. conformity with fact or reality; verity; *the truth of a statement.*

3. a verified or indisputable fact, proposition, principle, or the like; *mathematical truths.*

4. the state or character of being true.

5. actuality or actual existence.

The song continued to play as the key untwined its way. What was set in my past, now resonated in my present. The tune had reached its goal of now, but how?

How could I have forgotten to believe that I was so loved?
At last, it came back to heal me and my inner world I rose above.

I carefully collected all of my dolls and set them on a shelf. There were no more voices in my head because I had listened to each and every one, solving our problems one by one. I suppose they said everything there was to say, and I know I did because I gave my owl a name and I called it a

good judgment day!

I looked closer at my glass heart vase set a-glow…and what did I know?
It wasn't Pixie Pan and Teek in my vase at all!
It was a small thin boy standing tall blowing bubbles galore.
He stopped and said,

"My name is Bixby B. Mess, and I am possessed.
I have something to say...

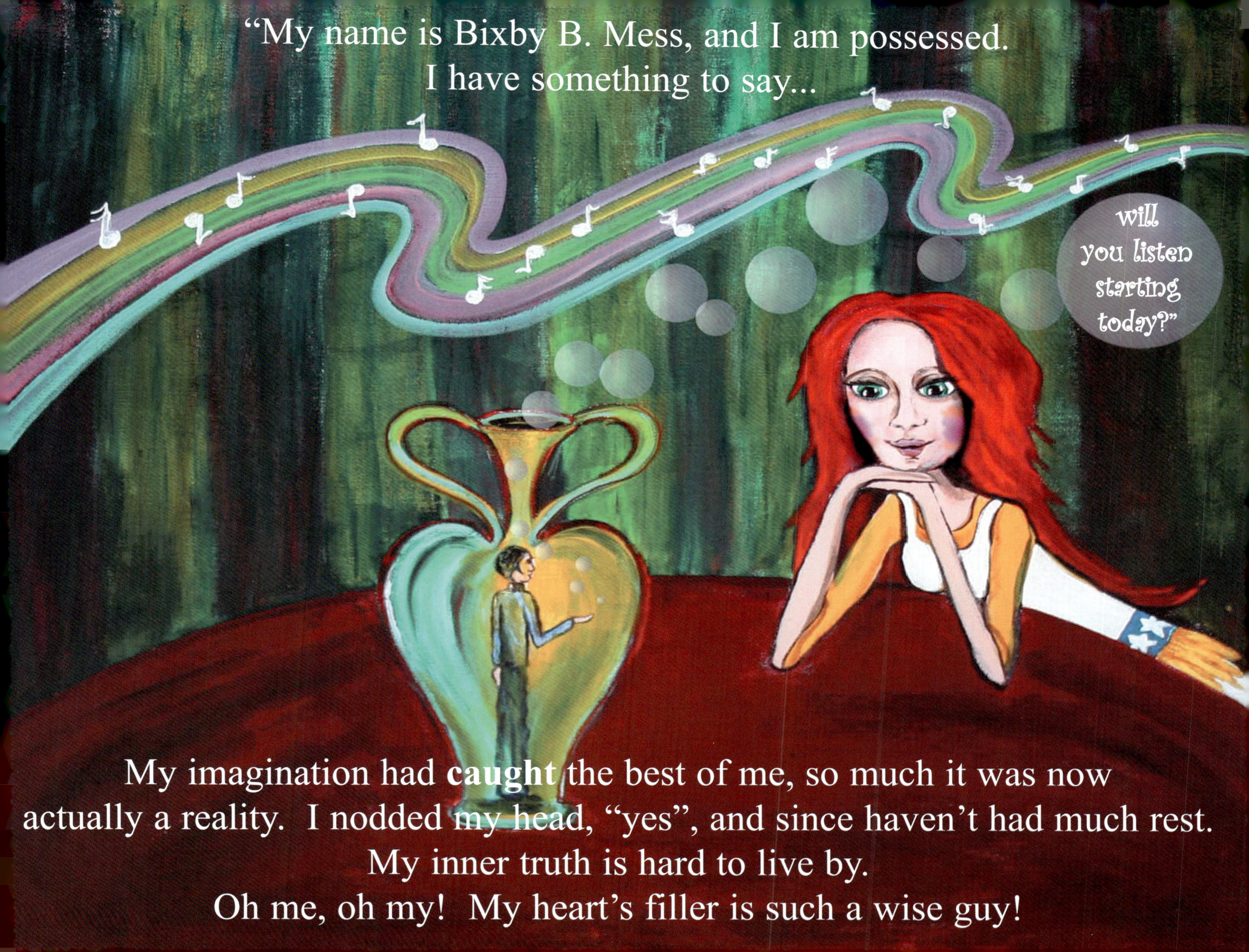

My imagination had **caught** the best of me, so much it was now actually a reality. I nodded my head, "yes", and since haven't had much rest.
My inner truth is hard to live by.
Oh me, oh my! My heart's filler is such a wise guy!

Coming Soon... *Bixby B. Mess Was Very Possessed*

possessed
adjective

1. influenced or controlled by something (as a spirit, a passion, or an idea).

2. MAD: CRAZED: urgently desirous to do or have something.

3. frenzied as if possessed by a demon; *the soldier was completely possessed, a possessed worker smashing windows.*

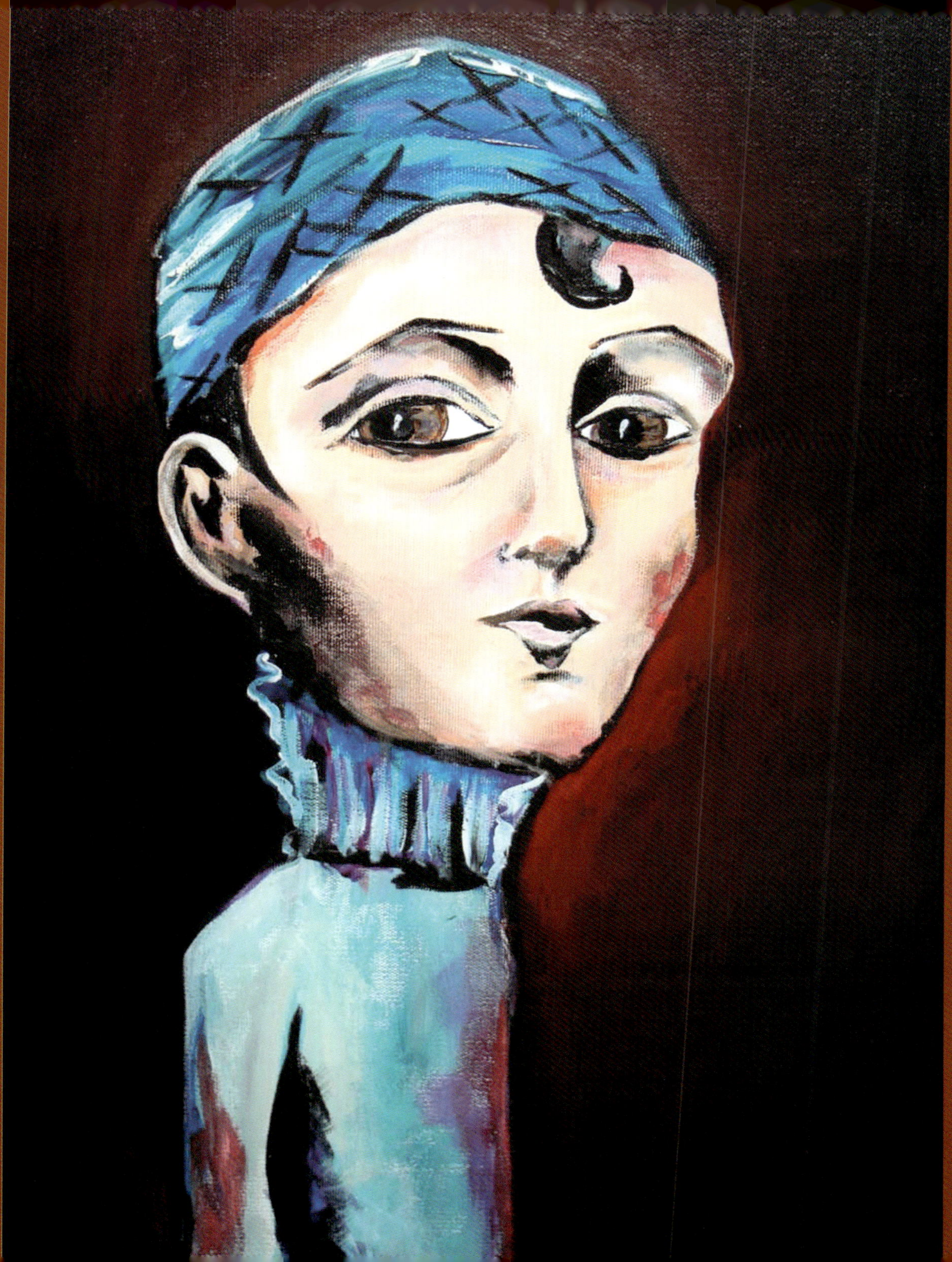

imagination
noun

1. the act or power of forming a mental image of something not present to the senses or never before wholly perceived in reality.

2. creative ability, ability to confront and deal with a problem; *use your imagination and get us out of here.*

3. the thinking or active mind; *stories that fired the imagination.*

4. a creation of the mind, an idealized or poetic creation.

I remembered what was never forgotten. My father sat next to me with his fingers upon the piano keys. He smelled of beer and sometimes I feared, but not tonight. He played whole-heartedly, impromptu, so beautifully. His raw soul laid down like a dog after a battle of deep bites, or a boxer who found his soul after loosing his last fight…loosing his rights to fight.

The tears streamed down his cheeks slowly, continuously. Wiping them, he didn't bother, although I am positive they bothered him. The piano's old keys were out of tune, now slippery with the sweat of his fingers and his cheeks tracked liquid sorrow. He played still through all of this, explaining for once…his apology.

The song was for me to hear, but not to be remembered in time. The music it created stayed intensely in the bottomlessness of my body, soul and mind. There were no words sung upon his lips. He broke down every time he did, attempting to sing that is.

I understand now after two ships passed in the night, he was telling his life's tragic story with his wounded heart and tortured mind. It was the best he could do to remember too…all of the black outs of responsibility unclaimed, all of the messes made. I too would later do the same.

His last tune came and it was drawn out in key C, much more uplifting. He turned his broken body around, facing the mirror which hung with no sound; its presence profound.

"We made each other crazy." He said with his eyebrows raised, staring in a daze. I had heard through the grapevine that in my early life this was true, just not from me, but my mother, who knew. In fact at times I have thought that the stupor he was in that night confused him, leading him to believe I was her and not me. He loved her too, more than a last breath whose wish is to live, but cannot endure.

His boney and gifted hands lay inward propped up on his knees, elbows out, ready for what I was not ready for. Silence, then up he went and crossed in front of me. His back to the mirror now, his back to me. Silence again. My heart pumped alive, alive, when it didn't want to be.

He turned around like a school boy who had done something terribly wrong. He wiped his face from the left to the right and looked into my eyes, then back to the floor. Into my eyes, then back to the floor…

"How can you ever forgive me for the things I've done?'

Not having received all of the forgotten keys to my memory, I spoke from hearsay, "I don't know dad, I just do…but can you forgive you?"

He stumbled towards me and held me tight. We danced as father and daughter should to his favorite song's lyrics and he walked me outside where I heard the gravel under our feet. Pointing at the full moon high in the starry sky, he put one arm around me and stared at this man in the moon.

"I'm like the moon, Sis (that was his nickname for me). I'm always watchin' out for you." He squinted his right eye. "No matter how far you are, I can see you just how you are. I'll scare all the boogie men away from you! I will!"
My father was adorable how he claimed to make the boogie men disappear as I recalled he was the one who created them for me when I was we-bit tall. None of that mattered now.

It was fall. Ten years of not speaking to my father went by. I had finally come to forgiveness for the righteous things I projected upon my father's choices in life. Little did I know the shoes he had walked in. I only knew the memories which surfaced shortly after our night round the piano. Dreadful forgotten memories remembered and made the meaning of fear terribly clear. Dark elements of the possession of my father's soul at times. His suicide attempts and running about with knives, a mother victim to his crimes…and me left watching, like the man in the moon unable to scare the boogieman away. Memories I had forgotten all again.

This particular fall it was a rainy and thunderous day in my mind and it was meant to stay…for a time. I reached out to my father and he answered me. I reached out again and silence fell. Oh, dad, how could you die? With no good-bye, only thirty days after I said mine.

Brian Lane, died on October 16, 2005 by way of plane crash…a plane he built with the genius of his mind and the skill of his hands. Yes, my father left me with memories of a dead-beat dad. Yes, he was mean and unreasonable and scary to me. He didn't mean to be. He too suffered brain disease. Even though it was healthy not to be in his company, I missed him all throughout my life.

Three years of Posttraumatic Stress and appropriate grieving went by. My bipolar was triggered here and there like a gun in the night. I did not see me winning this fight. The three golden keys kept me hanging in there, but it was the fourth key I had forgotten to believe, the key to my special memory. I went back and faced all the repressed memories in my head. Every age, every fear and created new outcomes for what I know he would have changed if he could find it possible, and one day that special memory became clear. Sacred and true, the colors ran through, the intangible communication just the same…of that precious memory of my father's apology brought to me through keys of black and white. What is wrong or right?

I choose to dedicate the my father's forgotten song to his one and only wife, once upon a time named Debra Lane, who misunderstood that she was not misunderstood. The trials she lived through were mine too.

I have been watching her mirror all throughout time, watching her image only to see mine, and her behind the mirror she reflects. I thank her for giving me that, backwards of course for all but me to see, how much she loved me…I just couldn't see, she just couldn't see, Lonely Miss C. was always me.

It took time to believe that my father always loved me. If only I could remember his now forgotten song. If only I could interpret all of what he said and felt while his hands moved across the keys…the keys. It is always in the keys. It lead to his apology.

Possessed by what he left me…memories and a song…I have an inner knowing that says I must move on. Bixby will question you with all of Skinny's heart, to make a change, to make a fresh start, and to allow the unknown song to move you as you begin to listen today, to what it is you've been trying to say.

GREAT GRATITUDE

I wrote this book because her story is one of the only things as it passed me that I missed, but understood. I remember seeing her, Skinny Miss S., as she blew past like a bubble breezes by in the twilight sky, reflecting every angle of her perfect self with my image coming back upon me. Ponder that…the two becoming one. For just a moment I knew her in her entirety, and still she holds on, as I remember her coming in to slip out. I suppose it's all we do when we are finally free. Connect…and cause a memory…which grows into a song or a story sometimes, depending upon how strong. It's not anything that should be understood, but because I do, sharing it may come out skewed. She is misunderstood by most, but my personal guide like a friendly ghost…another version of me. Acknowledged; pleased.

I salute all of those suffering, surviving, and befriending mental illness. When you stand in front of the mirror may you always see the saint you are intended to be. You are whole, you are clean, you are perfect as you are, and you will place yourselves where you are seen. The world will be more aware of the battles you conquer if you believe they can be lifted because you are so gifted. You are in charge of your win; now ask yourselves when to begin.

My appreciation and gratitude to all who inspired my experience with method writing. Life is a playground and I have tried all of the equipment. Round, going round…I've made my rounds with all who come in. So to all that come in…thank you, come again. Those of you who have stuck around to experience the glue, thanks for sitting in the shade and experiencing the day. You are the few who know I am true.

To my very true love, Dan Lang. Nights became early mornings containing our manic and bedazzled energy while we stayed course to complete page by page, box by box, and bubble by bubble. Architecting a home for Skinny Miss S. you've made one of your true joys, and to do it together! How simply marvelous! Without your dedication and selflessness I could not have breathed life into this child of mine. You are hands down the most intelligent and heart-filled person I have ever laid eyes upon. May you in all ways be acknowledged and acclaimed, my wonderful sweetheart. In my eyes you contain such fame. Did you know I love you so?

Mom, we have sailed the highest seas then plunged to the bottom to find pearls of treasure to please. Debra Hamilton, you are an enigma, a mystery. You are my favorite doll. I have listened to you from the time I was small. You highlight books because you love to learn. You chit and chat of experiences. You discern. You move on in times of trouble. You are the strongest part of strength. You are an underestimated power. Much I have learned from the study of you. A parent is the source…the origin of their child. I was with you from the start even when you combed your baby doll's hair, I would stop and stare…I was there. I was there, before I was here.

Thank you, Dad. David Brian Lane, you most definitely have come through. This book contains a fragment of your dynamic spirit; therefore, I celebrate it's coming to fruition in memory of you. Boo!

To my step-father, James Meier, who has undeniably supported and loved my brothers with a solid heart. You look at the issues of life and ponder their meaning. At the end of the day it isn't all what it seems…and you know what is the most important. Simply love, forgiveness, and acceptance. In that we see eye to eye; I remember each and every time either one of us has cried. I thank you for the times you have held me up and I am honored for the times you have allowed me to hold you up as well. All of the ups and downs unimportant to tell, and all of the love important to feel.

My brother, Joseph Meier, who is my beaming moon…thank you for being you. My Baby Bird, you are who you are, strong and discerning to the world around you. Your eyes are wise and wide open to the manifestations flying by. The music of your soul plays and I catch each and every tune. Your kindness for others is beyond evolved; your mind's questions…you are quick to solve. I admire your ability to see the good. I honor the look in your eyes as they watch the world spin 'round, hoping that you will never loose your faith in your truth. To you I am me and to me you are you; do we ever confuse the two? Yes, we do! I love you.

My brother, Samuel Meier, who is my shining sun…thank you for being you. Bone, we are connected in the most peculiar way and differently with each day. Some things have no rhythm or reason; they just are their own tune. You have all of it…and you will always have me. I look forward to seeing your dreams become reality, conversing about your loves in life, and quietly admiring you as I support your life's choices. Did I mention how brilliant your imagination is? Creative and true…always you. I respect the respect you have for yourself and may life invite you to indulge yourself! I love you.

London Lang, my sweet girl who is made of the finest of hearts! You are so smart. Thank you for sharing your hallway with me. It's seen days and months of color and clutter. You are oh so patient like no other! Without the space I would have not been able to paint. You have the patience of a saint! Thank you for being able to pass down what I think I know and teaching me when I don't. You have a way with your way and it is infectious because it comes from truth and integrity. Thank you also for loving my brother like no other <3!

I wish to admire Brandon Lang for his intense and creatively smart mind. I am proud of your enthusiastic drive for learning things and mastering games. I am so lucky to have you in my life to keep me on my toes, and who knows, maybe someday my OCD won't bother you or you'll make your bed…one of the two!

I am so fond of my dearest Nana Peggy Hamilton. Her example as a saucy, graceful, and witty woman has inspired me to be just the same. You are one of my favorite anti-depressants, for who could be depressed around the likes of you? You are sincerely one of my favorite people and I love to hear the stories of your past. I believe that every one of them will last. They will always exist to me, in my memory, and I will pass them on and on.

For my grandfather too. He was the most wise and honorable man who modeled such dignity. Willis Hamilton, you were a dream. Your death was unforgettable to me and even in your last breath, you taught me…everything. I love you still.

My Auntie Sandy, how life teaches us to grow. Sandra Hamilton, as a small girl you played teacher and I your faithful student. You always just know how to know. Your kind heart keeps giving and feels deeply. You are my auntie, older sister, and my friend until the end. You have held my hand in times of trouble. You have worried for me like no other.

Allison and Brian Shaneman! Your couple-hood is a platform for health, pure love, and example. You have been my family and my friends. Talking with each of you is effortless and vast. You have known me since I was a child and you raised me to always smile. You are my comfort and my place to rest after a long day of trying to be "this way" or "that". I have great gratitude for the two of you. It is because of you that I may one day say, "I do." Brian, you are a mentor, magician, and father to me. In that you are a Trinity! Alley, you are an absolute dream. Pillows so soft and a nurturer who knows how to make the pain stop. Thanks and gratitude to the two of you!

Many thanks and recognition to my friend of integrity, Christopher Ulrich, who strived to be a part, not apart from, Skinny Miss S. You have helped her get out of her mess. You have been my co-illustrator of corresponding styles which complement the same title. You have inspired me to continue on when I lost all direction or motivation to paint. You have "read" the book on a magical level and told me things even I did not hear Skinny saying. I feel more than blessed to have an artistic partner who is beyond talented, intuitive, and sensitive to the needs of this project. You are a brother to me and I am thrilled to be your "sis".

To Melinda Mascayano, who attended the circus in Vegas with me to hear the madness of my creations without judgment, only wonderment. You understand an unstable artist's soul for you are steadfast in your stability and take hold. You are a cure to all who you enter into your dreamy, but realistic realm. You are an artist whom I admire as you unfold. You are a beautiful rose whose story will not remain untold.

I send a tribute to my handsome, Dan Henneberger, for emulating your strong and color-filled self through your tree illustrations which mean so much to me. The book would not be the same without your spirit standing in it graced with the essence of your life. You live joyfully and playfully and are an example of filling your years with laughter, not tears. You are so important to me; more than you will ever know.

To Michelle Smart and Darlene Pina, my beautiful friends. Michelle, I have waited to put this baby in your hands and all along you have waited with patience for my process to find its destination. You are loyal and strong. One I feel more than fortunate to have along for the ride; one I look to with pride. Darlene, you believed in me from the start. Not only what I could do with Skinny, but you also believed in my heart. It takes one to know one is all I can say. You bring a light and calm to my days.

MORE GRATITUDE

Thank you, Sarah Bennett, my friend and my soul sister, who has walked beside me through most of our days of depression and obsession. We journeyed together, sorting out why and could never find just the right answer. You are very seriously one of my favorite people in the world. To watch you grow and all that you know has been one of the greatest gifts to me. You are truly my best friend till the end which will never end. No words can express how beautiful you are. You are a shining star.

To my dear, Tamera Partiss, who has cheered me through. Behind every writer there is a nurturing mother. Thank you for all of your sincere encouragement. And your voice…your voices…the voices in Skinny Miss S.'s head are all for you to bring to life. Such star talent you are. May your little twin stars fill your heart as manifesting them will encourage others to be passionate creators. Will we always be moving…and grooving? I hope only as long as we do it together. There is nothing better. Oh, I guess there is because there is Lee!

To my Terry Treves. How can I begin to thank you for all you have contributed and given to me from the kindness of your heart? Let me attempt to start. You understand humanity's need for a helping hand. You are a fighter for justice and truth, therefore I am a fan. I have much to learn from the realness of you. When I crashed you picked me up. You gave me a purpose and a list to cross each item off. You gave me direction and guidance of all the things you knew I could know too, given time. I was falling, but you didn't let that get to you. You never judged me or any of my episodes. You walked face to face beside me so that I was sure to know…I am never alone. You are never alone.

To my dearest and true Eleanor Francis. You are my friend, my strong-hold, and my sanctuary. If I grow to be half the grace of a woman that you are, I will know I do not need to return to reincarnate, for you are that evolved. Your voice, your glee, your friendly nature, your silent wisdom, and your entire personality are all things I look up to as a small girl looks up to a beautiful willow tree swaying in the breeze. You will always have your keys, because your home is happily yours now to fill with peace and I am grateful to help you fill it with joy! You are a class act and are adorned with beauty.

I thank myself for holding on. Holding on when the storm was strong. Bringing back my awareness to face the pain. Calling out to my highest of powers as I renounced their names. Recreating who I now know I can trust. Searching for what is beyond beliefs. Recreating myself to live life as I must. I thank myself each and every day, for showing up, just never the same. Believing in nothing means I'm not in a box. Believing in nothing means I experience all possibilities…blah, blah, blah…but true

In great appreciation to Dr. Charlene Crothers, my incredible psychologist who has treated me from the girlish age of 21. You know me like no other under the sun. I have securely placed my secrets in your hands, for not everyone would understand, but you do. You educate me too. You esteem me to live, inspire me because of what you give. The many who frequent your coach are under the utmost professional care. You give me rose colored glasses when it is only gray I see, and take them off when I need to see myself in reality. You are one of the only people I know I can trust who observes me objectively. Thank you for 16 years and counting of unconditional support, as I went through my memory's boxes in my closet I was determined to sort. You acknowledge my perceptions of how I remember the forgotten, still reminding me that I can always overcome. You snap me back in shape when I enter your office shapeless. Inspiring me to LIVE when it is death I think I fear, is my favorite challenge you've set for me. You make it crystal clear. I pose the question, "Can I make memories to heal?" and somehow I know you would support that deal.

I wish to acknowledge my excellent psychiatrist, Dr. Edward Jesalva. The magic you perform with the combination of your intuitive skills and ongoing increasing knowledge is to be more than noted. Medications are supplements to alter our behavior, thus a patient's reality. You take such care as you analyze what type and what dosage is the best cocktail for me. You know your stuff and that is worth a golden key. A bad psychiatrist could be the biggest harm to one's healing. A good psychiatrist knows to listen. You do more than listen; you ask the right questions. An excellent psychiatrist is intuitive and bright and takes pride in winning a mental fight. You just know how to make my head "right". I am thankful for your intelligence in managing my disorders with genuine care and the informed information you offer to share.

To Dr. Mary Kunz, my amazingly talented therapist specializing in eating disorders. You saved my life and taught me so many things during the two years of intense rediscovery of what it was that formed a block within me. You helped correct my relationship with food, but mostly you were just you…a wonder of love and compassion and care. You knew that LOVE cures all who choose not to self-care. You stood as a warrior as I remembered how to uncontrollably throw out my forgotten memories. You saluted my body memory's brilliant way to trigger my inner knowledge one cold December day. You protected me from the negative forces which still made their presence. How magical our time was, and did we not get our work done! Here's to being lost, then found. With you by my side, I landed with both feet on the ground.

TO THE FINEST IN THEIR FIELD

THE END NOTES

1 The National Suicide Prevention Hotline. <http://www.suicide preventionlifeline.org/>.

2 Wikipedia Online Encyclopedia. “DSM IV Medical Reference Book for Mental Disorders.” <http://www.wikipedia.com/> based on the external link to The American Psychiatric Association. <http://www.psych.org/MainMenu/Research/DSMIV.aspx>.

3 American Psychiatric Association. “Major Depressive Episode”. Diagnostic and Statistical Manual of Mental Disorders (Fourth Edition-Revised) DSM-IV-R.

4 American Psychiatric Association. “Generalized Anxiety Disorder”. Diagnostic and Statistical Manual of Mental Disorders (Fourth Edition-Revised) DSM-IV-R.

5 Wikipedia Online Encyclopedia. “Bibliomancy”. <http://www.wikipedia.com/>

6 American Psychiatric Association. “Schizotypal Personality Disorder”. Diagnostic and Statistical Manual of Mental Disorders (Fourth Edition-Revised) DSM-IV-R.

7 American Psychiatric Association. “Religious or Spiritual Problem”. Diagnostic and Statistical Manual of Mental Disorders (Fourth Edition-Revised) DSM-IV-R.

8 American Psychiatric Association. “Anorexia Nervosa”. Diagnostic and Statistical Manual of Mental Disorders (Fourth Edition-Revised) DSM-IV-R.

9 American Psychiatric Association. “Obsessive-Compulsive Disorder”. Diagnostic and Statistical Manual of Mental Disorders (Fourth Edition-Revised) DSM-IV-R.

10 American Psychiatric Association. “Attention-Deficit/Hyperactivity Disorder”. Diagnostic and Statistical Manual of Mental Disorders (Fourth Edition-Revised) DSM-IV-R.

11 American Psychiatric Association. “Primary Insomnia”. Diagnostic and Statistical Manual of Mental Disorders (Fourth Edition-Revised) DSM-IV-R.

12 American Psychiatric Association. “Delusional Disorder”. Diagnostic and Statistical Manual of Mental Disorders (Fourth Edition-Revised) DSM-IV-R.

13 American Psychiatric Association. “Agoraphobia”. Diagnostic and Statistical Manual of Mental Disorders (Fourth Edition-Revised) DSM-IV-R.

14 American Psychiatric Association. “Major Depressive Episode”. Diagnostic and Statistical Manual of Mental Disorders (Fourth Edition-Revised) DSM-IV-R.

15 Wikipedia Online Encyclopedia. “Inner Child”. <http://www.wikipedia.com/>

16 Wikipedia Online Encyclopedia. “Repressed Memory”. <http://www.wikipedia.com/>

17 Wikipedia Online Encyclopedia. “Side Effects”. <http://www.wikipedia.com/>

18 Wikipedia Online Encyclopedia. “Family Therapy”. <http://www.wikipedia.com/>

19 Wikipedia Online Encyclopedia. “Pillow Talk”. <http://www.wikipedia.com/>

20 Wikipedia Online Encyclopedia. “Support Group”. <http://www.wikipedia.com/>

21 American Psychiatric Association. “Bipolar Disorder”. Diagnostic and Statistical Manual of Mental Disorders (Fourth Edition-Revised) DSM-IV-R.

22 American Psychiatric Association. “Substance Abuse”. Diagnostic and Statistical Manual of Mental Disorders (Fourth Edition-Revised) DSM-IV-R.

23 American Psychiatric Association. “Transgender”. Diagnostic and Statistical Manual of Mental Disorders (Fourth Edition-Revised) DSM-IV-R.

24 Wikipedia Online Encyclopedia. “Transgender”. <http://www.wikipedia.com/>

25 American Psychiatric Association. “Dissociative Disorder”. Diagnostic and Statistical Manual of Mental Disorders (Fourth Edition-Revised) DSM-IV-R.

* All colored boxed definitions were referenced from The Merriam Webster Online Dictionary. <http://www.merriam-webster.com/>.